THE OHIO STATE UNIVERSITY
DEPT. OF PREVENTIVE MEDICINE
410 WEST TENTH AVENUE
COLUMBUS, OHIO 43210

EPIDEMIOLOGY AND COMMUNITY MEDICINE

EPIDEMIOLOGY AND COMMUNITY MEDICINE

SIDNEY L. KARK, M.D.

Professor and Chairman, The Haim Yassky Department of Social Medicine, The Hebrew University–Hadassah Medical School and Hadassah–Hebrew University Medical Center, Jerusalem, Israel

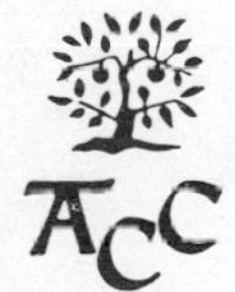

APPLETON-CENTURY-CROFTS/New York
A Publishing Division of Prentice Hall, Inc.

Library of Congress Cataloging in Publication Data

Kark, Sidney L
Epidemiology and community medicine.

Includes bibliographical references.
1. Hygiene, Public. 2. Epidemiology.
3. Community health services. I. Title.
[DNLM: 1. Community health services.
2. Epidemiology. 3. Public health.
4. Socioeconomic factors. WA100 K183e]
RA427.K29 362.1 74-12237
ISBN 0-8385-2220-3

Copyright © 1974 by APPLETON-CENTURY-CROFTS
A Publishing Division of Prentice-Hall, Inc.

All rights reserved. This book, or any parts thereof, may not be used or reproduced in any manner without written permission. For information address Appleton-Century-Crofts, 292 Madison Avenue, New York, N.Y. 10017

74 75 76 77 78 79 80 / 10 9 8 7 6 5 4 3 2 1

Printed in the United States of America

Cover design: Paula Wiener

Preface

Health care in the community is most often a service meeting the demands of individuals who turn to a practitioner or clinic for medical treatment or advice. Very often, and this is especially true in those countries in which services are provided on an insurance basis or directly by Government, the services are provided through health centers. During the past half-century or more the health center has become a major world-wide institution providing primary health care. Sometimes the service of such centers is predominantly curative, sometimes it is only preventive, and increasingly it combines preventive and curative services. In the main, its efforts, preventive and curative, are focused on the individual and sometimes on the family, and often one hears that community care is a function of the center, only to find that the deed does not match the word. Why do so many health centers fail to provide community-oriented care? The 'load of patients' demanding care at the center is often adduced as the reason for confining the health center's activities to care of ambulant persons who turn to it for help. This kind of part-truth is a block to advance of community medicine proper. The fact is that doctors and nurses and their substitutes in many countries, are not trained to practice community medicine. Their medical schools, built around teaching hospitals, have directed their orientation and skills towards individual care only and they have little competence in other fields which are no less important. This book is written in the hope that it will be both a guide and stimulus to the many medical, nursing, and other health practitioners in the community. It is also directed to those who are studying in undergraduate and graduate schools to enter such practice. Whether existing medical schools and other institutions training health professionals can provide the training needed for the practice of community medicine proper depends on their ability to modify their orientation and structure which are now so dependent on teaching hospitals. The investment by a university in exploring ways of developing new institutions for health care in the community is essential for the growth of community medicine as an added dimension of medicine.

This is especially needed in re-orienting and revitalizing primary health care to the newer demands for health and medical care of communities as well as of individuals and their families. In doing this, the university and its medical school in particular, can provide students with learning situations in the application of scientific methods to community medicine proper.

During the past 33 years my wife, Dr. Emily Kark, and I have been involved with a number of close associates in several experiments in community medicine, the feature of which has been the integration of public health practice and personal medical care in the community. Throughout this experience there has been a consistent evolution towards a form of medicine which I have referred to in the final section of the book as community medicine and primary health care. It has become increasingly apparent that the use of epidemiology in daily practice is essential for the successful development of community medicine in, and through, primary health care.

The focus of this book is on community health and what can be done about it. The health of a community is viewed as an interrelated network of somatic and psychologic processes associated with varying patterns of disease. The interacting triangle of disease and the somatic and psychologic characteristics of a community are presented as the starting point for epidemiologic description and for community diagnosis. A number of illustrations of this kind of thinking about health and disease are presented in the introductory section on community health. This is followed by sections on community determinants of health and disease and concepts of cause and effect using as an illustrative example the relationship between infection, disease and community health. Discussion on the concept of community health syndromes precedes the final section on community medicine and primary health care. This final section on community medicine and primary health care is a case illustration of the way in which community medicine is being integrated with primary health care in a university teaching health center. The framework needed for the practice which is outlined in this text is provided by a community health center established by the Hadassah Medical Organization as part of its program of services which it has developed in its association with the Hebrew University. I have been associated with it for over 20 years, first in its planning and inception and, since 1959 when it became a practising unit of the Department of Social Medicine. I would like to pay tribute to the Hadassah Medical Organization and in particular to Professor K. J. Mann, its director, for this evidence of their vision and faith in the future of medical practice in the community.

I am much indebted to many of my colleagues, present and past, for the opportunity of working with them in developing the use of epidemiology in this appraoch to community medicine and primary health care. The case illustration presented in Section 5 was written jointly with Noemy

Mainemer and is in effect a report of this team's joint efforts. The team has included family doctors, pediatricians, psychiatrists, epidemiologists, statisticians, community and family nurses and other public health professionals. I believe that continuity of care of an individual patient, a family or a local community, depends a lot on the stability of practitioners in the area. An outstanding feature of our departmental health center has been the continuous functioning together of a core of medical and nursing staff. Their long association with other faculty members of the Department of Social Medicine has been an important force in planning and exploring ways of integrating community medicine into daily primary health care.

It is not possible to name all members of the team, but among the many who have played a very important part in this development and who continue to do so are the following:

Epidemiology and Biostatistics Unit: *J. H. Abramson, L. M. Epstein, E. Peritz, I. Ronen, B. Adler*
Mother and Child Health Unit: *Z. Shamir, D. Flug, M. Gitlin, H. Palti*
Family Medicine Unit: *B. Gampel, C. Hopp, R. Avni, R. Cohen, Y. Halevi*
Health Education Unit: *H. Pridan, I. Cohen*
Surveillance and Care of Long-Term Illness: *S. Wartski*
Public Health Nursing Unit: *H. Derenburg, P. Karpf, R. Elishkovsky, G. Helman, H. Kosovsky, B. Lis*
Community Mental Health Unit: *I. Levav*

Among those who encouraged and by so doing helped me in writing this book, have been many students who have asked for a book of this kind to help them in their study of epidemiology and community medicine. Many of these students and former medical residents in our department have been involved in different aspects of various programs in the course of their specialization or in preparation of theses. The results of several of these studies have been included in the text, such as those by Mrs. H. Derenburg (Family spacing), Drs. L. Epstein and R. Avni (Physical growth in infants) and Dr. A. Posner (Analysis of an epidemic of influenza in family practice). Dr. A. Reshef, a former student and resident of this department and now Chief of the Division of Nutrition in the Ministry of Health, continues to make an important contribution as a nutritionist consultant to the public health programs of our department. Much of the text has been used and tested with students of various disciplines studying in the Department of Social Medicine. Students include Israelis attending regular courses as well as 'international' students, the course for whom has been sponsored by the Division for International Cooperation of the Ministry of Foreign Affairs. I would like to thank them for their encouragement and assistance in the preparation of the material for this book.

I am especially indebted to Noemy Mainemer for her help in the preparation of material, checking and reading of the text, and her joint authorship of Section 5. Others who provided critical comments of different sections were Dr. Eric Peritz, Biostatistician of our Department of Social Medicine, Dr. Kurt Deuschle, Professor of Community Medicine of the Mount Sinai School of Medicine of The City University of New York, and Dr. John Cassel, Professor of Epidemiology of the School of Public Health, University of North Carolina. Miss S. Pelz was of much assistance in editing and in various technical functions, and the secretarial work of Mrs. B. Slonim. Mrs. S. Elmaleah, and others of the secretarial staff have been invaluable. Finally, I want to thank my wife, Dr. Emily Kark, who not only encouraged me in writing but shared many of the ideas and was responsible for much of the work involved in critical review and editing.

Contents

1

Introduction: Epidemiology and Community Medicine

Social medicine has been defined in various ways, a cardinal feature being its concern with health and disease of population groups. It includes foundation disciplines such as epidemiology, as well as the study and evaluation of health care systems, and has application in practice which is focused on population groups. The groups may be single families, clusters of families in neighborhoods, friendship groups, occupational and student groups, and small communities, as well as wider groupings in cities, nations and multinational regions. In this context epidemiology and community medicine are important elements of social medicine.

EPIDEMIOLOGY

The function of epidemiology is to study health in population groups. Like other medical sciences it aims to describe health, whether normal or abnormal, and find causes for its variations. However, epidemiology's unit of observation is a population group and not the individual. The pioneer teachers of epidemiology, Wade Hampton Frost of Johns Hopkins University School of Hygiene, and Major Greenwood of the London University School of Hygiene and Public Health, differentiated it from other medical sciences in being a study of disease as a mass phenomenon in which the unit of observation is "the group, the herd,"[1] or "an aggregation of individuals making up a population."[2] The same definition is commonly in use today: "The unit of observation in epidemiology is the group, or 'population' as it is called, which may be the actual population of a country . . . or any other defined group of people."[3]

Like other sciences, the kinds of questions epidemiology raises are not related only to the more restricted body of knowledge that has developed within its own framework of study. They arise in the context of the prevailing philosophic outlook and scientific study of the nature of man, his adaptation to his environment, and to the changing conceptualization of health and disease. The origins of a science cannot easily be traced to a distinct time or to a particular person. Epidemiologic thought is well developed in the writings of Hippocrates but its development as a basic medical science began many centuries later. The distinguishing feature of these early studies of scientific epidemiology was the observation of disease in a population group on the basis of which causal inferences were made. In some cases hypotheses based on these inferences were tested by epidemiologic experimental studies.

The importance of Lind's[4] contribution to prevention of scurvy was not the observation that scurvy was a prevalent and a severe disease among sailors. This was common knowledge at the time. Following a review of earlier opinions and limited clinical tests which he made, he pointed to the value of oranges and lemons in its treatment and prevention. Similarly, the importance of Pott's[5] observation that cancer of the scrotum was more common in chimney sweeps was his association of irritant soot with cancer, and his proposals for its eradication by thorough body washing following exposure at work. Epidemics of disease in which large numbers of people are affected in a single episode dramatize the importance of protecting the whole population; it is hardly surprising that many of the foundation contributions were made in such situations. Baker's[6] investigation of "Devonshire colic" and his demonstration of its association with lead in the local cider, Snow's[7] classic studies of cholera, Budd's[8] study of typhoid, and Panum's[9] study of measles remain of interest to modern epidemiologists because of the way in which their studies led them to make inferences of value to the understanding and sometimes to the control of the disease.

The following features of epidemiology have been stressed by many workers. Frost stated:

> Epidemiology is never, in fact, developed as a purely descriptive science. In collecting facts about the distribution of disease, the purpose in view is always to arrive at a better understanding of its nature, sources, means of spread, and eventually its control.[2]
>
> Epidemiology at any given time is something more than the total of its established facts. It includes their orderly arrangement into chains of inference which extend more or less beyond the bounds of direct observation. Such of these chains as are well and truly laid guide investigation to the facts of the future; those that are ill made fetter progress. But it is not easy, when divergent theories are presented, to distinguish immediately between those which are sound and those which are merely plausible. Therefore it is instructive to turn back to arguments which have been tested by the subsequent course of events; to cultivate discrimi-

nation by the study of those which the advance of definite knowledge has confirmed.[10]

Later epidemiologists have all focused attention on these essential elements of epidemiology. Among the most succinct statements is the following: "Epidemiology may be defined as the study of the distribution of a disease or condition in a population and of the factors that influence this distribution."[11]

The consistent emphasis on both the descriptive and analytic aspects of the subject is illustrated in the following extract from a modern textbook on epidemiology which resembles the earlier statement by Frost.

> Epidemiology is the study of the distribution and determinants of disease prevalence in man. . . .
>
> . . . Two main areas are indicated in the definition. These are the study of the distribution of disease (descriptive epidemiology) and the search for determinants of the noted distribution (analytic epidemiology). The first, describing the distribution of health states in terms of age, sex, race, geography etc., might be considered an extension of the discipline of demography to health and disease. The second, involving interpretation of the distribution in terms of possible causal factors, is the special contribution of epidemiology. Definitions of epidemiology that consider only the descriptive phase do not indicate the unique component of the discipline.[12]

The importance of the analytic elements of epidemiology has been emphasized by Cassel and his associates.

> There has been a failure on the part of some investigators to recognize that the significant contributions made by epidemiology in the past have been those in which it has been applied as an analytic rather than as a descriptive science. . . . Too many current epidemiological studies content themselves with describing incidence and prevalence data by selected demographic variables. . . . Such conclusions as are derived are largely restricted to identifying high-risk population groups for case finding purposes or to estimate the volume and nature of service needs. Such studies have led to an unfortunate dichotomy in the minds of some between "epidemiological" and "etiological" investigations.[13]

Maintaining this emphasis on the need for inference as well as description in epidemiologic study, epidemiologists are bringing their science into line with scientific methods as a whole, of which Bertrand Russell wrote many years ago:

> Scientific method . . . is in essence remarkably simple. It consists in observing such facts as will enable the observer to discover general laws governing facts of the kind in question. The two stages, first of observation, and second of inference to a law, are both essential. . . . The man who says "unsupported bodies in air fall" has merely generalized, and is liable

> to be refuted by balloons, butterflies, and aeroplanes; whereas the man who understands the theory of falling bodies knows also why certain exceptional bodies do not fall.[14]

It is natural that epidemics of infectious diseases should have occupied such a prominent position in the development of scientific epidemiology from the 19th into the 20th century. Not only was this reinforced by the revolutionary discoveries throughout the age of bacteriology in which all attention was focused on microorganisms and their role as the causal agents of disease, but the very occurrence of an epidemic, especially an acute epidemic, directed attention towards the community at risk. In a literal sense, the community feels itself at risk and demands action at community level.

While there were many who confined their conceptualization of epidemiology to the mass phenomena or community aspects of infectious disease, early field epidemiologic investigations included noninfectious diseases as well. An outstanding example of these are Goldberger's studies on pellagra in the southern United States, which began in 1914.[15] However, it is probably true to say that Goldberger was selected for this task because the authorities at the time thought that pellagra was of infectious origin.

So important and stimulating were the advances made through microbiologic studies, that while epidemiology was always searching for more than just a specific causal microorganism of a particular disease there were times when this became an all-absorbing interest. John Gordon, who himself pioneered the epidemiologic study of accidents, has written of the reaction to this trend.

> In the minds of many a realization gradually took form that disease was no longer being studied, but rather parts of a disease; . . . that in pursuit of knowledge about the agents of disease, the main objective was being lost. . . . This movement did not originate precisely in 1920, nor in the years immediately following. . . . The return to a holistic interpretation of community disease, its consideration as a unified and total process had been under way for a number of years.[16]

COMMUNITY MEDICINE

A community's health is an expression and a consequence of interdependent characteristics of the community and its environment. Health itself must also be seen as determining community structure and behavior, as well as influencing the environment. The interdependence, or causal chain $\rightleftharpoons$, may be summarized in a triangle, shown in Figure 1-1.

Health care of a community may be directed to these various aspects simultaneously and in coordinated fashion, or it may focus on a particular

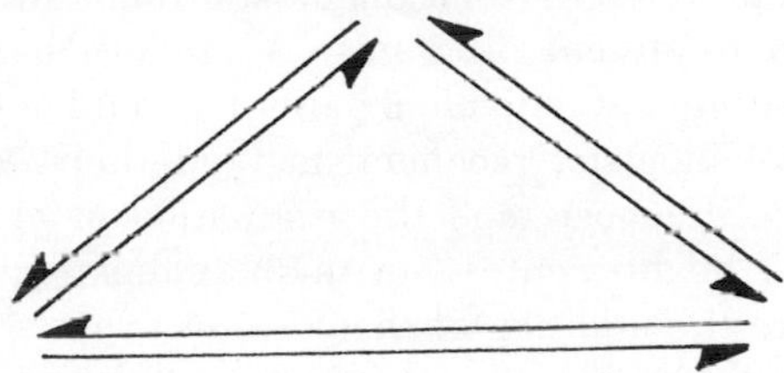

FIG. 1-1. Triangle of causal relationships between the state of health of a community, its environment and material resources, as well as its biologic, social, and cultural characteristics.

facet. In more developed societies and especially in industrial urban areas, community health care includes the following:

Direct personal health care—curative, preventive, and rehabilitative
Community organization and health education
Environmental surveillance and conservation, with sanitary control.

Within the scope of these three main areas of community health care a variety of services have come into being. With its focus on the health of the community as a whole, community medicine is interested in the integrative development of these various areas, while not necessarily having the expertise itself to carry out each element. Thus environmental conservation extends beyond community medicine and epidemiology to engineering as well as to the ecologic aspects of natural and social sciences. Similarly, community organization and health education embrace the quality of life in all its aspects, including the aesthetic and creative, economic, sociocultural, and educational aspects, each of which has implications for the community's health. Community medicine's function lies in understanding their meaning for the community's health and on this basis promoting and modifying their development.

Its difference from, and relationship with other branches of medicine lies in the fact that its interest is centered on the community and the groups of which the community is composed. The field of community medicine requires scientific foundations for action no less than does any other field.[17–19] Diagnosis of the state of health of a community is as important a foundation of community medicine and community health care in general as is careful diagnosis of the state of health of an individual patient seeking care. The personnel and tools required must be built into community health practice, if such diagnostic foundations are to be laid for the action and treatment programs. A modern hospital, concerned as it is with the treatment of individual patients, could not function without pathologists, microbiologists, biochemists, and their laboratories. They are essential to the diagnosis and the evaluation of change in patients' health. Community health centers, in their application of medicine to a community, require the addition of these same experts as well as others trained in community diagnosis, such as epidemiologists, biostatisticians, and social scientists, with their equipment and laboratories. There is need for research in the whole field of scientific development of community medicine. This will involve research into ways of diagnosing the state of health of a community and of measuring the impact of health services on it. Is there a value in such studies? The answer can only come from research into the usefulness of community diagnosis and evaluation of medical care. This will need extension of the research into experimental studies of different kinds of community health care.

The basic data for community health care include measures of the community's state of health, the etiologic factors related to it, and the nature of its health services. Epidemiologic inquiry is an integral part of the practice of community medicine, ensuring sound methods of data-gathering for description of the state of health of a community. It achieves this by study of the differential distribution of health characteristics and the probable causes of this distribution. Similarly, study of health care, professional and other, is a continual necessity for satisfactory development of community health services. Among other things it involves knowledge of the available services and their use in relation to the health service system as a whole, and the variations between different groups in their perceptions of health and of the health services that are provided.

Medical care in the community includes the following:

Individual care—primary health care as well as medical care to meet special needs of individuals.

Family medicine—family oriented medicine, or health care centered on the family as the unit; not all "family physicians" are family oriented but this does not detract from what should be the distinctive aspect of family practice.

Community medicine—focus on community and its subgroups is the essential function of practice.

The functions of these kinds of medical care may overlap and strengthen one another. On the other hand they may be, and very often are, separate.

Primary health care, as usually understood, involves the medical practitioner to whom a person first turns when ill, and has extended to include personal preventive care, such as immunization procedures, and advice on personal health matters. Although it is concerned with the needs of individual patients, it often involves meaningful others, such as the patient's family. It is provided by different kinds of practitioners and is organized in different ways in various communities. The traditional general practitioner of European medicine and other countries settled by Europeans is the first person that usually comes to mind. This particular system of practice, traditional to one society, has not been readily transposed to others. In many countries the traditional medical practice is of a different kind, but modernization of primary medical care is developing, based on varied teams of paramedical and auxiliary public health personnel.

At the same time, in more developed countries, the old-time solo practitioner is being replaced by teams of doctors working with other professional health workers, particularly nurses and laboratory and radiology technicians. In these countries too, auxiliary personnel are being used to extend primary health care.

The development of medical care to meet special needs of individual patients has perhaps been the outstanding feature of modern medicine. Specialization has raised the standards of care potentially available and at the same time created problems in distribution of primary medical care. Although specialization was originally distinct from primary medical care, this distinction is no longer always clear. Thus the specialist caring for a person with long-term illness may often be regarded as giving primary medical care and specialists working together in group practice or health centers may be correctly described as a primary health care team.

Individual care and family medicine are often found as practices in the community without any effective development of community medicine. However community medicine can and should function within primary health care. A major objective of this book is to outline an approach to the development of "community medicine and primary health care" as a unified practice. This would be an additional dimension of the health service system, added to the more established traditional "hospital" and "public health practice." With these objectives in mind the text has been arranged in the following five sections.

1. Community Health
2. Community Determinants of Health
3. Infection, Disease and Community Health: An Illustration of Changing Concepts of Cause and Effect
4. The Community Syndrome Concept
5. Community Medicine and Primary Health Care

REFERENCES

1. Greenwood M: Epidemiology—Historical and Experimental. The Herter Lectures for 1931. Baltimore, Johns Hopkins, 1932, p 2.
2. Frost WH: Epidemiology. In Maxcy KF (ed.): Papers of Wade Hampton Frost, M.D. New York, Commonwealth Fund, 1941, pp 494, 497.
3. Morris JN: Uses of Epidemiology, 2nd ed. Edinburgh, E & S Livingstone, 1964, p 3.
4. Lind J: A Treatise on the Scurvy. Edinburgh, Sands, Murray and Cochran, 1753. (Lind's experiment is quoted by Drummond JC, Wilbraham A: The Englishman's Food. London, Jonathan Cape, 1939, p 317.)
5. Pott P: Chirurgical Observations Relative to the Cataract, the Polypus of the Nose, the Cancer of the Scrotum, the Different Kinds of Ruptures, and the Mortification of the Toes and Feet. London, Hower, Clarke and Pollins, 1775.
6. Baker G: An Essay Concerning the Cause of Endemial Colic of Devonshire, 1767. Reprint. New York, Delta Omega Society, 1958.
7. Snow J: On the mode of communication of cholera. In: Snow on Cholera. New York, Commonwealth Fund, 1936.
8. Budd W: Typhoid Fever, Its Nature, Mode of Spreading and Prevention, 1873. Reissue. New York, Delta Omega Society, American Public Health Association, 1931.
9. Panum PL: Observations Made During the Epidemic of Measles on the Faroe Islands in the Year 1846. Translation by Mrs. A.S. Hatcher. In: Panum on Measles, New York, Delta Omega Society, 1940. American Public Health Association, 1940.
10. Frost WH: Introduction. In: Snow on Cholera. New York, Commonwealth Fund, 1936, p ix.
11. Lilienfeld AM: Epidemiologic methods and inferences in studies of noninfectious diseases. Public Health Rep 72:51, 1957.
12. MacMahon B, Pugh RF, Ipsen J: Epidemiologic Methods. Boston, Little, Brown, 1960, p 3.
13. Cassel J, Patrick R, Jenkins D: Epidemiological analysis of the health implications of culture change. A conceptual model. Ann NY Acad Sci 84:938, 1960.
14. Russell B: The Scientific Outlook. London, George Allen and Unwin, 1931, p 15.
15. Terris M (ed.): Goldberger on Pellagra. Baton Rouge, Louisiana State University Press, 1964.
16. Gordon JE: Evolution of an epidemiology of health. In Galdston I (ed.): The Epidemiology of Health. New York, New York Academy of Medicine, 1953, p 61.
17. McGavran EG: Scientific diagnosis and treatment of the community as a patient. JAMA 162:723, 1956.
18. Kark SL, Kark E: A practice of social medicine. In Kark SL, Steuart GW, (eds.): A Practice of Social Medicine. Edinburgh, E & S Livingstone, 1962, Chap. 1.
19. Kark SL, Community health research. Johns Hopkins Med J 124:258, 1969.

SECTION I
COMMUNITY HEALTH

The focus of medicine is on the investigation of disease and the treatment of sick people. As a medical science epidemiology shares this orientation and is the main foundation on which action is based for the protection of the community against disease and its effects. Nevertheless, attention is being paid by medicine as a whole to its role in promoting health and this has been reflected in epidemiologic studies of the well-being of groups,[1,2] such as studies concerning the relationship between the social status and physique of reproductive women in a community, the outcome of pregnancy, and the well-being of the children of these women.[3] It is such studies that extend our perception of the usefulness of medicine to the community as well as to individuals and their families, and at the same time widen its horizons to its potential for promoting community health in addition to its more established, traditional role in treatment of the sick and prevention of disease.

This section on community health focuses attention on concepts of health and disease. A model of community health is presented considering the somatic and psychologic characteristics as well as disease and disability. Lastly, the distribution of health and disease in the community is discussed in relation to some of the more common biologic and social groupings in communities.

2
Concepts of Health

GENERAL CONSIDERATIONS

All communities have their concepts of health integrated as part of the total culture. Associated with its values and beliefs about health, every community has its well-established ways of maintaining health, preventing disease, and treating the sick. Widely differing culture groups share the concepts of health as a state of balance and harmony, and of disease as a disturbance, imbalance, or disharmony. Kuper states that "health itself has long been recognized by the Hindu as more than purely physical well-being."[4] A Hindu physician said, "To the Hindu, health is harmony," and he described harmony as "being at peace with the Self, the community, God and the cosmos." Kuper presents a number of illustrations of this basic interpretation. The Hindu "show deep psychological insight into the importance of harmonious personal relationships in dealing with health. Every effort is made to "match" a young couple psychologically as well as physically, in order to produce healthy children." With the concept of harmony goes that of equilibrium, *sattva,* a desired quality which is continually being challenged by other qualities.

The Navajos of America are described as having very similar concepts of health.

> Religion is concerned with the here and now. It has as its focus the maintenance of balance between the individual and his total physical and social environment, as well as the maintenance of balance between the supernatural and man. When these forces are in a state of balance, good health is the result; an upset in this equilibrium causes disease.[5]

In English the word "health" is derived from the Old English, "hal," or "hâel-th"—hale means whole, as does "heal," to make whole, which has a common teutonic origin as in Dutch, "heelen," and German, "heilen."[6] In Hebrew the concept of wholeness and peace is expressed in words which have a common root: שלם (the letters *sh*, *l*, *m*). The word "shalem," meaning whole, is also used to mean healthy, without disease and without injury,[7] as in "ויבא יעקב שלם עיר שכם" — "And Jacob came well to the city Shechem"—Genesis 33:18. Similarly, "shalom," meaning peace, is also used in the sense of the condition of well-being as in "לך נא ראה את שלום אחיך ואת שלום הצאן" —"Go, please, see if it is well (shalom) with your brothers and well (shalom) with the flock"—Genesis 37:14. These words are still used in this sense, as in the everyday greeting "מה שלומך," that is, "mā sh'lom-cha" (*ch* as in Ba*ch*), "how is your peace," meaning, how are you?

To many, health and disease are distinctive processes with different basic qualities.

The Pioneer Health Centre, Peckham, London, epitomized the beliefs of its founders, Innes Pearse and Scott Williamson, in its focus on "health" as distinct from "sickness." They perceived health as a condition of mutual response between an organism and an everchanging environment [8–10] and designed their health center to promote health in this sense, by having facilities and equipment for a wide range of leisure activities to accommodate a health center community of 2,000 families. Their concepts on health and the action needed for health were developed in a pilot health center which they began in 1926, and then established in a building especially designed for the promotion of health. The kind of health observations they made regarding the members of the health club expressed those concepts involving "an attempt to estimate the physical efficiency of the family and all its members, and their capability for: (1) individual life; (2) family life; (3) social life."[10]

Their observations thus included periodic physical examinations with laboratory investigations, social observations of people in their various activities in the community of the health center, and family consultations in which the health of the family was reviewed and discussed between the "biologists" (physicians) and the family. In writing of their experience they emphasize the importance of including an appraisal of function in a *health* examination.

> It will be clear that the health examination, or biological overhaul as we prefer to call it, cannot end in the consulting-room. It is continued in observation of each family acting in the social milieu of the Centre. To see individuals at a social gathering, swimming, dancing, skating; at whist or billiards; at dramatic, musical, or other activity, provides us with essential data which serve to modify or enlarge observations made in the consulting-room. It is becoming more and more apparent as we proceed that the ground in which the seeds of disease are sown is that of disfunction and disability.[9]

Emphasis on health as an entity in itself and its more inclusive meaning is written into the constitution of the World Health Organization which states that health is "a state of complete physical, mental, and social well-being and not merely the absence of disease or infirmity."[11] The focus on health as a distinctive entity directs attention to the potential for promotion of health beyond the more readily known specific preventive and therapeutic measures against disease. By including the social as well as the physical and mental attributes of health, this definition embodies a broader concept of health than is usual at present, many years after the World Health Organization was constituted.

Similarly, disease can be perceived as something more than mere deviation from health, each disease being an entity with distinguishing qualities in its distinctive pathologic processes, its typical clinical appearance, and often its characteristic epidemiologic pattern of distribution in time, place, and community. True and useful as this perception is, it is only a part of the whole. The common or shared characteristics of many diseases are at least as striking as their distinguishing features.

Early in his career, Selye[12] was impressed with the fact that distinctive or characteristic signs and symptoms of specific diseases are relatively uncommon when compared with the large number of signs which are common to many diseases. These latter he referred to as nonspecific and he writes of the "syndrome of just being sick," i.e., having a group of signs and symptoms "that characterized disease as such, not any one disease," and which were the "nonspecific reaction" of the body to damage of any kind. In infectious fevers the nonspecific signs include fever; pain in the body and joints; headache; coated tongue and red throat; loss of appetite; loss of weight; enlargement of the spleen or liver; confusion; delirium; and local reaction such as inflammation. He deemed this nonspecific response to a pathogenic agent a "general adaptation" syndrome. "Many diseases are actually not so much the direct results of some external agent (an infection, intoxication) as they are consequences of the body's inability to meet these agents by adequate adaptive reaction."[12]

The dichotomy between health and disease may be more a matter of degree than is at first apparent. The distinctive qualities which differentiate them may well be extremes of a continuous variation from optimal health to serious disease. The milder the disease or the more border-line the health, the more difficult it is to differentiate between health and disease.

The Hippocratic concept of health and disease stressed the relation between man's nature and his environment, the essential unity of mind and body, and the natural causation of disease. It postulated man's nature as consisting of four humors, each having the following characteristics which likened it to one of the four elements which, according to Aristotle, made up all matter.

Blood, hot and moist, like air
Phlegm, cold and moist, like water
Black bile, cold and dry, like earth
Yellow bile, hot and dry, like fire

Health (eukrasia) prevailed when the four humors were balanced or in equilibrium and when the balance was disturbed disease (dyskrasia) was the result. The body was assumed to have powers of restoration of humoral equilibrium, and it was the physician's primary role to assist in this healing process. While the specific elements of the humoral theory of Hippocrates were based on inadequate and incorrect foundations, the general concept of psychobiologic balance and the innate capacity of responding to disturbance in the equilibrium that constitutes health is highly relevant to modern epidemiology and community medicine.[13,14]

There are men who, with a comparatively limited number of facts, are able to postulate generalizations which stimulate subsequent generations to new lines of investigation and to enlarge and modify the original generalization on the basis of these fresh observations. Claude Bernard[15] made such a contribution to biologic science in his development of experimental medicine and his concept of an inner environment.

> The conditions necessary to life are found neither in the organism nor in the outer environment, but in both at once. Indeed, if we suppress or disturb the organism, life ceases, even though the environment remains intact; if, on the other hand, we take away or vitiate the environment, life just as completely disappears, even though the organism has not been destroyed. . . .
>
> . . . In living beings the internal environment, which is a true product of the organism, preserves the necessary relations of exchange and equilibrium with the external cosmic environment.[15]

Many years later Cannon[16] used the term homeostasis (from the Greek homoios: like, similar status, position, or standing) to describe the ability of living beings to maintain relative constancy of their inner environment in the face of a changing outer environment. He extended the concept to consideration of the regulatory mechanisms involved in maintaining homeostasis, and suggested the possible usefulness of the concept in the study of "social homeostasis."

REGULATION OF IRON BALANCE: AN EXAMPLE OF HOMEOSTASIS

The study of iron metabolism is illustrative of the role of homeostatic regulations in maintaining iron balance. Red blood cells have a natural survival period (± 120 days), at the end of which they are destroyed, their hemoglobin being broken down into its constituent parts. The iron is liberated into the plasma and is thus again available for use. In the normal adult male very limited quantities of iron are excreted and the main need for iron is met by this endogenous cycle. There is thus little need for absorption of dietary iron, the bulk of which is excreted. In women, menstruation involves iron loss, and in pregnancy, while the loss through menstrual bleeding is halted, fetal demand, especially in the last trimester, and blood loss during delivery depletes their iron stores. The need for absorption of dietary iron is thus greater than in men.

Control of the absorption of iron is a major factor in maintaining the amount of iron in the body at a more or less constant level.[17-21] The main site of iron absorption is the proximal part of the small intestine, the amount absorbed being determined by the mucosa. The way in which the mucosal cells control the process of absorption is not yet clear but there is evidence that the iron concentration in these cells is important. Depletion of the concentration of iron in the cells leads to increased absorption of iron from the digested dietary content of the intestinal lumen, whereas saturation of the cells with iron blocks further absorption. The degree of iron saturation of the mucosal cells is determined by the iron balance of the plasma. The plasma is the main channel through which iron moves from one part of the body to another, and while the plasma iron turnover varies considerably according to demand, its iron concentration varies within much narrower limits. Thus sudden increased demand, as might be caused by bleeding, leads to some reduction in plasma iron concentration, but this is soon reflected in depletion of iron in the cells of the intestinal mucosa, which in turn is accompanied by increased absorption of iron.[22] In this way, as well as through absorption from storage depots, the plasma iron concentration is rapidly returned to its level before bleeding.

In response to chronic blood loss the plasma iron concentration may remain unchanged, with a steady supply of iron to the bone marrow being brought by plasma transportation from storage depots or intestinal mucosa. With increase in the amount of iron by absorption and by control of loss, the plasma makes good the storage deposited. Anemia may not become apparent in this whole process, depending upon the amount of stored iron and the availability of iron for absorption. Thus it is not anemia as such which causes increased absorption of iron from the intestinal lumen, but rather the plasma iron balance which affects the degree of saturation of iron of the intestinal mucosal cells.

Of epidemiologic interest in community medicine are the processes which promote optimum functioning of the various homeostatic mechanisms involved in iron metabolism, those which put an added strain on the system, and those which interfere with homeostatic mechanisms with resultant states of imbalance (Table 2-1).

Epidemiologic investigation of iron balance involves measurement of these processes as well as the health conditions which reflect the functioning of the regulating mechanisms of iron metabolism. The latter may include study of the red blood cells, hemoglobin, and iron stores, as well as

TABLE 2-1. Processes Influencing Homeostatic Regulating Mechanisms of Iron Metabolism

PROCESSES WHICH PROMOTE SATISFACTORY FUNCTIONING OF HOMEOSTATIC REGULATING MECHANISMS	PROCESSES WHICH CHALLENGE THE FUNCTIONING OF THE HOMEOSTATIC MECHANISMS	PROCESSES WHICH INTERFERE WITH HOMEOSTATIS, WITH EVIDENCE OF IMBALANCE
Satisfactory amounts of dietary iron available for absorption in the small intestine	Pregnancy—the additional requirements both for the fetus, and the loss of blood during delivery—requires high levels of iron stores during early pregnancy to ensure availability when most needed, as well as dietary or prophylactic iron for absorption	Any factors which interfere with the processes listed in the first column including inadequate amounts of available iron in the diet, malabsorption syndromes, various causes of increased hemolysis of red blood cells, continuing blood loss as in hookworm infestation and schistosomiasis, or bleeding from peptic ulcer.
An intact mucosa of the small intestine with satisfactory absorptive capacity		
An iron transportation system, involving stable plasma iron concentration, suitable amounts of stored iron, a rate of red blood cell breakdown consistent with its steady replacement, and a satisfactorily functioning bone marrow	Growth and development, with increased demand for iron especially during phase of growth when red cell volume is increasing rapidly as part of increase in circulating blood volume	An accumulation of abnormally large quantities of iron in the liver and other storage tissues, as in the very common form of siderosis in Africans of southern African[25–27] and in less common conditions such as hemochromatosis,[17,28] aplastic anemia,[17] thalassemia,[29] and cystic fibrosis of the pancreas[30]
A rate of loss of iron from the body readily replaced by increased absorption and transportation to bone marrow	Chronic blood loss as in menstruation, especially menorrhagia, with need for additional iron available for absorption and erythropoiesis	

signs and symptoms associated with severe anemia. Anemia is the common manifestation of iron deficiency that is of epidemiologic interest. The community picture may be analyzed on the basis of the qualitative and quantitative observations. Qualitative observations are commonly made in medical diagnosis, i.e., whether the person has the condition. In this case the decision as to whether a person has anemia is usually based on the hemoglobin level. Various levels have been suggested as cut-off points for the diagnosis of anemia. Thus in 1968 an Expert Committee of the World Health Organization recommended the following.[23]

Children aged 6 months to 6 years: 11 g/100 ml
Children aged 6 to 14 years: 12 g/100 ml
Adult males: 13 g/100 ml
Adult females, not pregnant: 12 g/100 ml
Adult females, pregnant: 11 g/100 ml
At all ages the normal mean corpuscular hemoglobin concentration should be 34 g/100 ml

This represented a change from a previous expert committee's opinion which recommended that in pregnancy a hemoglobin level of 10 g/100 ml or less should be regarded as anemia. Thus a quantitative observation is used to separate those who have anemia from those who do not. Quantitative observations may be arranged in the form of a frequency distribution. This frequency distribution may be tabulated or presented as a histogram. Table 2-2 is a tabulation of the frequency distribution of hemoglobin levels

TABLE 2-2. Distribution of Hemoglobin Level in 50 Parturient Women (in g/ml)

Hb LEVEL	NO. OF WOMEN
6.0–6.4	1
6.5–	0
7.0–	2
7.5–	4
8.0–	0
8.5–	20
9.0–	20
9.5–	51
10.0–	67
10.5–	114
11.0–	81
11.5–	69
12.0–	28
12.5–	32
13.0–	5
13.5–	5
14.0–	0
14.5–14.9	1

in a consecutive series of 500 parturient women, in a community in which a mild degree of anemia in pregnancy was common, and which has been reported on elsewhere.[24]

Using a cutoff point of 11 g to define anemia, the figures in Table 2-2 suggest the occurrence of anemia in 56 percent of the women. Using a cutoff point of 1 g lower this picture changes considerably—less than 20 percent of the women would be regarded as having anemia. Since both qualitative and quantitative observations are commonly used in clinical and epidemiologic investigations, and since quantitive observations are also used to define the presence or absence of diseases by the use of cut-off points, the health of population groups will now be considered further.

THE HEALTH OF A POPULATION GROUP

The usual way to consider the health of a population group is in the summation of the health of its individual members. Even in the most limited sense it is seldom, if ever, that the health of all members of a community is known. The most commonly used indices are those which measure the physical and mental condition of a community, such as growth and development of children, including measures of intelligence and physical growth, or physique and efficiency in, for example, pregnant women or workers in industry.

When investigating the occurrence of a particular health condition in a community, it is often useful to separate those who have the particular condition or attribute from those who do not, as if they were distinctly different groups with markedly differentiating qualities. This is the main method of describing the occurrence of disease. Contrasted with this is a more quantitative method of differentiating the health qualities of people in a community. There are a number of these qualities, such as blood pressure levels and hemoglobin counts, which have a continuous distribution in population groups; measures of the distribution itself may often be very helpful. Both the "qualitative" and "quantitative" ways of describing a community's health are commonly used.

The occurrence or frequency of a disease is most often expressed as a ratio or proportion of those who have the disease *(D)* and the total or exposed population *(P)*, i.e., D/P, which is calculated as a rate per unit of population (per 1,000; 10,000; or per 100,000) depending on convention and convenience. Two kinds of rates are in general use in describing the frequency of disease: incidence and prevalence.

The *incidence rate* of a disease measures the number of new cases of that disease which occur during a defined period of time per unit of population, and is expressed as follows:

$$\frac{\text{Number of new cases of the disease during a particular period of time}}{\text{Population exposed during that time}} \times 1{,}000;\ 10{,}000;\ 100{,}000$$

The *prevalence rate* of a disease measures the total number of cases of that disease at a particular time per unit of population, and is expressed as follows:

$$\frac{\text{Total number of cases at a particular time}}{\text{Population at that time}} \times 1{,}000;\ 10{,}000;\ 100{,}000$$

Duration of disease is an important aspect when considering these rates. A disease with a relatively low incidence may yet be common in a community at a particular time if it is of long duration. Diabetes mellitus, with modern methods of treatment, is such a disease. However, diseases which may have a high incidence, and which occur in short epidemics, with high mortality rates or high rates of complete recovery, may have a low prevalence unless the rate is measured at the height of the epidemic, as in epidemics of influenza or measles.

There are a number of refinements of both rates but it is perhaps helpful to look more closely at the basic components of the ratio *D/P*. *D*, the number of cases of the disease, is in fact a figure of those known to have the disease or to have had it over a defined period. Much will therefore depend on the way *D* is ascertained. It may be restricted to cases diagnosed in hospital, as in many studies of mental diseases and in the establishment and maintenance of cancer registers. In more developed countries, the hospitalization rate of cancers as a whole will undoubtedly be more reflective of the frequency of the disease than will hospitalization data of mental diseases. When the number of cases, *D*, is confined to known hospitalized cases, this vital information should always be shown as "Hospitalized Cases of the Disease."

Another common means of determining incidence is through a system of notification of cases to a health authority. The compulsory reporting of various infectious diseases was an early development of public health practice and has been extended to include other conditions in different countries, such as industrial diseases and work injuries, and nutritional diseases, e.g., pellagra. Severity of disease and its consequences, as in formidable epidemic diseases, and social and health legislation affecting compensation and treatment, as in work injuries and compensatable diseases, will obviously influence the reporting of cases. Here, too, the numerator *D* should be clearly stated to be "Notified or Reported Cases of the Disease." Yet another approach to the determination of *D* might be surveillance of a total population or representative samples of the population. Again it is obvious that the methods used in such surveys will have to differ markedly as between the case finding in short-term acute illness (e.g., acute tonsillitis associated with hemolytic streptococcal infection) and that in long-term disabling disorders. In many of the latter, which have become important public health problems, it is often difficult to determine the time of onset of the disease and hence incidence rates are less reliable.

The denominator P is composed of D plus those not known to be diseased *(ND)*. The ratio D/P is thus $D/(D + ND)$, and the way in which ND is determined is obviously of as much importance as is that of D. Surveillance by continuing community health surveys is not yet a routine, The figure for the total population is used and both incidence and prevalence rates are determined by the numerator of known cases and the denominator of the estimated population. The population might be the whole population, or particular segments of it, e.g., age and sex groups, or those exposed to the particular condition under investigation. Implicit in such rates is the assumption that the community can be divided into those who have the disease and those who do not.

Increasingly, various criteria for the diagnosis of a disease include cutoff points on a line of a continuously varying attribute. One example of this in the diagnosis of anemia has already been mentioned. Another is in the diagnosis of hypertension. In this case, a World Health Organization Expert Committee[31] recommended the following levels of blood pressure in the diagnosis of hypertension.

1. A systolic blood pressure below 140 mm Hg and a diastolic blood pressure below 90 mm Hg—normal range.
2. A systolic blood pressure of 165 mm Hg and above or a diastolic blood pressure of 95 mm Hg and above—abnormal (hypertensive) range.
3. The in-between readings, systolic blood pressure 140–164 mm Hg, and diastolic blood pressure 90–94 mm Hg, are classified as borderline hypertension.

This grouping by cutoff points separates normotensive and hypertensive persons by a relatively wide range of blood pressure, introducing a category of borderline hypertension, as first used in the Framingham Study.[32]

The problem of substituting a high blood pressure level or a low hemoglobin count for diseases such as hypertension and anemia requires further discussion, more especially in their translation as epidemiologic foundations for community health diagnosis.

Certainly there are many diseases defined by measurements that are regarded as deviating sufficiently from a so-called normal range as to warrant their being used as criteria for diagnosis of disease. The introduction of such cutoff points is an attempt to quantify diagnosis and, in so doing, to make it more scientific. At the same time it introduces the arbitrary decision that a quantitative attribute like blood pressure does in fact represent a disease when it reaches a certain level.

Critical thought is needed in the use of such cutoff points for community medicine, with special regard to the purpose of the epidemiologic investigation. The diagnosis of hypertensive disease may require certain clinical findings as well as specified raised blood pressure levels. A program in a community in which coronary artery disease and hypertensive disease are both common would obviously include such people. However, epidemiologically, the association between blood pressure level and subsequent clinical coronary artery disease has been shown at blood pressure levels below those that might be regarded as representing hypertensive disease itself (Fig. 2-1).

An increase in the ratio of actual to expected death rates from cerebrovascular disease in relation to blood pressure level has also been noted in men and women.[33]

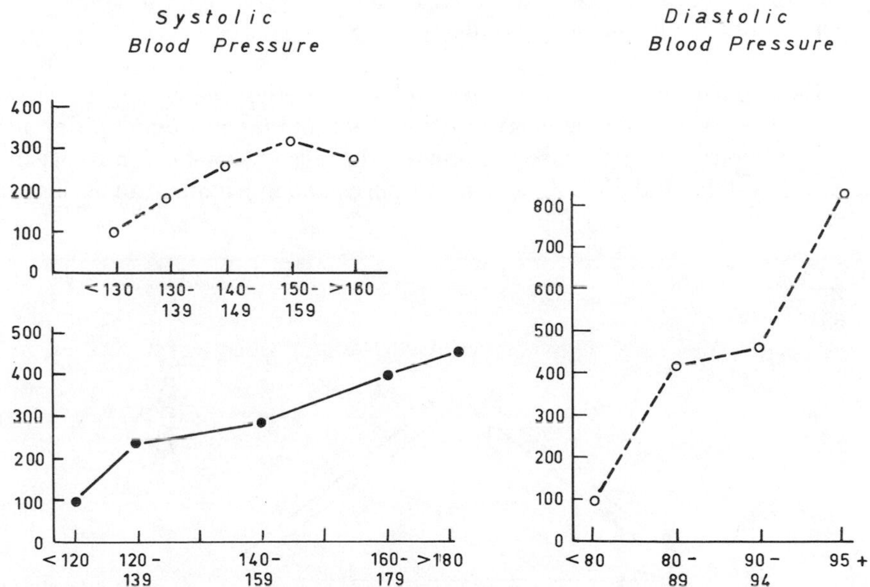

FIG. 2-1. Relative risk of coronary heart disease in men according to initial blood pressure. ●———● : The findings of the Framingham Study, in men aged 30–59—10 years' follow-up after initial examination. o----o: The findings of study of men aged 40–59 in the Peoples' Gas, Light, and Coke Company, Chicago—3.3 years follow-up after initial examination. (Adapted from Stamler.[33])

It would seem that the more we seek measurable variables of health status and function, the more blurred become the distinctions between adjacent points along the line of continuous variation. The quantitative estimation of health variables includes both somatic and psychologic characteristics and is a foundation of epidemiology and diagnosis of community health. It is not always necessary to introduce cutoff points along these lines to make the epidemiologic picture fit the clinical diagnosis of a disease. The state of health of a community can be better described by recognizing that there are different ways of doing this. The framework can include traditional clinical concepts of dichotomous separation of the diseased from the well or healthy as well as a continuum in the distribution of a health-relevant attribute. The measurement of the community's health should therefore be based on both qualitative and quantitative observations, as represented by the following:

Disease and disability: the incidence and prevalence rates of various diseases and disabilities.

Somatic characteristics: the frequency distribution of measured somatic characteristics like physique, growth, and physiologic variables, e.g., blood pressure

Psychologic characteristics: the distribution of psychologic attributes of personality, behavior, and intelligence

Interdependence between these characteristics or variables is of central interest in epidemiology. We now know that in communities in which coronary artery disease is common, there is an association between levels of systolic and diastolic blood pressures and subsequent experience

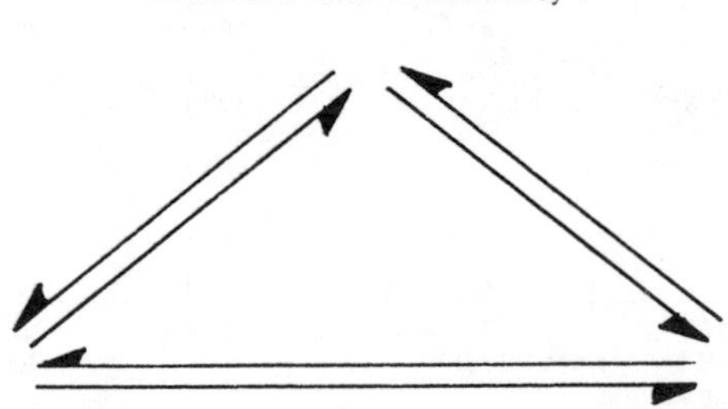

FIG. 2-2. A diagram of interdependent indicators of community health based on qualitative and quantitative observations.

of myocardial infarction. The consistency of this finding has led to high blood pressure being regarded as one of the main risk factors for myocardial infarction in such communities. The possibility of association and causal relationship between such specific elements of the three broadly defined qualities is the essence of many hypotheses tested in epidemiologic investigations. Associations found between the distribution of these health attributes in a community become the foundation for understanding community health and may be diagrammatically represented as a triangle of interacting or interdependent components (Fig. 2-2).

There are also meaningful associations within each component itself, such as clusters of diseases, somatic variables in somatotypes, and the combination of various personality traits into personality-types. Each of these three components of the triangle will be considered more fully in the next chapters of this section.

REFERENCES

1. Merrell M, Reed LJ: The epidemiology of health. In Galdston I (ed.): Social Medicine, Its Derivations and Objectives. New York, Commonwealth Fund, 1949.
2. Galdston I (ed.): The Epidemiology of Health. New York, New York Academy of Medicine, 1953.
3. Baird D: Variations in fertility associated with changes in health status. In Sheps MC, Ridley JC, (eds.): Public Health and Population Change. Pittsburgh, Univ of Pittsburgh Press, 1965.
4. Kuper H: Indian People in Natal. Pietermaritzburg, Natal Univ Press, 1960, p 242.
5. Adair J, Deuschle KW: The People's Health: Medicine and Anthropology in a Navajo Community. New York, Appleton, 1970, p 4.
6. The Concise Oxford English Dictionary. London, Oxford Univ Press, 1944.
7. Even-Shushan A: A New Dictionary, in Hebrew, Vol. 5. Jerusalem, Kiryat Sepher, 1952.
8. Pearse IH, Williamson GS: The Case for Action. London, Faber and Faber, 1931.
9. Williamson GS, Pearse IH, Noll A, et al: Biologists in Search of Material. An Interim Report on the Work of the Pioneer Health Centre, Peckham. London, Faber and Faber, 1938, p 48.
10. Pearse IH, Crocker LH: The Peckham Experiment. London, George Allen and Unwin, 1943, p 83.
11. WHO: The first ten years of the World Health Organization. In The Constitution of the World Health Organization. Geneva, Palais des Nations, 1958, p 459.
12. Selye H: The Stress of Life. New York, McGraw-Hill, 1956, p 15.
13. Sigerist H: Civilization and Disease. New York, Cornell Univ Press, 1945.
14. Dubos R: Man Adapting. New Haven, Yale Univ Press, 1967.
15. Bernard C: Introduction to the Study of Experimental Medicine, 1865. Translated by Henry Copley Greene. New York, Collier Books Edition, Abelardschuman, 1961, p. 92.

16. Cannon WB: The Wisdom of the Body, 2nd ed. New York, Norton, 1939.
17. Bothwell TH, Finch CA: Iron Metabolism. Boston, Little, Brown, 1962.
18. Crosby WH: Intestinal response to the body's requirement for iron. Control of iron absorption. JAMA 208:347, 1969.
19. Crosby WH: Control of iron balance by the intestinal mucosa. Blood 22: 441, 1963.
20. Conrad ME, Crosby WH: Intestinal mucosal mechanisms controlling iron absorption. Blood 22:406, 1963.
21. Weintraub LR, Conrad ME, Crosby WH: Regulation of the intestinal absorption of iron by the rate of erythropoiesis. Brit J Haematol 11:432, 1965.
22. Weintraub LR, Conrad ME, Crosby WH: The significance of iron turnover in the control of iron absorption. Blood 24:10, 1964.
23. WHO Expert Committee: Nutritional Anemias. Geneva, WHO Tech Rep Ser No. 405, 1968.
24. Kark SL, Peritz E, Shiloh A, et al.: Epidemiological analysis of the hemoglobin picture in parturient women of Jerusalem. Amer J Public Health 54:947, 1964.
25. Strachan AS: Haemosiderosis and Haemochromatosis in South African Natives, with a comment on the Etiology of Haemochromatosis. Thesis for MD degree, Glasgow, Scotland, 1929.
26. Walker ARP, Arvidsson UB: Iron "overload" in the South African Bantu. J Trop Med Hyg 47:536, 1953.
27. Gillman J, Gillman T: Perspectives in Human Malnutrition. New York, Grune & Stratton, 1951.
28. Sheldon JH: Haemochromatosis. London, Oxford Univ Press, 1935.
29. Weatherall DJ: The Thalassemia Syndromes. Philadelphia, Davis, 1965.
30. Andersen DH: Cystic fibrosis of the pancreas and its relation to celiac disease. A clinical and pathological study. Amer J Dis Child 56:344, 1938.
31. WHO Expert Committee: Hypertension and Coronary Heart Disease. Classification and Criteria for Epidemiological Studies. Geneva, WHO Tech Rep Ser No. 168, 1959.
32. Dawber TR, Moore FE, Mann GV: Coronary heart disease in the Framingham study. Amer J Public Health 47(2):4, 1957.
33. Stamler J: Lectures on Preventive Cardiology. New York, Grune & Stratton, 1967.

3
Disease and Disability

Scientific study of disease in population groups requires a system of classification in which various individual syndromes of illness with their many names may be grouped according to certain common characteristics. Along with this development is the need for standardizing criteria and methods of examination for recognition of these diseases, as well as appreciation or measurement of their variation in severity and expression.

PROBLEMS IN CLASSIFICATION OF DISEASES

The most recent international classification of diseases[1] indicates many of the problems involved in their classification. Inconsistencies are inevitable in grouping diseases which encompass a wide variety of conditions. They differ in their causes, in the main systems affected, in their clinical appearance, and in their severity. Of the 17 categories of disease in the classification, eight are grouped according to the body systems mainly involved,* and even other categories grouped together on a different basis make reference to the systems involved, such as "Congenital Anomalies" and "Neoplasms," which are subclassified according to the systems and particular organs affected.

Several groupings are arranged according to cause, including "Infective and Parasitic Diseases," and "Avitaminoses" and other nutritional deficiencies. "Accidents, Poisonings, and Violence," are categorized in a dual manner, i.e., by external causes and the nature of the injury. The category concerned with "Certain Causes of Perinatal Morbidity and Mor-

*These include diseases of the blood and blood-forming organs, the nervous system and sense organs, circulatory system, respiratory system, digestive system, genitourinary system, skin and subcutaneous tissue, and the musculoskeletal system and connective tissue.

tality" directs attention to cause within a particular age-group of the population, extending from the 28th week of gestation to the seventh day of life.[1] Another section concerned with a particular category of people is that of "Complications of Pregnancy, Childbirth and the Puerperium." "Mental Disorders" are classified separately, including those already known to be caused by or associated with physical conditions of the brain. The category "Symptoms and Ill-defined Conditions" is of much potential value to classification of disorders of patients in primary medical care. There is a considerable proportion of patients turning to doctors with symptoms for which no satisfactory classifiable diagnosis can be made. There is often the temptation to refer to such conditions as "neurotic" or "functional." For epidemiologic and community diagnostic purposes it is better to analyze the symptoms in this special category, thereby assuring that neuroses are diagnosed on the basis of positive findings, rather than merely by process of exclusion of physical findings which might explain a symptom.

Only a few of the problems involved in such a multiple system of classification will be demonstrated.

Section I, "Infective and Parasitic Diseases," is restricted to diseases generally recognized as "communicable" or "transmissible" and yet excludes many such conditions. Thus communicable staphylococcal infections, such as boils, carbuncles, and cellulitis, are classified in the category "Diseases of the Skin and Subcutaneous tissue" and not in Section I. Similarly, many respiratory infections are not included in Section I, e.g., common cold, acute pharyngitis, acute tonsillitis, acute bronchitis, influenza, and pneumonia, but are included in "Diseases of the Respiratory System." However, Section I includes conditions such as septic or streptococcal pharyngitis, septic tonsillitis, or any acute upper respiratory infection specified as due to streptococcus.

This type of problem and several other issues requiring decision by compromise are discussed in the introduction to the first volume of the *International Classification of Diseases*.[1] While the classification of diseases is far from perfect, the advantages of its use are as obvious now as they were when William Farr wrote the following, after his appointment in 1837 as first medical statistician to the General Registrar Office of England and Wales.

> The advantages of a uniform statistical nomenclature, however imperfect, are so obvious, that it is surprising no attention has been paid to its enforcement in Bills of Mortality. Each disease has, in many instances, been denoted by three or four terms, and each term has been applied to as many different diseases: vague, inconvenient names have been employed, or complications have been recorded instead of primary diseases. The nomenclature is of as much importance in this department of inquiry as weights and measures in the physical sciences, and should be settled without delay.[2]

A three-digit system is used in the *International Classification of Diseases* which involves the use of numbers to represent particular diseases, placing them within a category. These categories refer to qualitative differences. Only in rare cases does the classification refer to quantitative criteria. The introduction of measurements of intelligence is one of these cases in which the classification specifies measurable criteria for diagnosis of mental retardation. Another example is that of blindness in which measures of central visual acuity and visual field are specified.

In general the *International Classification of Diseases* does not pretend to set criteria for diagnosis of disease, nor to represent the severity of disease in quantitative terms, whether of duration, outcome, or interference with functioning. To the epidemiologist in community medicine and in community diagnosis these considerations are vital.

There are limitations in evaluating the morbidity status of a community through the use of a classification of diseases in various categories. Limited knowledge about cause, pathology, and effects of diseases must inevitably be reflected in classification. Simplicity is the essence for the world-wide usefulness of a disease classification, as is intended in the *International Classification of Diseases*. There are several important questions about morbidity which the classification does not answer, one of which is the variation in expression of diseases.

VARIATION IN EXPRESSION OF DISEASE

Both qualitative and quantitative differences in the expression of disease are of relevance to perception of morbidity. Examples of qualitative variation are the diverse clinical manifestations of many disease entities themselves as well as the different syndromes that result from the association of several disease processes in the same individuals. Thus the various manifestations of syphilis and tuberculosis are well known and are included in some detail in the international classification.

In many communities diabetes is a more common disease than is tuberculosis or syphilis and has at least as serious implications for community health. The international classification makes provision for diabetes mellitus as a whole. Its many possible manifestations suggest the need for the more specific subclassification that has been done in various countries, e.g., the Israeli extension.[3]

The importance of recognizing the different expressions of a disease extends beyond its immediate relevance to correct diagnosis and care of a patient. The fact that the same disease expresses itself differently in different population groups or communities is well known and the factors determining these differences in form are of epidemiologic relevance. This is illustrated in the different manifestations of diabetes mellitus in two ethnic groups, the Indian and Zulu of Natal.[4] Comparing the complications in 133 Zulu diabetic patients with 207 Indian patients, of whom 19.5 and 15.9 percent, respectively, had had the disease for over 5 years, the prevalence of the main cardiovascular and renal complications was very much higher in the Indian group, as was retinopathy. This clinical study suggests that diabetes mellitus, whatever its incidence and prevalence in these ethnic groups, has a different meaning for the health of the two groups.

Quantitative variation in the expression of disease has also been given much attention by epidemiologists and geneticists. The concept of a "gradient of infection" provides for inclusion of all infections in the study of an outbreak of an infectious illness, ranging from the infected asymptomatic carrier of a microorganism to cases of serious illness. Epidemiologic studies of infectious disease must extend beyond the seriously ill cases who may be found at clinics, in hospital, or on autopsy examination. Recognition of the iceberg phenomenon in infectious disease epidemiology is essential if transmission of the infecting agent is to be understood and traced. The submerged mass of cases, asymptomatic carriers or mild cases, have an important role in infection. Restriction of diagnosis of poliomyelitis to cases with paralytic or other serious complications only, or of infectious hepatitits to those with jaundice, limits understanding of the way in which infections of these diseases are spread and of their differential distribution in various population groups.

Similarly, in genetic studies the concept of variation in expression of genetically determined diseases has been described by the term "expressivity." It is not always clear how the term is used, as the differences in expression may be qualitative or quantitative. However, there are some who confine its use to "the variability in severity of a genetic trait."[5]

Cystic Fibrosis–A Case Illustration of Variation in Expression

The genetic transmission of particular defects or errors does not result in their uniform expression. Cystic fibrosis is an example of variability in expression of a disease. The three characteristic features of this disease are malabsorption syndrome; chronic pulmonary disease; and an increase of sodium, chloride, and, to a lesser extent, potassium in the sweat.[6–9]

Cystic fibrosis was first reported in 1936 in Switzerland[10] and subsequently described more fully and differentiated as an independent pathologic and clinical entity in 1938 by Andersen.[11] It is inherited as a recessive autosomal genetic disorder, the parental heterozygotes showing no manifestations of disease nor of abnormal electrolytes in sweat.

Before its recognition the vast majority of cases must have died from effects of malabsorption or pulmonary disease, but with its recognition and helpful replacement therapy as well as antibiotic prophylaxis and treatment for the pulmonary complication, it has become a chronic disease with a rising prevalence. Its chronicity has been manifested in differences in degree and kind of syndrome.

The variation in expression of this condition is summarized in Table 3-1. In addition to the complications outlined, a number of others have been found in cases who have survived through adolescence to adulthood.[12]

TABLE 3-1. The Main Variations of Expression in Cystic Fibrosis

ALIMENTARY DISORDERS	RESPIRATORY DISORDERS
Malabsorption syndrome —expressivity ranges from apparently normal digestion to very marked evidence of malabsorption with steatorrhea	Pulmonary disease with much variation in its severity and rate of development.
Intestinal obstruction of newborn known as meconium ileus	Upper respiratory infection in children over 5 years of age—sinusitis, allergic rhinitis, and polyps may develop
Rectal prolapse	
Cirrhosis of liver with siderosis	

The factors that determine variation in expression of different conditions will be considered subsequently. One of these, which will be discussed more fully later, will be mentioned here. It is usual to speak of a clinical syndrome as consisting of a number of related signs and symptoms. Extending the use of this term to the description of disease in a community, we may speak of a community syndrome. The importance of this concept for our present consideration is that the expression of a particular disease is often determined by the other diseases or health variables which occur concomitantly, e.g., the difference in meaning of hypertension between its occurrence in a community where coronary atherosclerosis is also common, and its occurrence in one in which the latter condition is not marked. In the former, it is a high risk factor for acute myocardial infarction, whereas in the latter it is not. This is discussed in Section 4, Chapter 21.

DISABILITY

A grading of severity of illness is very common in all aspects of medical practice, whether based on observation of the state of health of the patient or on the prognosis as to outcome of the illness. The observations may be quantitatively expressed as individual biologic measurements such as serum levels of glucose, proteins, cholesterol, hemoglobins, or packed red cells. On the other hand the severity of an illness may be graded by the disability which it causes. Heart disease has been graded in this way and the New York Heart Association classification is an example of such a grading.

Functional Capacity of Patients with Heart Disease

Class I: Patients with cardiac disease but without resulting limitations of physical activity. Ordinary physical activity does not cause undue fatigue, palpitation, dyspnea, or anginal pain.

Class II: Patients with cardiac disease resulting in slight limitation of physical activity. They are comfortable at rest. Ordinary physical activity results in fatigue, palpitation, dyspnea, or anginal pain.

Class III: Patients with cardiac disease resulting in marked limitation of physical activity. They are comfortable at rest. Less than ordinary physical activity causes fatigue, palpitation, dyspnea, or anginal pain.

Class IV: Patients with cardiac disease resulting in inability to carry on any physical activity without discomfort. Symptoms of cardiac insufficiency or of anginal syndrome may be present even at rest. If any physical activity is undertaken, discomfort is increased.[13]

Different Ways of Looking at Disability

Role Oriented. People differ in their daily functioning, their status and roles, and in the way they relate with one another. Inability to fulfill normal expectations in these respects, whatever the expectations are for different people in various communities, is often a reflection of illness. In fact a wider and wider range of disabilities are recognized as disease or being caused by disease. Thus it is only in comparatively recent times that alcoholism as such, and not only its complications, has been considered a disease, and similarly aspects of delinquent and criminal behavior are being recognized as disease or expressions of disease.

The concept of being sick is something different from that of disease as used, for example, in the *International Classification of Diseases*. Being sick involves recognition of not feeling well or not being able to carry out regular daily or expected functions. Recognition of disability, present and actual or potential, is an essential element of being sick. The recognition is not only by the individual himself, but by his family, formal and informal network of associates, and his community or society as a whole. Recognition involves certain demands of the sick person, such as the need to seek medical care, which in turn gives social sanction to the disability of the individual. A theoretical framework which furthers our understanding of the sick role was developed by Parsons in his study of modern medical practice in the United States as a case illustration of his conceptual scheme of "the social system."[14]

He outlines four aspects to recognition and acceptance of the special position of being sick and the expectations of the role of the sick person:

1. First, is the exemption from normal social role responsibilities, which of course is relative to the nature and severity of the illness. . . .
2. The sick person cannot be expected by "pulling himself together" to get well by an act of decision or will. . . .
3. The third element is the definition of the state of being ill as itself undesirable with its obligation to want to "get well". . . .
4. The obligation—in proportion to the severity of the condition, of course—to seek *technically competent* help, namely, in the most usual case, that of a physician and to *cooperate* with him in the process of trying to get well.[14]

Morbidity Oriented. Another concept relevant to consideration of disability is that of morbidity outlined by the United States National Center for Health Statistics in its health survey procedures.[15]

1. Morbidity is basically a departure from a state of physical or mental well-being, resulting from disease or injury, of which the affected individual is aware. Awareness connotes a degree of measurable impact on the individual or his family in terms of the restrictions and disabilities caused by the morbidity. Morbidity includes not only active or progressive disease but also impairments, that is, chronic or permanent defects that are static in nature, resulting from disease, injury, or congenital malformation. The existence of morbidity in an individual caused by a particular disease, injury, or impairment is called a "morbidity condition," or simply a "condition."
2. During the course of this condition there may be one or more periods which the affected individual considers himself to be "sick" or "injured." These periods are spoken of as episodes of illness. The period or periods of illness may coincide with the period during which the condition exists, or they may cover only a part of that period. A condition may involve no illness, in the usual sense of the word. Hence, illness is only one form of evidence of the existence of a morbidity condition. Other evidence might be a decrease in, or complete loss of ability to perform various functions, particularly those of the musculoskeletal system or the sense organs; or a change in the appearance of the body, such as a rash or lump, believed to be abnormal by the person affected.
3. For the purposes of this survey the concept of a morbidity condition is usually further limited by specifying that it includes only conditions as a result of which the person has taken one or more of various actions. Such actions might be the restricting of usual activities, bed disability, work loss, the seeking of medical advice, or the taking of medicines.

Motivation Oriented. Whatever devices may be introduced to measure disability, the motivation of the disabled person is an important factor in determining the amount of disability associated with the disease or injury. Positive or negative motivation of affected individuals may have an important influence on whether they get well. Apart from these psychologic aspects, there are often material considerations from which the patient and, in addition, his immediate dependents benefit. Accident insurance, injury or illness resulting from work, or sickness as a reason for absence from work may all tend to encourage an exaggeration of the disability.

CRITERIA FOR MEASURING DISABILITY

When measuring the kind and degree of disability as an indicator of severity of disease, the following elements may be helpful: (1) the specific disabling condition; (2) disability in fulfillment or performance of various roles; and (3) limitations and disturbances in relationships.

The Specific Disabling Condition

The impact of acute illness may vary from an extreme situation with more or less severe disabilities to minor inconvenience. Differing from an acute condition are many chronic illnesses or disabilities which may be progressive.

The degree of disability will obviously be related to the nature of the disability, as well as its cause and possibility for treatment or correction. Thus visual disability must be assessed in relation to correction, and disability from loss of a limb in relation to functional ability with prostheses. Similarly, the disability resulting from Stoke-Adams syndrome, or heart block with inadequate cardiac output, must be related to the potential or actual effect of the insertion of electronic pacemakers.

Disability in Fulfillment or Performance of Various Roles

The normal or expected role behavior is the standard against which disability must be measured. Among the more readily assessed limitations in role-functions are those relating to work, homemaking or housekeeping, study at school or university, recreation of all kinds, and play in children. A less readily assessed, but often very important, role-function is sexual activity.

Measurement of disability arising in association with chronic disease was outlined and used by the Commission on Chronic Illness (USA).[16] They included three kinds of measures: "Activities of Daily Living," "Overall Functional Capacity," and "Usual Activities."

Since then community health surveys have increasingly focused on disability in chronic disease. Some aspects of its measurement are considered further.

Limitation in Mobility. Limitation in mobility is a general measure resulting from various disease conditions and can be assessed with the diagnosis of the condition itself. The National Center for Health Statistics of the United States defines four categories[15] to describe chronic mobility limitation:

1. Confined to the house—confined to the house all the time except in emergencies.
2. Cannot get around alone—able to go outside, but needs the help of another person in getting around outside.
3. Has trouble getting around alone—able to go outside alone but has trouble getting around freely.
4. Not limited in mobility—not limited in any of the ways described above.

Limitation in Major Activity. Four categories of chronic limitation of major activity have been defined according to the extent to which activities of people are limited as a result of chronic conditions.[15]

1. Persons unable to carry on major activity for their group. . . .
2. Persons limited in the amount or kind of major activity performed. . . .
3. Persons not limited in major activity but otherwise limited. . . .
4. Persons not limited in activities.

Major activity refers to the usual activities of persons. Thus in the case of preschool children the criterion is their participation in ordinary play with other children, in schoolchildren it is going to school, in housewives it is keeping house, and among workers and all other persons it is their ability to go to work.

Limitations in Activities of Daily Living (ADL). Activities of daily living include dressing, bathing, and feeding oneself; going to toilet; getting out of bed or up from a chair; remaining continent; speaking; reading; and writing.

The general consideration of limitation in mobility and activities needs to be extended and refined in grading impairment of major functions in patients with severe disorders. This includes the kind and severity of the disabilities associated with disease and injuries, as in cerebrovascular disease and stroke, cerebral palsy, arthritis, and fractures. The widening range of rehabilitation services has been the main stimulus in this, the

TABLE 3-2. The Characteristic Ordered Pattern of Dependence in Activities of Daily Living in Chronically Ill Elderly Persons

NUMBER OF ACTIVITIES OF DAILY LIVING		DEPENDENCY					
Dependent	**Independent**	**Bathing**	**Dressing**	**Going to Toilet**	**Transferring**	**Continence**	**Feeding**
0	x						
1		x					
2		x	x				
3		x	x	x			
4		x	x	x	x		
5		x	x	x	x	x	
6		x	x	x	x	x	x

(Adapted from Katz et al.[19]*)*

rehabilitation potential being an important guide to programming with the individual case and the change in function being the main means of evaluation of such care. As might be expected a number of indices have been used for this purpose.[17–22] Simplicity is the essence of the usefulness of such indices, especially if they are to be applied in community health appraisal as measures of the prevalence of disabling chronic illness or evaluation of community programs of care.

One such index of ADL, which was originally developed in the study and care of fractured-hip cases in the aged, was extended to other chronically ill, middle-aged, and elderly people,[19] including patients with cerebral infarction, neurologic disorders, multiple sclerosis, paraplegia or quadriplegia, and other neurologic diseases. The majority of the cases had more than one chronic disease. An ordered pattern of disability rating was found to include the vast majority of the patients. Eighty-six percent of all cases (1,001) could be graded within this basic pattern, which is represented in Table 3-2.

The framework of the index used by Katz and co-workers at the Benjamin Rose Hospital are shown in Table 3-3. The potential usefulness of such indices in epidemiologic investigation of chronic illness and in community health care of such illness in the aged warrants much attention.

While of considerable use in the study of older persons, evaluation of independence in activities of daily living has wide application in investigation of chronic disorders. In a national study of cerebral palsy in adolescence and adulthood in Israel, it was noted that, with increasing complexity in the kind of activity of daily living, a greater proportion of the group classified as spastic-type cases lost their full independence than did the athetotic group, among whom there was little change (Fig. 3-1).[23]

TABLE 3-3. Index of Independence in Activities of Daily Living*

A:	Independent in feeding, continence, transferring, going to toilet, dressing, and bathing
B:	Independent in all but one of these functions
C:	Independent in all but bathing and one additional function
D:	Independent in all but bathing, dressing and one additional function
E:	Independent in all but bathing, dressing, going to toilet, and one additional function
F:	Independent in all but bathing, dressing, going to toilet, transferring, and one additional function
G:	Dependent in all six functions
Other:	Dependent in at least two functions, but not classifiable as C, D, E, or F

**The index of independence in activities of daily living is based on an evaluation of the functional independence or dependence of patients in bathing, dressing, going to toilet, transferring, continence, and feeding. Specific definitions of functional independence and dependence appear with the index in the original text of Katz et al. (From Katz et al.[19])*

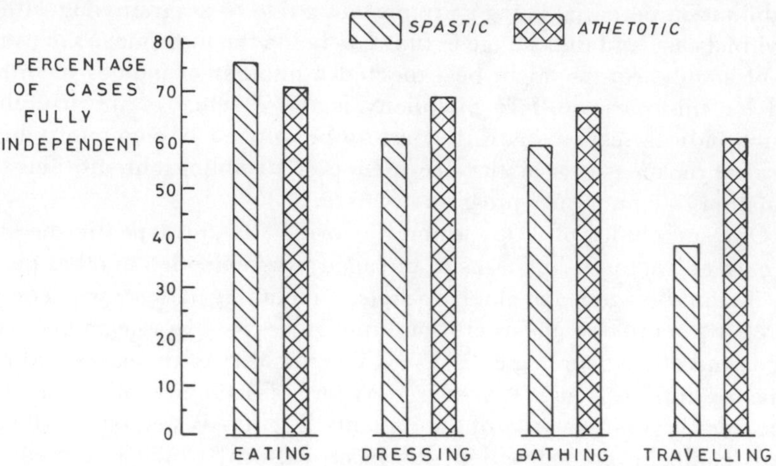

FIG. 3-1. A comparison of activities of daily living (ADL) of spastic and athetotic groups of Israeli adolescents and adults with cerebral palsy. (Adapted from Margulec.[23])

Limitations and Disturbances in Relationships. Disease and the disability it causes have so far been reviewed as relatively discrete or different attributes of morbidity. Thus interference with role functioning or role failure has been viewed as the result of disease, such as interference in the major activities of work, housekeeping, schooling, and self-care. More specifically, relational aspects are often a central feature of the disability which is manifested in chronic illness, especially in mental disorders. The autistic child may be recognized in early infancy by the mother who becomes concerned at the child's absence of response to the most elementary social situation, i.e., an inability of the children affected "to relate themselves in the ordinary way to people and situations from the beginning of life."[24]

The concept of withdrawal from close relationships is more applicable to those who have expressed such relationships with other people but tend to or actively withdraw from them. Isolation and aloneness may range from the "alone" autistic child; through psychotic persons, as in many cases of schizophrenia; to people who live alone by virtue of their social situation, such as many elderly people, especially women, in cities of Western societies. Whatever the cause, whether underlying personal disease or social situation, the individuals with limited social interactions manifest varying degrees of limitation in their relationships with others. This kind of disability is of considerable relevance in community health care, and although its measurement is difficult, this does not detract from its potential usefulness as an index of disability.

There is pathologic relational behavior in which underlying mental illness may be diagnosed in only a proportion of cases. Juvenile delinquency, expressed in different antisocial acts can, whatever the cause, be a major disability in many communities. Its prevalence among adolescents of slum communities in cities compels the attention of health services. It is true that in many countries "health" services and "welfare" services are separate functioning units and the problem of dealing with delinquency is not included in the functions of health services. Whatever opinions may be on this way of providing service, delinquent behavior is an important index of disability as manifested in relational failure or functioning.

Whether the behavior disturbance is the condition or disorder itself, or a disability secondary to or resulting from another disease, its measurement contributes to our appreciation of disease and disability in the community. The common conditions include personal abnormal behavior, such as juvenile delinquency; adult crime; prostitution; alcoholism and drug addiction; suicide and attempted suicide; as well as disturbances in family living, desertion, and divorce.

Antisocial behavior is in fact a diversity of behaviors rather than a specific entity, often greatly depending on the mores of the community and its definition of deviant behavior. The community's ways of dealing with deviants are determined by their offensiveness to mores and the challenge they pose to the physical or social security of those exposed. The social consequences lead to punishment and protective measures against the criminal. Neither "public health" nor "medicine" has as yet accepted full obligation for the treatment of antisocial behavior as such, as distinct from its personal health aspects. When the deviant behavior is an expression of a recognized illness, as in episodes of violence of some psychotics or in abnormal behavior associated with chromosomal abnormality,[25,26] the medical responsibilities are more readily definable. Recognition of some antisocial behaviors as diseases has no doubt resulted from their health implications for the deviant himself over and above their meaning for others. Thus alcoholism itself is recognized as a disease (303) over and above its effect on the alcoholic, and addiction or dependence on various drugs (304) is similarly included in the *International Classification of Diseases* in the section on mental disorders.

Inclusion of various disorders in the *International Classification of Diseases* does not necessarily imply their recognition by health authorities as health problems. The classification includes sexual deviation (302), and under the title of "Behavior Disorders of Childhood" (308) such behavior as "truancy" is listed. The deviant at home and in the neighborhood is a concern of the health or welfare worker, community physician, nurse, or social worker. This is so not only because of the implications of the deviant's behavior for his own health, but because of its potential epidemiologic significance for the health of others. Striving towards active adaptation and social homeostasis is as relevent for the public's health as are activities directed towards other aspects of the community and its environment.

The Need for an Associated Classification of Disease and Disability

Disease classification by itself is becoming less useful as an indicator of illness or morbidity in a community. This is especially so where chronic disease is common, where elderly people comprise a large proportion of the population, and where a considerable number of people survive serious conditions. An associated classification of diseases and disability in functioning is needed. It has been suggested and tested in groups of cases with chronic disease[27] but to the best of our knowledge has not yet been used in describing morbidity of a total community. Interference with expected role functioning, inability to carry out activities of daily living, and limitation in mobility are among the indices of disability which are associated with disease. The extent of the disability is not always directly correlated with the duration or more apparent crippling effects of the main disease diagnosed. There are those whose disability is more severe than would result from the stage of the disease itself, and there are those in whom the apparent severity of the disease would lead to the expectation of more severe disability in functioning. Such observations are common in persons with chronic disease and in persons with after-effects of injuries. Personality and social factors have been shown to be important determinants of the prognosis of various illnesses and of the functional capacity of people with long-term illness.[28–30] The fact that it is not "the disease" alone that explains the extent of disability in functioning reinforces the case for widening international and other classifications of disease to include functioning capacity and indices of disability.

REFERENCES

1. WHO: International Classification of Diseases, 1965, Revision Vol. 1. Geneva, WHO, 1967, p xxvii.
2. Farr W: Registrar General of England and Wales. London, First Annual Report, 1839, p 99. (Also quoted in ref. 1, p x of Introduction.)
3. Central Bureau of Statistics Health Section: International Classification of Diseases and Causes of Death—Israeli extension, 8th revision. Jerusalem, 1969.
4. Cleave TL, Campbell GD: Diabetes, Coronary Thrombosis, and the Saccharine Disease. Bristol, Wright, 1966.
5. McKusick VA: Medical genetics. In Harvey AM, Cluff LE, Johns RJ,

et al. (eds.): The Principles and Practice of Medicine, 17th ed. New York, Appleton, 1968, Sect. 6.

6. Professional Education Committee: Guide to Diagnosis and Management of Cystic Fibrosis. New York, National Cystic Fibrosis Research Foundation, 1963.
7. di Sant 'Agnese PA, Talamo RC: Pathogenesis and physiopathology of cystic fibrosis of the pancreas. New Engl J Med 277:1287, 1344, 1399; 1967.
8. di Sant 'Agnese PA, Darling RC, Perera GA, et al.: Sweat electrolyte disturbances associated with childhood pancreatic disease. Am J Med 15:777, 1953.
9. Kopito L, Shwachman H: Studies in cystic fibrosis. Determination of sweat electrolytes in situ with direct reading electrodes. Pediatrics 43: 794, 1969.
10. Fanconi G, Uehlinger E, Knauer C: Das Coeliakiesyndrom bei angeborener zystischer Pankreasfibromatose and Bronchiektasien. Wien Med Wochenschr 86:753, 1936.
11. Andersen DH: Cystic fibrosis of the pancreas and its relation to celiac disease. A clinical and pathological study. Am J Dis Child 56:344, 1938.
12. Shwachman M, Holsclaw DS: Complications of cystic fibrosis. New Engl J Med 281:500, 1969.
13. Criteria Committee of the New York Heart Association: Diseases of the Heart and Blood Vessels. Nomenclature and Criteria for Diagnosis, 6th ed. Boston, Little, Brown, 1964, pp 112–113.
14. Parsons T: The Social System. Glencoe, Ill, Free Press, 1951, p 436.
15. National Center for Health Statistics: Health Survey Procedure. Vital and Health Statistics. Public Health Service Publication No. 1,000, Series 1, No. 2. Washington, DC, US Dept. of Health, Education, and Welfare, 1964, pp 4, 46.
16. Commission on Chronic Illness: Chronic illness in a large city—the Baltimore study. In Chronic Illness in the United States, Vol. 4. Cambridge, Commonwealth Fund, Harvard Univ Press, 1957.
17. Staff of the Benjamin Rose Hospital: Multidisciplinary studies of illness in aged persons. II. A new classification of functional status in activities of daily living. J Chronic Dis 9:55, 1959.
18. Staff of the Benjamin Rose Hospital: Multidisciplinary studies of illness in aged persons. III. Prognostic indices in fracture of the hip. J Chronic Dis 11:445, 1960.
19. Katz S, Ford AB, Moskowitz RW, et al.: Studies of illness in the aged. The index of ADL. A standardized measure of biological and psychosocial function. JAMA 185:914, 1963.
20. Mahoney FI, Barthel DW: Functional evaluation. The Barthel Index. Md State Med J 14:61, 1965.
21. Feldman DJ, Lee PR, Unterecker J, et al.: A comparison of functionally orientated medical care and formal rehabilitation in the management of patients with hemiplegia due to cerebrovascular disease. J Chronic Dis 15: 297, 1961.
22. Sokolow J, Silson JE, Taylor EJ, et al.: A new approach to the objective evaluation of physical disability. J Chronic Dis 15:105, 1961.
23. Margulec I (ed.): Cerebral Palsy in Adolescence and Adulthood. Project No. OVR-6-61, sponsored by Vocational Rehabilitation Administration—US Dept. of Health, Education, and Welfare, and the American Joint Distribution Committee Services in Israel ("Malben"). Jerusalem, Academic Press, 1966.

24. Kanner L: Autistic disturbances of affective contact. Nerv Child 2:217, 1943.
25. Jacobs PA, Brunton M, Melville MM, et al.: Aggressive behavior, mental subnormality, and the XYY male. Nature 208:1351, 1965.
26. Court Brown WM: Males with an XYY sex chromosome complement. J Med Genet 5:341, 1968.
27. Katz S, Ford AB, Downs TD, et al.: Chronic-disease classification in evaluation of medical care programs. Med Care 7:139, 1969.
28. Querido A: Forecast and follow-up. An investigation into the clinical, social, and mental factors determining the results of hospital treatment. Brit J Prev Soc Med 13:33, 1959.
29. Moos RH, Solomon GF: Personality correlates of the degree of functional incapacity of patients with physical disease. J Chronic Dis 18:1019, 1964.
30. Wittkower ED, Durost HB, Laing WAR: A psychosomatic study of the cause of pulmonary tuberculosis. Amer Rev Tuberc 71:201, 1955.

4
Somatic Characteristics

There are many somatic characteristics which are used in measurements of health and as indices in diagnosis of disease. These characteristics may vary considerably in a population group and within wide limits the variation may neither reflect a state of well-being or health nor of disease or "abnormality." Somatic characteristics may vary either qualitatively or quantitatively. Qualitative or discontinuous variation involves the distribution of a distinctive attribute throughout a community, there being those who have the attribute and those who do not. In contrast to this is variation of a quantitative kind, in which all people have the characteristic, differing from one another in a quantitative dimension.

DISCONTINUOUS VARIATION

The following are examples of characteristics with discontinuous variation of epidemiologic interest.

1. Genetic variations. Blood groups—ABO, Rh. Hemoglobins—A and various abnormals, including sickling, and thalassemia α and β.
2. Cell growth and transformation.[1]

> The division of normal cells is self-limiting and their growth orderly, while that of tumour cells is uncontrolled and haphazard leading to ever-increasing numbers of cells. . . . Thus it may be said that tumour cells appear to arise as a result of a genetic transformation, a change which heritably endows them with the properties of virtually unlimited propagation and the ability to grow as cancers in animals.

3. Internalization of a microbial agent and other substances, as in infection and poisoning.

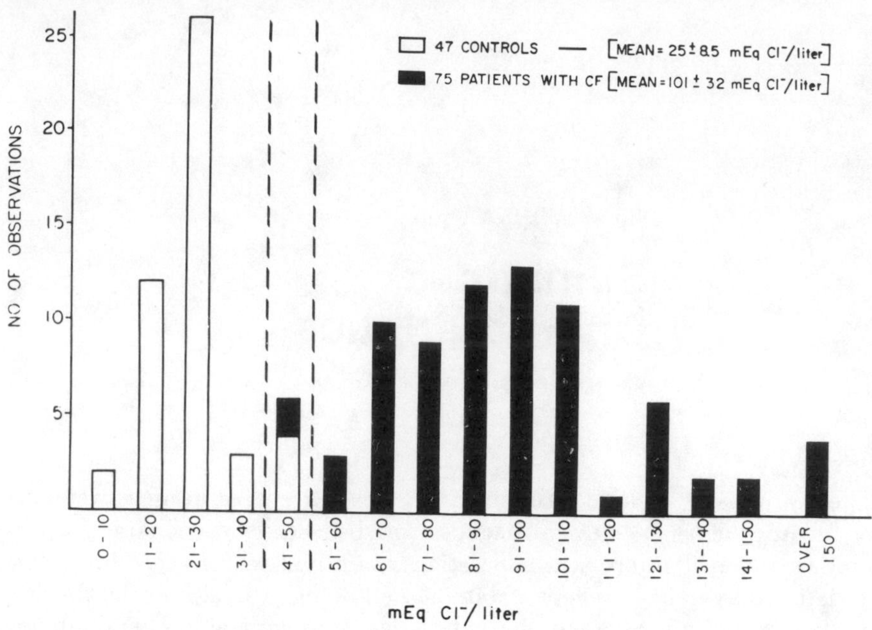

FIG. 4-1. The sweat chlorides in cases with cystic fibrosis and normal controls. (From Kopito and Schwachman.[2])

An example of qualitative variation is illustrated in the sweat changes which are found in cases of the genetically determined disorder, cystic fibrosis. A high sodium, chloride, and potassium content of sweat is a feature of this condition. Sweat tests have a high specificity and sensitivity, presenting a bimodal curve as seen in Figure 4-1.[2]

CONTINUOUS VARIATION

Continuous variation is characterized by polygenic inheritance through multiple "small" genes and multifactorial causation through life experience and environmental factors. It includes characteristics which are measured in the following ways.

Anthropometric measurements: e.g., height, weight, skinfold thickness
Physiologic-clinical measurements: e.g., blood pressure, respiratory capacity, exercise tolerance, physical performance
Laboratory examinations: blood cell measurements, blood chemistry.

Differences in physique between population groups may be shown in differential rates of growth, age of maturation, or adult stature and form. In a relatively homogenous community, with stable or unchanging conditions of living, the distribution of variables which measure physique can be expected to be of a continuous kind, with graded differences between individuals. The height distribution of individuals of comparable age and sex will tend to be a "normal" or "Gaussian" curve. This finding suggests that a multiplicity of factors, rather than any one single factor, determine such a variable as height. The genetic influence is polygenic rather than a single genetic factor and the influence of life experience is also probably multifactorial. Differences in diet, nutrition, and disease occurrence are among the more important determinants.

However, where there are marked differences between various component groups of a total population, it is to be expected that these differences will be reflected in their physical appearances. The differences between the groups may be in their genetic constitution or in their levels of living and nutritional or health status. The height distribution in such heterogeneous population groups will in fact be made up of several differing distributions. While there is usually a considerable overlap in the curves of height of such differing groups of people, the average person of one group may be relatively tall or short compared with the other (Fig. 4-2).[3]

Differences in height distribution of various groups are common and their interpretation as indicators of health in different communities is of importance. Case studies of the problems involved in making such inferences will be discussed with respect to several common measurements made in clinical medical practice and in epidemiologic investigations: measurements of height, weight, and blood pressure.

WEIGHT AND HEIGHT

Differences in physique of various peoples are well known and height and weight differences are among the most readily noted. The tall, relatively thin, Nilotic peoples of southern Sudan and the Tutsi of Ruanda[4] are well known examples of linear build. Thus the average height of 279 Dinka men studied was 188.67 cm, standard deviation (SD) 6.02 (71.47 inches, SD 2.41), with a mean weight of 58.3 kg, SD 5.9 (128.29 lbs, SD 13.00).[5] The ponderal index: height (inches)/ $\sqrt[3]{\text{weight}}$ (pounds) (14.2, SD 0.41) demonstrates their linearity (Fig. 4-3). The ponderal index is one of the indices of height/weight which is also used as a measure of adiposity in many epidemiologic investigations.

Similarly, comparing weight and height of the Tutsi and Ba-Hutu of Ruanda, Hiernaux[4] found the height and weight of the average adult

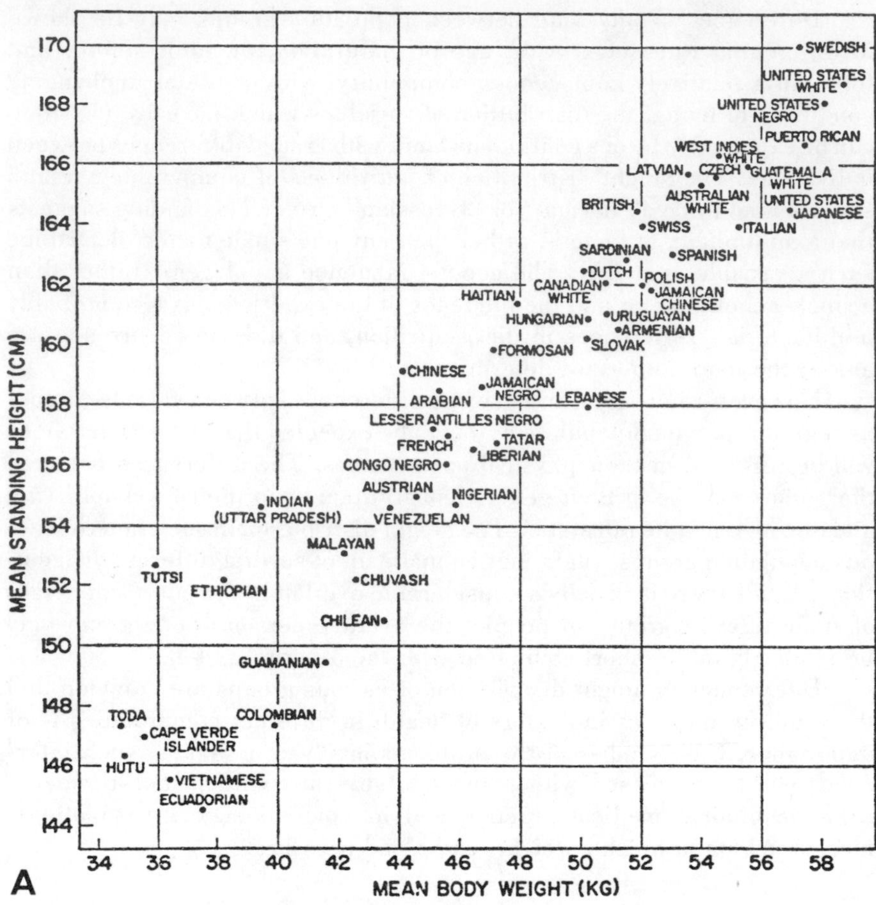

FIG. 4-2. The relation of mean body weight and mean standing height in boys and girls from different parts of the world. A: Boys aged 15 years. (From Meredith.[3])

Tutsi man to be 176 cm and 57 kg, in contrast to that of the Hutu, 167 cm and 58 kg. The age of maturation in these two Ruandan peoples was similar, 93 to 94 percent of adult height being reached by age 17 years, and in girls of both groups the menarche age was estimated to be 16.5 years. The difference in adult height is a result of differences in the growth rate and not because of a longer period of growth in the Tutsi.

Differences in the weight growth of infants of various communities and social classes are also widely recognized. Despite this fact there is a widespread practice of using standard curves of growth in infants and children established on the basis of studies in particular communities.

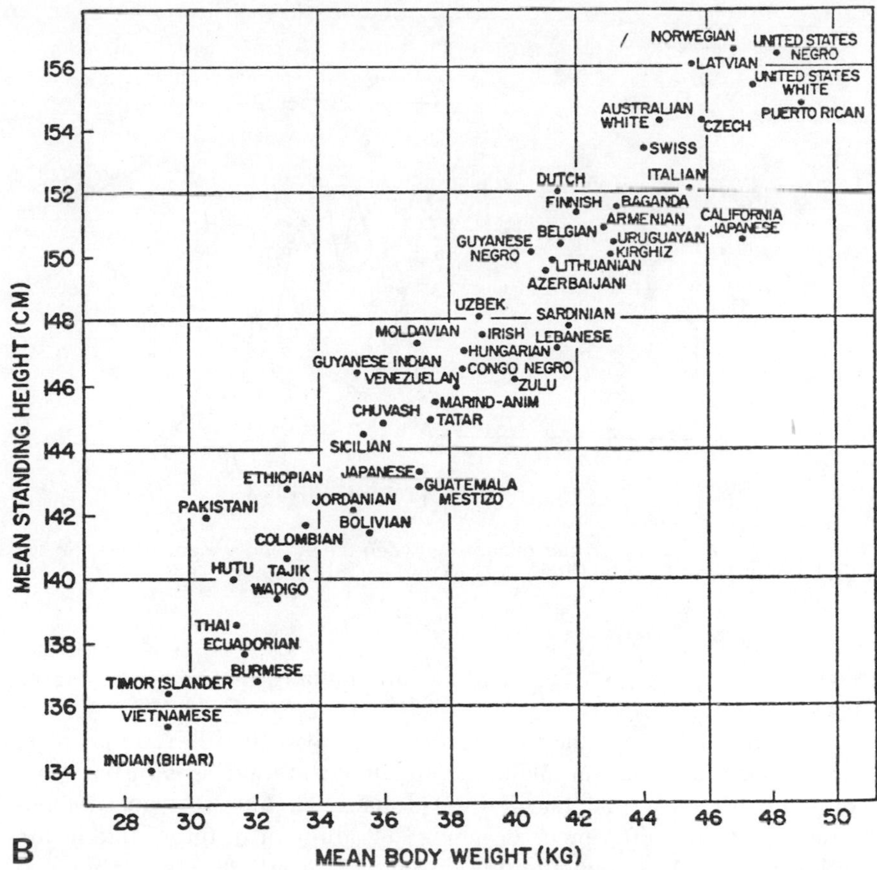

FIG. 4-2 (cont.). B: Girls aged 13 years. (From Meredith.[3])

Among the better known of these are the percentile curves of growth prepared by Stuart[6–8] from his longitudinal long-term investigations of Boston children. These have been, and still arc, utilized in many maternal and child health centers in various parts of the world. These studies have made an important contribution to child health practice but their use as standards should be critically tested in different settings. Not only are there differences between peoples, but secular changes, i.e., changes over time, in different groups, outdate the basic data, making it necessary to establish growth curves applicable to particular communities at different times. These will help establish more realistic guidclines in community health work. Examples of the need for this are presented in Figures 4-4 4 6.[9–11] It will be noted in Figure 4-4 that the differences in weight

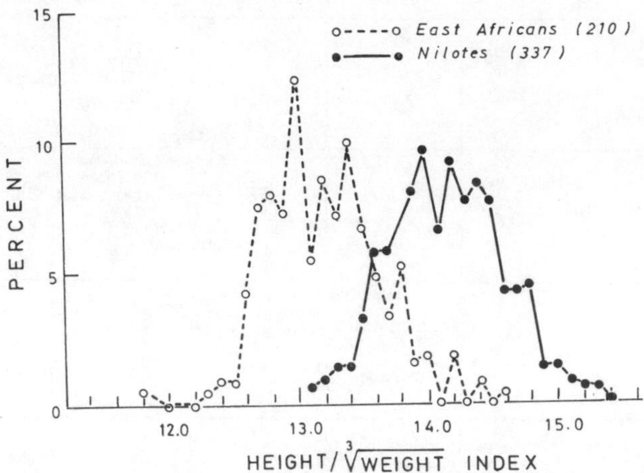

FIG. 4-3. The differences in the relation between height and weight of men in two African populations. (Adapted from Roberts and Bainbridge.[5])

growth of the Indian and African infants are not only differences of degree but also of kind.

Not only are there marked differences between different peoples, but variations in stature of men and women of different ages in the same community may be a reflection of secular change. Acheson[12,13] has demonstrated significant differences in heights of adults of different age in the Rondda Foch mining communities of South Wales. The mean height of younger adult men, and to a lesser extent that of younger women, was greater than that of older persons. In contrasting this secular increase with that of the British national average, as estimated by Tanner,[14] he draws attention to the considerable improvement in social conditions in this mining valley (Fig. 4-7).

The secular trend in increased stature in more developed countries has been associated with an even more striking secular change in age of maturation and rate of growth in childhood. Data available on maturation, easily obtained and a useful standard, is the age of girls at menarche. As with height and weight, considerable differences have been found in this characteristic in girls of different communities and in different social classes; remarkable secular changes have also been reported. The secular trend in Europe and America has been analyzed by Tanner.[14,15] He has shown that over the period 1830–1960 the average age of menarche has decreased well over 4 years. It is in communities of these continents that a secular increase in height has been noted. Reaching adult stature in

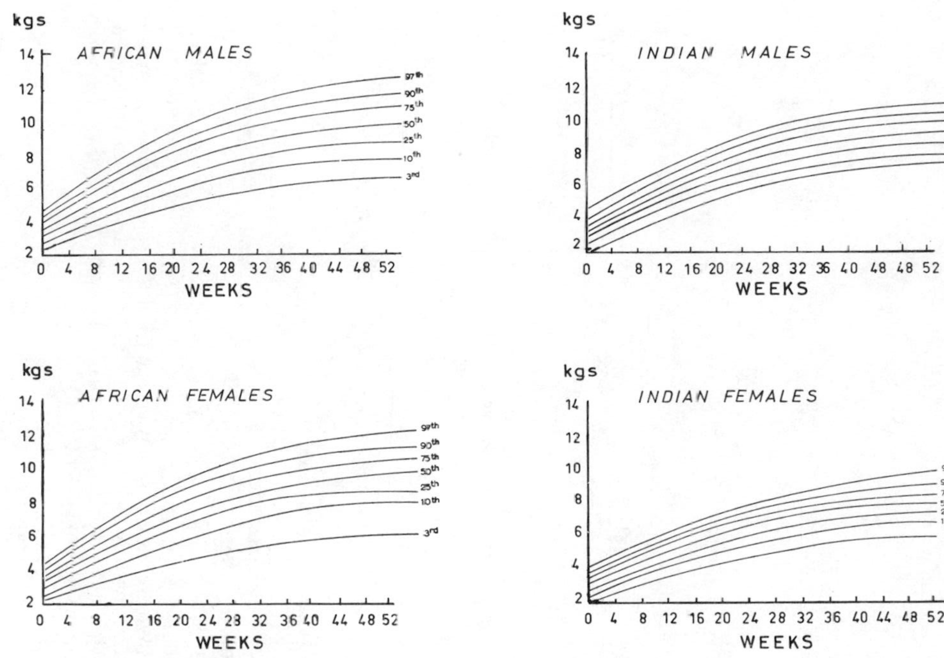

FIG. 4-4. The percentile distribution of infant weights at different ages in two communities. Note the different shape of the curves of the two communities. (From Kark and Kark.[9])

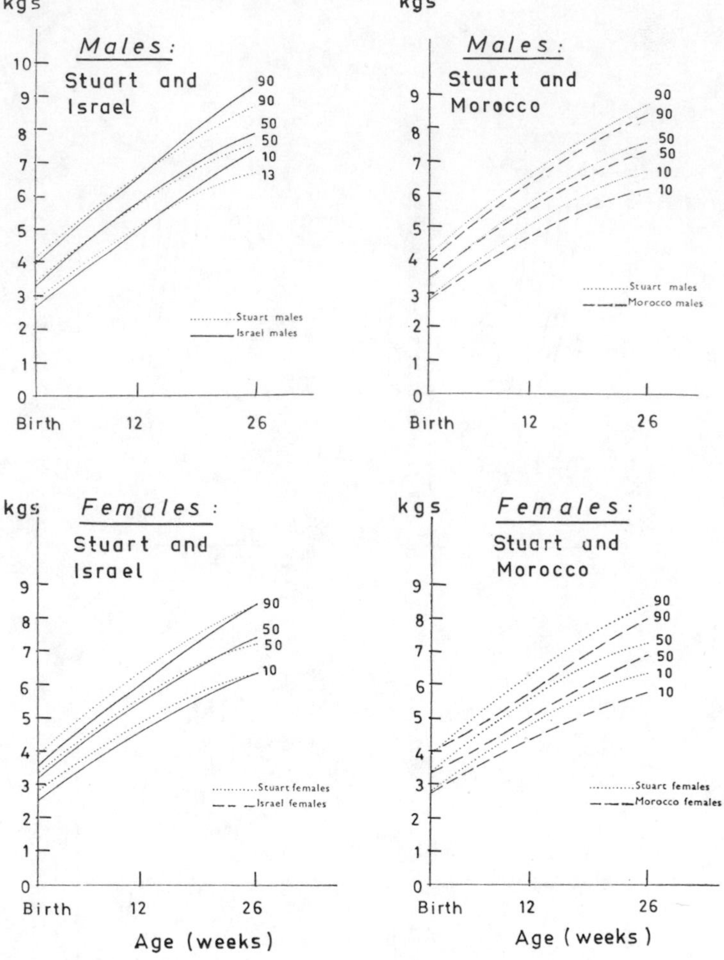

FIG. 4-5. Weight growth of Jewish babies of Jerusalem, Israel, from birth to 6 months of age. A comparison of babies of Israel-born parents with those of Moroccan-born parents. The Stuart percentile curves of growth[8] are used as a basis for comparing the two groups. (From Epstein.[11])

a much shorter period means a considerably increased rate of growth through childhood and this too is well documented in many of the communities. These secular changes have not been found in all parts of the world, but the absence of data on many communities precludes the possibility of generalizing about secular trends for the greatest part of the world's population.

There is evidence that this secular trend is ending in some communities.[16] Studies of upper-class groups of infants, children, and entrants to colleges indicate no change in growth. Comparing boys from "private" schools (upper-class boys) on admission to Harvard University in the 1930s with the entrants of 1958–1959 (an interval of some 25 years), there was no significant difference in height—177.8 cm (71.1 inches) versus 178.5 cm (71.4 inches). Among slightly less privileged boys from public schools who were Harvard entrants, the change in this period of time was from a mean of 173.8 to 177.5 cm. A comparable analysis of a group of college entrants to a women's college indicated that the stature of girls from both private and public schools had not changed since the 1930s, indicating

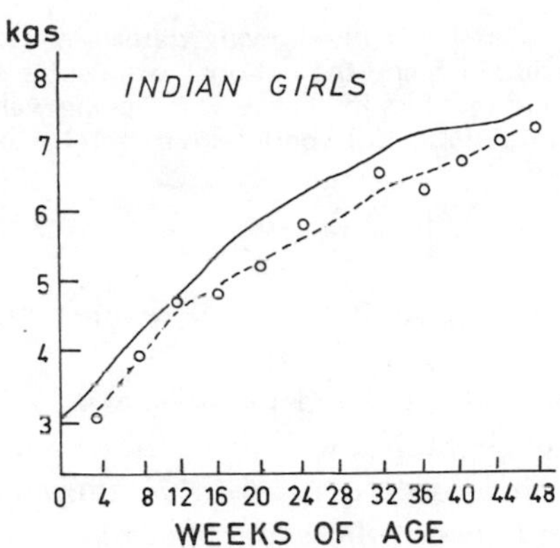

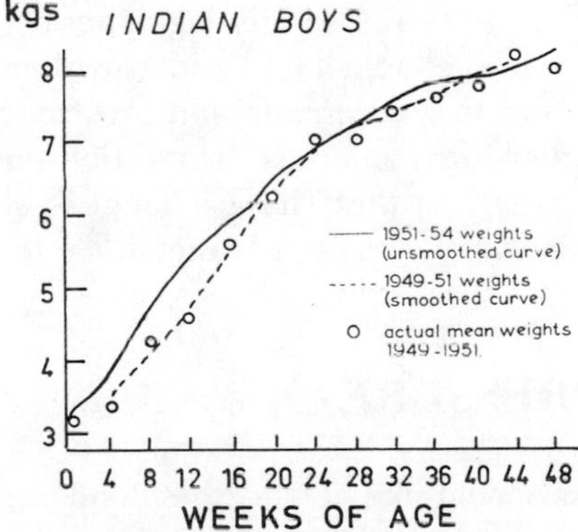

FIG. 4-6. Change in the weight curve of infants associated with a community health program. (From Abramson.[10])

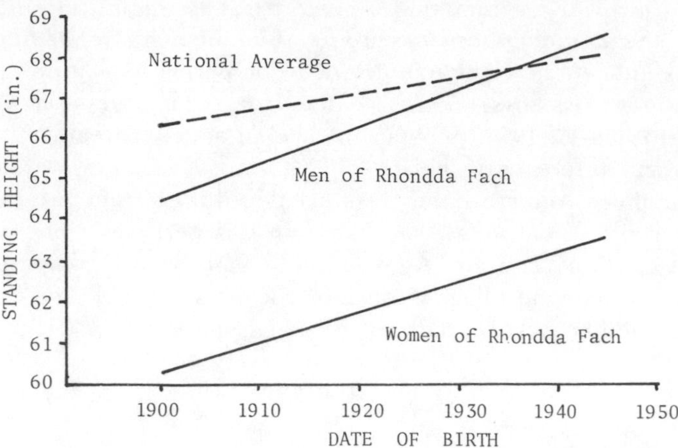

FIG. 4-7. Secular trend in adult height, showing stature by date of birth for the men and women of the Rhondda Fach and the national average (as estimated by Tanner.[15]) It should be borne in mind that loss in stature with ageing will contribute to a minor extent to the smaller stature of the older people. (From Acheson.[12])

that the average stature of such girls had reached the maximum by the 1930s.

Among poor and less educated peoples, with a high rate of disease and malnutrition throughout life, well-directed action might effect change in health and, hence, in growth (Fig. 4-6). It is, therefore, of special importance to discriminate between the aspects of physique and growth which are more readily influenced by disease and nutritional status and those features of a people which are related to their genetic constitution. In his discussion of this subject Tanner[17] distinguishes between rate of growth, growth in size, growth in skeletal shape, and growth in tissue composition. Variations in shape and tissue composition are frequently the effects of different genetic composition, whereas "starvation seems usually to cause effects in a certain order, so that shape changes seldom, if ever, occur before size and rate changes are far advanced."

BLOOD PRESSURE

In contrast to a measurement like height, the blood pressure of individuals varies considerably at different times of the day, when asleep or awake, when resting or active. ". . . It is a value at a point of time of a very

TABLE 4-1. Examples Showing Variation in Blood Pressure Readings During a 24-hour Period

	Female Aged 27	Female Aged 62	Male Aged 33
Basal	110/70	132/82	152/109
Lowest hour	86/47	102/61	123/78
Highest hour	126/79	172/94	153/107
Casual	108/64	155/93	157/109

(Data from Richardson et al.[21]*)*

changeable character. . . ."[18,19] Because of the considerable variation, there has been much discussion on the meaning of a casual measurement of blood pressure. A number of workers have sought for ways and means of measuring a so-called basal pressure and Smirk[20] describes in some detail his method of doing this. The subject sleeps in the institution, and early in the morning, before eating and while the room remains darkened, a blood pressure reading is taken. This is done by a physician with whom the subject is familiar, with every attempt being made to spare the individual any disturbance. Pickering is critical of these attempts to seek a basal pressure and questions what indeed the basal pressure represents. In the study of a series of individuals over a 24-hour period he, as a member of a team with Richardson,[21] showed the considerable variation that exists in the same individual, in people of various ages, and with various levels of blood pressure.

Table 4-1 is a summary of some of the cases which they present, showing the variation in blood pressure readings during a 24-hour period.

A considerable variation in single readings of blood pressure no doubt has much meaning for clinical investigation but in itself does not necessarily vitiate population studies. However, another kind of variation, namely that between consecutive readings of blood pressure, may do so. During population studies in which the same population is examined after a period of time, it has been shown[22,23] that blood pressures which were initially high tended to be lower on the second examination and those which were relatively low at first tended to become higher. The direction of change tends towards the mean. This should be borne in mind when analyzing change of a health variable such as blood pressure in a population.

Additional problems in investigating blood pressure in population groups are the differing ways in which blood pressures are read and the differences between observers (observer variation). Thus there is a preference for the every tenth zero reading, which in a population study can influence the mean level. Furthermore, the preference may be differently applied by observers.

It is customary to use particular guidelines of systolic and diastolic pressures above which a person is regarded as having hypertension. The cutoff point which divides normality (normotensive) from abnormality (hypertensive) may be decided in different ways.[24] There are definitions based on a statistical model of the "normal" curve of pressure—measurements which deviate sufficiently from the mean are regarded as abnormal. The danger in this is the assumption that the mean blood pressure in a population group represents a measure of health. In some groups the mean may be high and the whole distribution may tend to higher levels of blood pressure.

Cross-sectional Studies

Many community studies[22] have shown considerable change in blood pressure with increasing age. The mean systolic blood pressure not only increases, but the shape of the distribution curve changes. In younger ages there is a large central tendency, a dome-shaped and relatively steep curve with slight skewing. With increase in age, and especially after 45 years, the distribution of the blood pressure not only shifts to higher levels but the central tendency is smaller with a flatter, more widely dispersed, curve.

Diastolic pressure increases with age, but the pattern of distribution changes much less, the central tendency being large at all ages, with relatively steep sloping curves.

These findings are illustrated in Figure 4-8 from Winkelstein and Kantor's[25] analysis of a blood pressure study in Bergen, Norway.[26]

It has been thought that higher pressures are "normal" (not unhealthy) in older age groups[27] because such pressures are so common. However, the usual is not necessarily normal in a health sense. Epidemiologically, we need to know the morbidity and mortality associated with different levels of blood pressure at different ages. Stamler[28] has shown the usefulness of this type of analysis, in which increase in blood pressure is associated with increase in risk for coronary heart disease in United States investigations. Figure 1-1, in Chapter 1, illustrates the importance of considering the rise in blood pressure as a whole and not only the cutoff points which divide the population into "well" (healthy) and "not well" (diseased) persons.

In considering stature, growth, and maturation, it is clear that there are considerable differences between the peoples of various parts of the world and even between those living in the same country. Recognition of this fact inhibits a too facile generalization of criteria for "normal" age of maturation or physique, and compels a careful appraisal of the

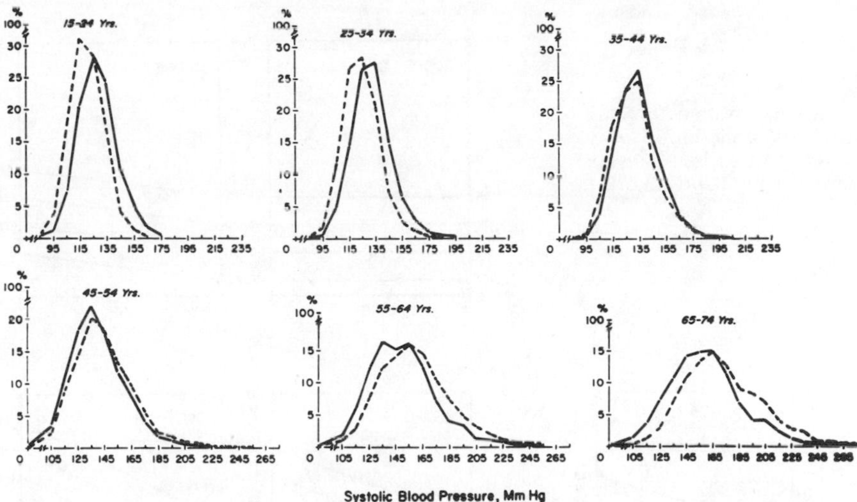

FIG. 4-8. Frequency distributions of systolic blood pressure measurements according to sex and age, Bergen. Males are represented by the solid line, females by the broken line. (From Winkelstein and Kantor.[25])

usual features of a particular community. This leads in turn to consideration of factors determining differences between communities. Similarly, differences in blood pressure levels and variations with age can be expected. However, there are a number of communities in which there is very little or no change in blood pressure with increase in age.[29–33]

Comparison between blood pressure levels and age-trends in a number of different communities is a difficult task which has been made easier by an ingenious and simple grid devised by Epstein and Eckoff.[34] Five different grids include slope and level of blood pressure. The slope ranges from no change of blood pressure with age (slope 0) to increasing degrees (slopes 1 to 4) of blood pressure rise with age. The levels are represented by three channels beginning with systolic blood pressure ranges of 105 to 115 (channel a), 115 to 125 (channel b), and 125 to 135 mm Hg (channel c) among children. They tested its use in a comparison of a number of populations (Fig. 4-9). Henry and Cassel[35] have also discussed these important differences in blood pressure levels with age in different communities (Fig. 4-10). These data indicate that the often-quoted generalization—blood pressure increases with age—needs modification and when not qualified is both incorrect and misleading. The fact that communities differ so markedly suggests the need for reexamination as to whether the rise in blood pressure with increasing age is true for all people in those societies in which the general trend is an increase.

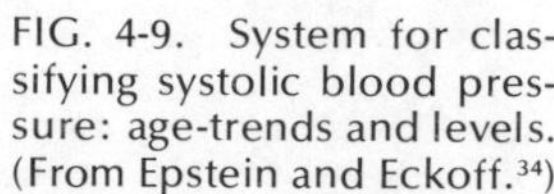

FIG. 4-9. System for classifying systolic blood pressure: age-trends and levels. (From Epstein and Eckoff.[34])

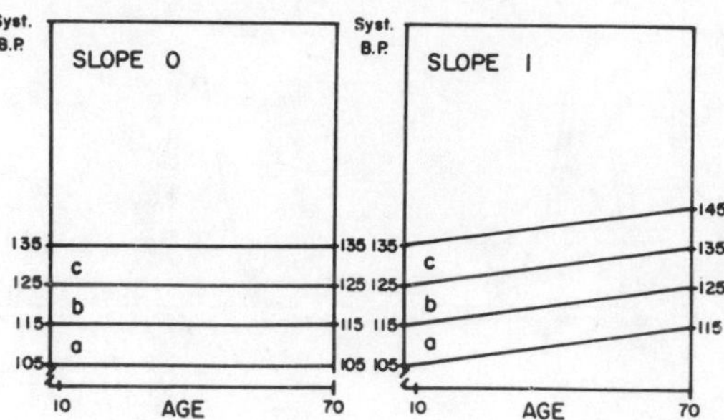

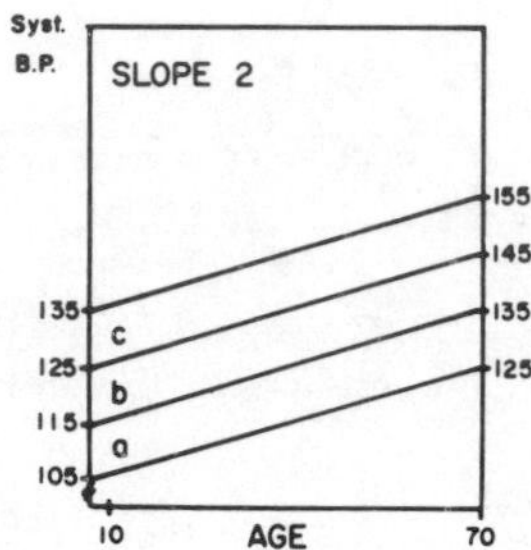

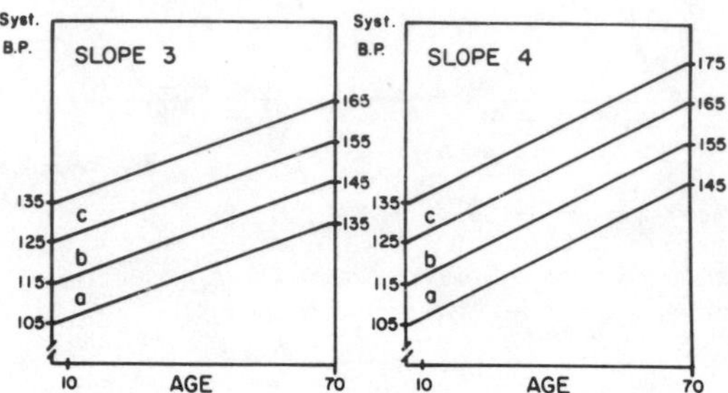

Winkelstein and Kantor[25] in their analysis of the Bergen study show that when the blood pressure distribution at different ages is analyzed by percentiles, a marked difference is noted in the change of systolic pressure between younger and older men and women. Findings that resemble these Bergen trends are also noted when the data on Israeli civil servants aged 40 to 44 and 55 to 59 are compared (Table 4-2).[36]

This kind of cross-sectional data of a population at a particular moment in time poses a challenging question—whether young men with low blood pressure will tend to be those with lower blood pressures in later life. This is a vital question needing an answer which only long-term epidemiologic investigations can provide. The existence of such men whose blood pressures do not rise with age, and who are more healthy because of it, has been recognized for many years. Sir Thomas Lewis, pioneer English clinical researcher in cardiology, expressed this clearly.[37] "The average blood pressure rises with age; this is not to say that rising blood pressure is normal, for many vigorous and long-lived men retain low blood pressure; it is good that an otherwise healthy but aged man should show a pressure below the average for his years."

Data on blood pressure of a group of men aged 50 to 59 employed in a Chicago utility company were available, going back in one group of men for 20 years and in another for 30 years. The general trend showed

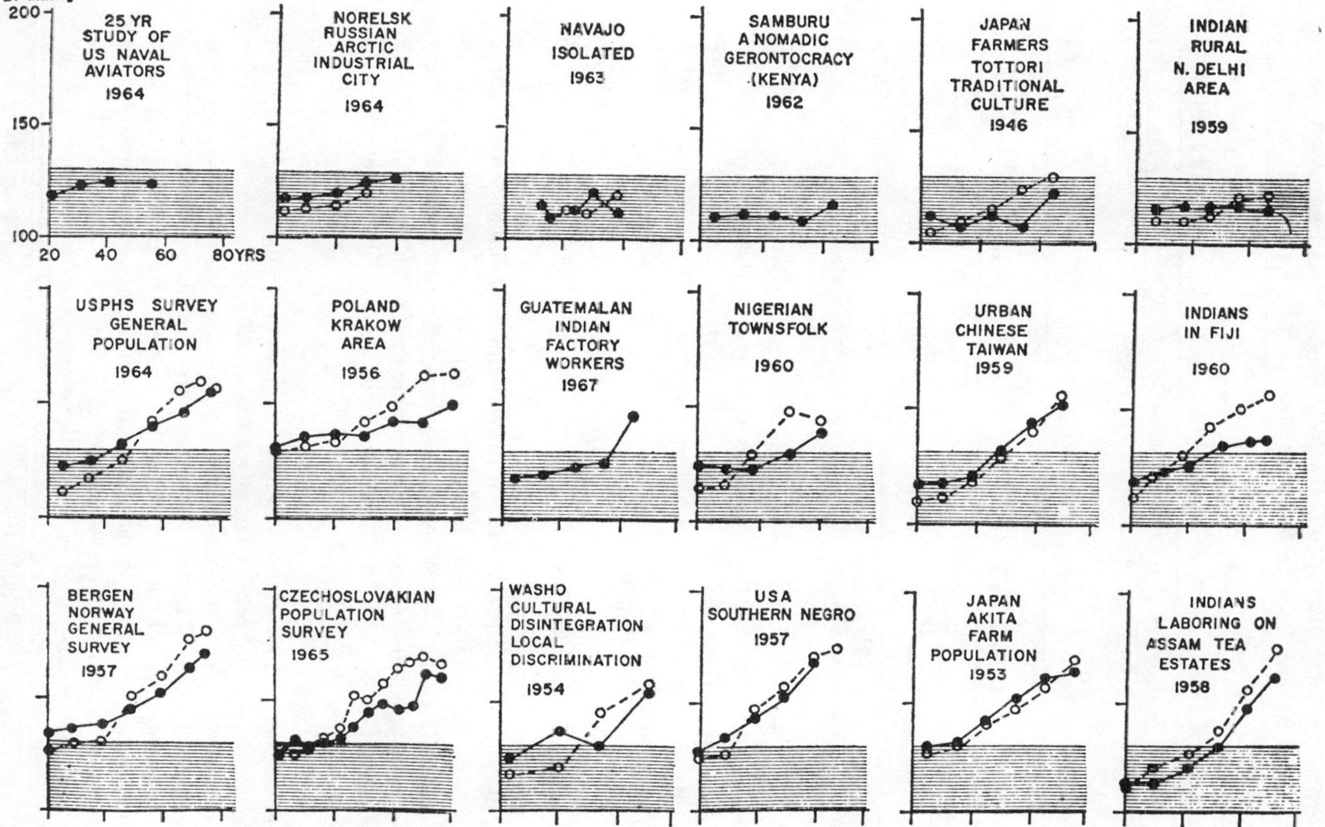

FIG. 4-10. Contrasting the change of blood pressure with age in different communities of the same race. Note the communities in which no change with age was found. (From Henry and Cassel.[35])

TABLE 4-2. The Difference in Systolic Blood Pressure in Men of Different Ages, in Bergen, Norway, and in Israel*

BERGEN

Age	5th Percentile	50th Percentile	95th Percentile
20	113	135	153
75	125	168	222
Percentage difference	11	24	37

ISRAELI CIVIL SERVANTS

Age group	5th Percentile	20th Percentile	50th Percentile	80th Percentile	95th Percentile
40–44	108	117	128	141	161
55–59	113	124	141	162	186
Percentage difference	5	6	10	15	16

*Systolic blood pressure in mm Hg, per percentile.
(Data from Bergen adapted from Winklestein and Kantor;[25] data from Israel adapted from Medalie et al.[36])

a rise in blood pressure for the groups as a whole, but there was a segment of men that showed no significant rise in blood pressure throughout the period; this was especially noted in those who initially had a low normal diastolic pressure.[38]

Prospective Studies

Prospective studies of the same cohort have helped elucidate some aspects of this association that are well illustrated in reports of a study of a group of men extending over a period of 24 years.[39,40] Survivors of a cohort of young men selected for naval flight training in 1940 in the United States were reexamined in 1951–1952 and again in 1957–1958. A summary of the findings is presented below.

1. Blood pressure distribution changed with increasing age. The mean systolic pressure increased slightly from age 20 to age 35, after which there was even less or no change. The changes during the age span 20 to 35 of this cohort resemble the findings reported on men of a Welsh mining valley[41] in which, as the authors noted, there was "a plateau in the 20- to 40-year age group," but it is unlike the Welsh study and others that showed a steep rise in systolic blood pressure after the age of 40. The mean diastolic pressure in the aviator cohort of men increased with age between the age groups of 20 to 40 years, the increase being somewhat more marked than was that of the systolic blood pressure.

In both systolic and diastolic pressure the curves reflect quantitative variation in each age group, and with increasing age central tendency becomes less marked with flattening of the curve. The resemblance to the Bergen study findings is striking, as well as to those[22,41] of earlier investigations which led Pickering to believe that blood pressure was a continuously distributed variable in a population and that the concept of essential hypertension, as a single qualitatively different disease entity, was incorrect.

2. The men tended to maintain their relative standing in the distribution of blood pressures in the cohort as they passed through different ages. Thus men in the upper blood pressure category, i.e., those having a pressure greater than the mean plus 1 SD in the original examination, were on the whole in a similar relative position 12 and 18 years later. While there was an increase in the mean blood pressure of the group as a whole, this study indicates the possibility of two distinctive groups. The first group consists of the majority of men in whom there was little or no consistent change during the 24-year period; the second group is smaller, consisting of those men whose blood pressure increased consistently. This group consisted of men who had greater weight increase with age and whose parents were shorter lived. Thus despite the fact that the general distribution curve of systolic blood pressure among these men is continuous, there is a small group who do seem to differ qualitatively from the majority.

The grid of classification of levels and slopes devised by Epstein and Eckoff for comparing different population groups may well be helpful in categorizing individuals whose records will become increasingly available as repeated periodic health examinations become more common. The differences between populations might then be expressed in a more refined way than the change in the mean blood pressure, by recording the proportion of population in each grid. Such comparisons must await further long-term longitudinal measures of blood pressure in communities and other "normal" population groups.

There is considerable disagreement about the interpretation of the distribution of blood pressure in communities. The main schools were well represented by the opinions of Platt[42] on the one hand and Pickering[43] on the other. Platt has contended that hypertensives are a distinct entity. He considers hypertension to be determined by single gene recessive inheritance,[44] thereby including it among the disorders which we would classify as having qualitative or discontinuous variation. Segregating the population into distinctive groups has been based upon an interpretation of the nature of the curve of distribution, a bimodal curve. This received some support in a study by Morrison and Morris,[45] who compared the frequency distribution curve of blood pressure of 90 London transport drivers, of whom at least one parent had died in middle age, with that of those whose parents were alive or had died at a later age. The former group had a higher blood pressure distribution. This finding is in accord with that of the 1,000 cohort study reviewed above.[40]

In contrast to this view Pickering[43] and his associates have consistently demonstrated quantitative continuous variation to be a characteristic feature of the population groups they have studied.

The following is a summary of Pickering's views, recorded by Pickering himself.[18,19]

> The qualitative approach is still very much a habit of mind of all who have had a medical education. It stems from the emphasis on diagnosis and the vital question, Has the patient a disease or not? And so characteristics associated with "disease" tend to be divided into normal and abnormal, physiological and pathological, good and bad. Medicine in fact can count up to two. Elevated arterial pressure is no exception. Blood-pressure is classed as normal or abnormal, normotension or hypertension. Those with hypertension have the disease, those with normotension have not. . . . We now know that there is no dividing-line. To create one is nothing more or less than to create an artifact, and the resulting classification is nothing more than a set of secondary artifacts.

In discussing variation in height, it was emphasized that it was a product predominantly of the interaction of a multiplicity of factors, involving both polygenic factors and subsequent life experiences. Discontinuous and continuous variation may be found in the distribution of a single characteristic. While the distinction between these kinds of variation is important, its "either-or" application to all attributes is incorrect; too rigid a classification of characteristics in this way would lead to false conclusions. Height may be seen as a case where the distinction between continuous and discontinuous characteristics is not always so clear. Shortness may be a result of a genetic mutation as in achondroplasia, but it has been shown that "some pathologic dwarfs may be taller than the shortest of normal people."[46] Thus there is some overlap between the two kinds of short people. At the other extreme there may be a very limited number of cases of gigantism, such as those resulting from pituitary tumors secreting an excess of growth hormone.

In contrast to the cases of dwarfism and gigantism, which are distinctive abnormal entities, is the height distribution of the mass of individuals in a population.

Similar considerations may be true of the distribution of blood pressure in a community. There is need for further epidemiologic investigation which may help to prove that both quantitative and qualitative variation are relevant to its distribution in a population, and hence in the occurrence of hypertension.

REFERENCES

1. Bendich A, Borenfreund E, Honda Y, et al.: Cell transformation and the genesis of cancer. Arch Environ Health 19:157, 1969, p 157.
2. Kopito L, Shwachman H: Studies in cystic fibrosis. Determination of sweat electrolytes in situ with direct reading electrodes. Pediatrics 43: 794, 1969.
3. Meredith HV: Body size of contemporary youth in different parts of the world. Monogr Soc Res Child Dev 34:1, 1969.
4. Hiernaux J: Weight/height relationship during growth in Africans and Europeans. Hum Biol 36:273, 1964.
5. Roberts DF, Bainbridge DP: Nilotic physique. Amer J Phys Anthropol 21:341, 1963.
6. Stuart HC: Studies from the Center for Research in Child Health, Harvard University. I. The center, the group under observation, and studies in progress. Monogr Soc Res Child Dev 4:1, 1939.
7. Stuart HC, Meredith HV: Use of body measurements in the school health program. Am J Public Health 36:1365, 1946.
8. Stuart HC, Stevenson SS: Physical growth and development. In Nelson WE (ed.): Textbook of Pediatrics, 7th ed. Philadelphia, Saunders, 1959. Graphs and percentile tables from Studies of Child Health and Development, Maternal and Child Health, Harvard School of Public Health.
9. Kark S, Kark E: Growth of African and Indian babies in the first year of life. In Kark SL, Steuart GW (eds.): A Practice of Social Medicine. Edinburgh and London, Livingstone, 1962, pp 164–165.
10. Abramson JH: The "Marshlands" health service. In Kark SL, Steuart GW (eds.): A Practice of Social Medicine. Edinburgh and London, Livingstone, 1962, p 355.
11. Epstein LM: Standards for weight growth of Israeli-born babies. J Trop Pediatr 15:4, 1969.
12. Acheson RM, Fowler GB: Sex, socioeconomic status, and secular increase in stature. Brit J Prev Soc Med 18:25, 1964.
13. Acheson RM: Maturation of the skeleton. In Falkner F (ed.): Human Development. Philadelphia and London, Saunders, 1966.
14. Tanner JM: The trend towards earlier physical maturation. In Meade JE, Parkes AS (eds.): Biological Aspects of Social Problems. Edinburgh, Oliver and Boyd, 1965, p 40.
15. Tanner JM: Growth at Adolescence, 2nd ed. Oxford, Blackwell Scientific, 1962.
16. Bakwin H, McLaughlin SM: Secular increase in height. Is the end in sight? Lancet 2:1195, 1964.
17. Tanner JM: Growth and physique in different populations of mankind. In Baker PT, Weiner JS (eds.): The Biology of Human Adaptability. Oxford, Clarendon, 1966, p 47.
18. Pickering G: Hyperpiesis: high blood pressure without evident cause: Essential hypertension. Brit Med J 2:959, 1965.
19. Pickering G: Hyperpiesis: high blood pressure without evident cause: Essential hypertension. Brit Med J 2:1021, 1965.
20. Smirk FH: High Arterial Pressure. Oxford, Blackwell Scientific, 1957.

21. Richardson DW, Honour AJ, Fenton GW, et al.: Variation in arterial pressure throughout the day and night. Clin Sci 26:445, 1964.
22. Hamilton M, Pickering GW, Fraser Roberts JA, et al.: The aetiology of essential hypertension. I. The arterial pressure in the general population. Clin Sci 13:11, 1954.
23. McKeown T, Record RG, Whitfield AGW: Variation in casual measurements of arterial pressure in two populations (Birmingham and South Wales), re-examined after intervals of 3–4.5 years. Clin Sci 24:437, 1963.
24. Geiger HJ, Scotch NA: The epidemiology of essential hypertension. I. Biological mechanisms and descriptive epidemiology. J Chronic Dis 16: 1151, 1963.
25. Winkelstein W, Kantor S: Some observations on the relationships between age, sex, and blood pressure. In Stamler J, Stamler R, Pullman T (eds.): The Epidemiology of Hypertension. New York and London, Grune & Stratton, 1967.
26. Boe J, Humerfelt S, Wedervang F: The blood pressure in a population. Blood pressure readings and height and weight determinations in the adult population of the city of Bergen. Acta Med Sc and (Suppl) 321:1, 1957.
27. Master AM, Garfield CI, Walters MB: Normal Blood Pressure and Hypertension. Philadelphia, Lea and Febiger, 1952.
28. Stamler J: Lectures on Preventive Cardiology. New York, Grune & Stratton, 1967.
29. Donnison CP: Blood pressure in the African native. Lancet 1:6, 1929.
30. Lowenstein FW: Blood pressure in relation to age and sex in the tropics and subtropics. A review of the literature and an investigation in two tribes of Brazil Indians. Lancet 1:389, 1961.
31. Maddocks I: Possible absence of essential hypertension in two complete Pacific Island populations. Lancet 2:396, 1961.
32. Shaper AG: Blood pressure studies in East Africa. In Stamler J, Stamler R, Pullman T (eds.): The Epidemiology of Hypertension. New York and London, Grune & Stratton, 1967.
33. Shaper AG, Wright DH, Kyobe J: Blood pressure and body build in three nomadic tribes of Northern Kenya. East Afr Med J 46:273, 1969.
34. Epstein FH, Eckoff RD: The epidemiology of high blood pressure. Geographic distributions and etiological factors. In Stamler J, Stamler R, Pullman T (eds.): The Epidemiology of Hypertension. New York and London, Grune & Stratton, 1967.
35. Henry JP, Cassel JC: Psychosocial factors in essential hypertension. Recent epidemiologic and animal experimental evidence. Amer J Epidemiol 90:171, 1969.
36. Medalie JH, Kahn HA, Neufeld HN, et al.: Selected measurements on 10,000 Israeli males. Physicians Fact Book. Jerusalem, Israel Ischemic Heart Disease Study, 1968.
37. Lewis T: Diseases of the Heart. London, MacMillan, 1933, p 231.
38. Stamler J, Lindberg HA, Berkson DM, et al.: Epidemiological Analysis of Hypertension and Hypertensive Disease in the Labor Force of a Chicago Utility Company. Mimeograph Report, 1959.
39. Harlan WR, Osborne RK, Graybiel A: A longitudinal study of blood pressure. Circulation 26:530, 1962.
40. Oberman A, Lane NE, Harlan WR, et al.: Trends in systolic blood pressure in the thousand aviator cohort over a 24-year period. Circulation 36: 812, 1967.

41. Miall WE, Oldham PD: A study of arterial blood pressure and its inheritance in a sample of the general population. Clin Sci 14:459, 1955.
42. Platt R: The nature of essential hypertension. Lancet 277:55, 1959.
43. Pickering G: High Blood Pressure, 2nd ed. London, Churchill, 1968.
44. Platt R: Heredity in hypertension. Lancet 1:899, 1963.
45. Morrison SL, Morris JN: Epidemiological observations on high blood pressure without evident cause. Lancet 277:864, 1959.
46. Fraser Roberts JA: An Introduction to Medical Genetics, 5th ed. London, Oxford Univ Press, 1970, p 247.

5
Psychologic Characteristics

Measurements of behavior, personality, and intelligence should provide a picture of variation in mental health of a population group which goes beyond the incidence and prevalence of mental diseases. Basic to such measurements is an understanding of behavior development and the underlying maturation of personality and growth of intelligence. In contrast to the relative simplicity of measurement of physical attributes, e.g., height and weight, the assessment of various components of mental health is complicated and the definition of what is being measured is not always clear. In considering the psychologic attributes of health apart from the physical aspects there is no intention of denying the biologic foundations of mental functioning. It is rather to ensure consideration of psychologic characteristics even when the related biologic processes are not yet known.

Embryologic studies have established the fact that growth and development of form and function follow an orderly sequence of differentiation in which each phase of development depends upon the satisfactory unfolding of preceding phases. The results of interference with these epigenetic processes will obviously depend on the phase of growth during which the interference operates. Thus in fetal infection with rubella the effects vary with the growth phase during which the fetus is infected.

The epigenesis of brain and nervous system growth has its functional expression in behavior and intellectual performance in infancy and early childhood as well as later in life. Among the well-known tests that have focused on this area are Gesell's developmental examinations of motor characteristics, adaptive behavior, language, and personal-social behavior.[1,2] They have been used extensively, more especially in infants and young children.[3] By comparing the actual development of a child with that expected at his age a developmental quotient (DQ) is expressed.

INTELLIGENCE

As with the distribution of height, intelligence scores have a continuous variation. In his original thinking on the subject of hereditary genius, or as he later preferred to call it, "hereditary ability," Francis Galton[4] postulated a symmetrical distribution of men according to the grade of their natural ability. He based this on Quetelet's[5] analysis of the actual distribution of physical measurements, such as the height and chest girth of men, in relation to his tables of the expected distribution of deviations from an average. Arguing by analogy Galton stated: "Now, if this be the case with stature, then it will be true as regards every other physical feature—as circumference of head, size of brain, weight of grey matter, number of brain fibres, etc; and thence, by a step on which no physiologist will hesitate, as regards mental capacity."[4] As Penrose[6] pointed out, Galton's assumption of an exactly symmetrical distribution is not correct. There are proportionately many more idiots and imbeciles than there are eminently gifted men.

The continuous distribution of intelligence test scores suggests a multiplicity of determinant factors operating through the population group, i.e., polygenic inheritance and manifold additive experiences. This quantitative distribution of intelligence will naturally include a number of persons of low intelligence without specific pathologic associations. However, there are a number of distinctive conditions causally associated with mental deficiency. These include chromosomal abnormalities of which Down's syndrome (mongolism) is well known, as well as less common genetic defects such as the recessive condition phenylketonuria, or rare dominant trait disorders such as epiloia. Other well-defined entities associated with mental retardation are various kinds and degrees of brain damage due to birth trauma; prenatal infections such as syphilis, rubella, and toxoplasmosis; or postnatal infections involving encephalitis or meningitis.

Less severe mental retardation, as measured by intelligence scores or as reflected in educational backwardness, is a widespread condition associated with social factors.[6,7] The retardation is not a distinctive condition in the sense of being able to define those who have it as compared with those who do not. It is rather a group of individuals occupying a range of positions on the continuous curve of distribution of intelligence. It is one of the very few conditions classified in the *International List of Diseases* by quantitative criteria, including the Intelligence Quotient (IQ).

The intelligence of an individual can, and does, change under altered circumstances and in relation to variations in his health state. This is evidenced by the improvement which has been demonstrated in the intelligence of subnormal children when they are removed from adverse conditions.[8] There is also the decline in intelligence which occurs in the aged, which may be associated with other changes in health. An example of this has been presented by Wilkie and Eisdorfer in a study of change in intelligence in individuals first examined between the ages of 60 and 69 years and followed-up for 10 years. Decline in intelligence was significantly associated with hypertension, defined as a diastolic blood pressure over 105 mm Hg at the initial examination.[9] This decline was not found in individuals of the same age group whose diastolic blood pressure at the first examination was normal, 66 to 95 mm Hg, or borderline hypertensive, 96 to 105 mm Hg.

The fact that intelligence is changeable, and does vary with social class, suggests that health services might fruitfully focus attention on its stimulation or promotion as a central feature of community health care, especially in maternal and child health services, as well as exploring ways of preventing its decline in middle-aged and older persons.

PERSONALITY

Effective integration of personality assessments in epidemiologic investigations presents a challenge of particular importance at the present time owing to the considerable expansion of the interests of epidemiology and the activities of community health care. Personality is not only central to the concepts of mental health and mental disease, but its relationship with somatic characteristics can be the core of our understanding of processes connecting the social and biologic features of population groups. And yet it is often ignored. The comment which Cattell[10] directed to his psychologist colleagues some 25 years ago might be as forcefully directed to many of us in epidemiology and community medicine today.

> *The ignoring of a problem.* Although the endless variety and colorfulness of human personality intrigue the artist and challenge the ingenuity of the scientist who function together harmoniously in the mind of any good psychologist, many psychometrists have nevertheless fled from this richness of human nature as from some fearsome incubus. They have left reality to the novelist, and escaped into the cloistered order of the laboratory, where the husk of measurement may be exhibited even when the kernel is lost.

The challenge from which so many shrink is both conceptual and technical. What does personality mean and, more especially, what is its meaning for health? What is a healthy personality? What are the ways in which personality is assessed, and what are the problems in personality assessment which continue to make suspect those studies in which it is an important element?

There are various ways of viewing behavior and personality, depending upon the purpose of the investigation and the approach. An interview of an applicant for a vacancy will obviously be oriented towards an assessment of his suitability for the particular job, with the appraisal of his health being directed towards its influence on the functions expected of him. Adequacy in personal relationships may be top priority for one situation; for another, capacity for decision making in emergencies; in others physique and physical strength may be the major influence. When the focus of interest is not so much on ability to fulfill the requirements of a specific function in a work situation but rather on health or health care, different orientations are needed.

Personality has been viewed in the context of widely differing theoretical foundations. It is expressed in behavior, thoughts, and feelings involving the way people fulfill their varied social roles in relations with one another, and in their overt reactions to different situations of day-to-day living—at home, work, or at play; in crisis or sudden change; and in stressful circumstances. It involves less objective elements such as perception of self, of others, and of the environment; moods, motives, and interests; value-attitudes; and sentiments and abilities. It is at once a myriad of traits and yet a composite whole with consistent behavior. It is these aspects of personality that have allowed the novelist and playwrite to capture the whole and present us with more complete pictures than have yet been possible by the use of scientific descriptive method.

One generality that is helpful in defining the everyday meaning of personality is the following statement by Vernon.[11]

> . . . Colloquially, personality means—what sort of a person is so-and-so, what is he like? At the same time we usually restrict the term to the relatively permanent emotional qualities underlying the person's behavior, his drives and needs, attitudes and interests, and distinguish it from his intellectual and bodily skills and cognitive characteristics.

Just as in the distribution of somatic and intellectual characteristics, it is likely that personality characteristics may also be of a graded continuous distribution throughout a community, or possibly the community may be sharply divided between those who have the particular characteristics and those who do not, i.e., discontinuous distribution. The distribution of personality characteristics is probably of the continuous kind, but it is possible that particular elements of personality may yet be linked to single gene inheritance or other highly specific causal factors.

Various approaches to the phychologic component of mental health have been reviewed by Jahoda.[12] An important aspect of her review of the different ideas of many leading workers and their relevance for community health is its extension of the concept of mental health well beyond the presence or absence of mental disease. She groups the various ideas of different workers into 6 main approaches which she indicates overlap to some extent.

1. Attitudes of the individual towards himself, including such feelings about himself as self-acceptance, self-esteem, and self-respect; the correctness or objectivity of his self-concept; his sense of identity and awareness of a variety of important aspects of self, such as his interests, desires, obligations, and actions.
2. The degree to which a person realizes his potentialities through action. This involves his self-concept as well as his intellectual and other abilities, his striving and motivational processes focusing on goals outside of himself, with interests and activities associated with other people, ideas, or things.
3. Integration of personality. This broadly defined criterion of mental health includes both of the above criteria. It goes further in its focus on the concept of balance of personality factors involving emotional qualities of resistance to stress, the tolerance of anxiety and not the mere absence of anxiety, as well as more intellectual integration as represented by a unifying outlook on life.
4. Autonomy, or the individual's degree of independence of social influences, involving his capacity to conform to these influences or not, in terms of a set of standards within himself.
5. How the individual sees the world around him. This involves both social sensitivity and a "relative freedom from need-distortion," a phrase which Jahoda uses in discussing healthy perception of reality, meaning "a process of viewing the world so that one is able to take in matters one wishes were different, without distorting them to fit these wishes—that is, without inventing cues not actually existing."[12]
6. Environmental mastery, involving successful behavior and processes of adaptation and change of oneself and the environment. The relevant literature is reviewed in relation to various aspects of functioning, e.g., the ability to love; adequacy in love, work, and play; adequacy in interpersonal relations; efficiency in meeting situational requirements; capacity for adaptation and adjustment; and efficiency in problem-solving.

This emphasizes functioning as a cornerstone concept of mental health involving effective relational behavior and fulfillment of social roles. Proposing that ". . . the crucial test of psychological fitness is the test of performance—the individual's capacity to enact meaningful social roles, . . ." Steuart and Wilson regard ". . . functional efficacy, rather than the lack of symptoms, as a key criterion of mental health. . . ."[13]

A number of workers have adopted a multiple criterion approach. Jahoda herself is one of them, ". . . proposing active adjustment (environmental mastery), integration, and perception as jointly constituting mental health."[12]

In the Midtown Manhattan Study assets and liabilities were included in the psychiatric interview and the questionnaire. The first two criteria of mental health were freedom ". . . from various gross symptoms and from disabling inner tensions, . . ." and the others were capacities such as ". . . ease of social interaction, capacity for pursuit of realistic goals, [having] a satisfying sense of social belonging and a sensitivity to the needs of others, and having a feeling of adequacy in social roles (particularly sexual)."[14]

It is clear that there is not one distinctive personality type that constitutes the mentally healthy segment of a population group. There are obviously many personality attributes or traits and behavior characteristics that are combined in different and distinctive ways within the individuals of the group. The measurement of each factor may, like many other biologic variables, have a continuous distribution in a relatively homogeneous community, but the varied combinations of these personality factors will inevitably result in a diversity of expression of mental health. Steuart and Wilson emphasize that their

> . . . idea of positive health or competent social phychological functioning does not imply a unitary model of effectiveness. As there are many illnesses, so there are many healths. Mental health entails no magical or narrowly construed ideal of behavior, but rather recognizes alternative and varied patterns suited to the varieties of individual and group characteristics."[13]

PERSONALITY PROFILES AND DISEASE SUSCEPTIBILITY

The belief that people with particular kinds of personality are prone to specific disease syndromes is as old as medicine itself. In more recent times Dunbar developed and applied the concept of personality profiles and their relations with particular diseases.[15–17]

Dunbar's personality profile is not a summary diagnostic label, it is a comprehensive picture as indicated by the extract of the profile of coronary occlusion given in Table 5-1.

The specificity of such associations has been questioned often. To meet this criticism directed against the view that definite types of person are more likely to develop certain diseases, Dunbar stressed

> . . . the personality profile indicates the illness pattern to which a given personality may be particularly susceptible. . . . The personality profile is useful merely as indicating an area of susceptibility. . . . everyone

whose personality profile fits the pattern of the coronary or the accident prone, for example, does not develop coronary disease or the accident habit.[17]

Her concepts require more discussion here because of their potential impact on epidemiologic thinking about personality and disease. The implication for particular groups of people who have similar personality profiles is that they will also share susceptibility to certain diseases or disease patterns.

In epidemiologic studies it is not practical to carry out comprehensive testing at each level in order to reach an ultimate picture of the distribution of personality types in a population. Hence the attraction of shortcuts, such as the use of questionnaires and inventories in health screening.[18–24]

Because of the important bearing that advances in measurement of personality can have on epidemiology this topic will be discussed further, making reference mainly to Cattell's Personality Factor analysis.[10] Allport and Odbert prepared a list of some 4,500 words in the English language which were descriptive of personality traits.[25] "By throwing together terms which any average user of the language would consider synonyms,"[10] and by adding descriptive terms which had been used in technical psychology, Cattell prepared a comprehensive list of 171 traits. Most of them were listed in the form of pairs of polar opposites, e.g., the opposite of the trait "responsive" is listed as "aloof." In reviewing previous research, he found that many of the traits overlapped, allowing a reduction to 50 nuclear clusters. Thus the trait, responsive-aloof, becomes one trait of a nuclear cluster—sociability, sentimentalism, warmth versus independence, hostility, aloofness. Following factor analysis of various studies, Cattell developed a more limited number of factors which he called "source traits of personality."

Despite their limitations, the importance of questionnaires is their usefulness and their practicability, and his questionnaire, "Cattell's 16 PF Test"[26] is his own contribution to shortcut methods of personality measurement and has been used in several epidemiologic studies.

The concept of a personality profile being associated with particular disease syndromes has been used in a number of studies of coronary heart disease. Various personality tests and descriptions have been used by different workers. These are discussed more fully in Chapter 22. Here we will deal with one of these investigations: Caffrey's use of Cattell's 16 Personality Factor test in tests of different groups of monks.[27]

If certain behavior-patterns and personality characteristics are associated with a disease it might be expected that these characteristics would be more common in those communities in which the particular disease is relatively common. Comparative epidemiologic studies of communities of monks of different monasteries have indicated important differences in rates of coronary heart disease and have provided the opportunity for comparing their personality characteristics.[27] The lacto-vegetarian diet of Trappist monks was compared with the typically American, varied diet of the Benedictines. The Trappist diet provided a lower percentage of total calories from fat (26 versus 45 percent), of which there was a lower proportion from animal sources (43 percent of total fat versus 75 percent), and a correspondingly higher proportion of fat from vegetable sources (57 versus 25 percent). The Trappists also had a higher proportion of total calories from carbohydrates (64 versus 42 percent) with little difference in calories from protein and in total calories. If anything, the vegetarian Trappists had a higher calorie diet (3,203 versus 2,896 calories). Earlier studies[28,29] of monks in Trappist and Benedictine monasteries had shown that the different diets of the two orders were associated with differences in cholesterol and other lipid levels, and yet on an individual basis the serum lipid levels could not be directly correlated with fat intake alone. In their report Barrow and his associates concluded that ". . . on an individual basis there appear to be factors other than age and dietary fat which affect serum lipids."[28]

Differences in rates of myocardial infarction and angina pectoris were later reported within subgroups of these monks,[30] in which it was apparent that Benedictine priests had very much higher rates than did Benedictine brothers or Trappist priests and brothers. Benedictine priests had the same cholesterol level (223 versus 225 mg) but a higher triglyceride level (130 versus 100 mg) than the Benedictine brothers. They were heavier (172 versus 159 lbs) although their calorie consumption was somewhat less, indicating that they were a less physically active group than the brothers. While the diet of the Benedictine brothers was different from that of the Trappists, they resembled the Trappists in having a low coronary heart disease rate and in several risk factors, serum triglycerides and weight, but their cholesterol levels were higher (225 versus 206 and 203 mg of Trappist priests and brothers, respectively).

Based on these findings of Barrow et al., Caffrey[27] postulated that the group with the highest rate of coronary heart disease, the Benedictine priests, would have a relatively distinct personality profile, elevated on the following scales of the Cattell 16 Personality Factor test. He did not expect differences in scales C (emotionally stable, realistic, calm, patient versus neurotic), L (suspicious, self-sufficient, withdrawn versus trustful), O (worrying, lonely, sensitive versus self-confident), and Q_4 (conflict).

The Benedictine priests were significantly elevated in 9 of the 12 predicted scales (A, B, E, F, H, I, M, N, and Q_3) when compared with the other three groups of monks combined.

The implication of the various findings is perhaps best stated as follows: In communities in which coronary heart disease is common, episodes of myocardial infarction or angina pectoris occur more frequently in persons

TABLE 5-1. Personality Profile of Patients with Coronary Occlusion

GROUP STATISTICS	INDIVIDUAL PICTURE
Family History	**General Adjustment**
Cardiovascular disease in parents and siblings about average for the groups studied (42 percent). Accident history for parents and siblings about 9 percent. Exposure to cardiovascular disease or to sudden death in about 90 percent of the cases.	Education: Marked tendency to complete educational unit undertaken. Planned career. Work record: Sticking to one job, working to the top. Income: Highest of all groups studied. Vocational level: Characteristically class II (executives and officials). Social relationships: Generally respected. Tendency to dominate. Argumentative with men, attentive to women. Sexual adjustments: Role of exemplary husband (and father) combined with frustration and often secret promiscuity: high venereal disease rate. Emphasize sexual problems (overt anxiety). Attitude towards family: Hostile toward father, passive though often hostile and fearful toward mother. With wife and children—attempt to be boss and "carry the burden" combined with demand for care and attention.
Personal Data	**Characteristic Behavior Pattern**
Both parents usually lived beyond the patient's majority, the father usually died first. Both parents typically strict. High marriage rate. Many children, few divorces.	Compulsively consistent action. Tendency to work long hours and not take vacations. Tendency to seize authority; dislike of sharing responsibility. Conversation an instrument of domination and aggression. Tendency to attach emotions to ideas and goals. Articulte about feelings. Living for future.

Health Record	**Neurotic Traits**
Bad previous illness history with predominance of vegetative symptoms and many operations. Anginal symptoms frequent. Tendency to self-neglect. Women, poor pelvic histories.	Few early neurotic traits, tendency to brood and keep their troubles to themselves. In later life inner tension and a tendency to depression which is rarely admitted to others, together with compulsive asceticism and drive to work.
	Addictions and Interests
	Tendency to take stimulants to help keep on working (overwork). Little interest in sports, few hobbies. Skepticism about religion. Marked interest in philosophy.
Injuries	**Life Situation Immediately Prior to Onset**
Rarely more than one injury. Rate for one accident above average but these accidents were of a specific type: result of action by another person, typically cutting, shooting, or stabbing; few childhood accidents.	Exposure to shock—especially in job or in relinquishment of authority.
	Reaction to Illness
	Tendency to minimize symptoms and self-neglect.
	Area of Focal Conflict and Characteristic Reaction
	Authority—attempt to be and subdue authority; identification with authority and authority concepts.

(From Dunbar.[17])

who have certain personality traits and behavior patterns that may be defined in personality tests such as the Cattell 16 Personality Factor test.

Personality, Asthma, and Chronic Disease in Children

While clinical impressions are often the stimulus for further investigation they are not in themselves sufficient foundations for conclusions as to the association of different characteristics. Many reports have been made about the asthmatic child, presenting a picture of a particular type of personality and a family life situation characterized by overprotectiveness by the parents, especially the mother. From their study of a small group of cases with "asthma-eczema-prurigo syndrome" Rogerson et al.[31] summarized the following characteristic features of what they spoke of as "an asthma-prurigo personality": ". . . high intelligence on verbal tests with poor performance ability, marked overanxiety and lack of self-confidence, considerable latent aggressiveness, and egocentricity."

They also stressed that "the children were fussed over and overprotected by their parents to a pathologic degree." Using different words and sometimes extending the personality description of these children, many reports have been made with similar characteristics as to the core of a particular personality type in children with asthma. A review of this picture suggests the need for caution in its acceptance.[32] There are many questions that need answering before such important clinical impressions are accepted as part of the body of knowledge of medicine, validated epidemiologically and applicable to community medicine. One question concerns the consistency of an association between a particular personality type and asthmatic children in whom the disease varies in severity, frequency of attack, and response to treatment. Are there in fact particular types of personality in whom asthma develops more readily? Do asthmatic children have a different personality profile from other children with other chronic illnesses?

If these are associations of the kind postulated from clinical observations, are they causal in nature? If so, in which direction does the causal process operate? Does asthma produce a certain type of personality or do particular types of personality produce a susceptibility to allergies and infections which is manifested in asthma? These questions are not meant to cast doubt on the interaction between respiratory functioning in general and emotional factors, nor on the interaction between the specific respiratory dysfunction of asthma and emotional disturbance. They question the concept of specific personality types or profiles being more susceptible to asthma.

In a personality study of asthmatic and cardiac children Neuhaus[33] tested the hypothesis as to whether asthmatic children have a specific personality profile. His results include the following observations.

1. Asthmatic children and their well siblings did not differ in response to projective tests of personality.
2. Cardiac disease children had a similar picture to that of asthmatic children.
3. The well siblings of cardiac disease children did not differ from the sick children.
4. Both groups of children in families in which at least one child had asthma or cardiac disease differed from children in families in which all children were well.

This clearly suggests that asthmatic children do not have a particular personality profile, but it is possible that children in families in which there is at least one child with a chronic disease do manifest a personality picture differing from that of children in families in which no child has a chronic illness.

The personality characteristics of children in families in which there were asthmatic or cardiac cases were found by Neuhaus to be consistent with that regarded by other researchers as specific to asthma.

Yet another approach to the study of childhood asthma and personality was an inquiry into the relationship between the family situation, personality adjustment, and asthma in children.[34]

A significant association was found between many of the variables measuring family situation and personality adjustment of the children. An unexpected finding was that the course of the asthma was not found to be affected by these factors. No significant association was found between severity of the disease or response to treatment and family situation or the children's personal adjustment.

The psychiatric investigators examined their own earlier views by reviewing their earlier material "in an attempt to understand the reasons for our apparently unfounded assumptions." The following remarks are some of their stated conclusions:

> . . . As psychiatrists, we had tended to generalize from a highly selected group of asthmatic children, those with intractable asthma or severely disturbed children with coincidental asthma. We are probably much more prone than we at times realize to over-generalize from selected samples in our psychiatric work and it is probable that this had led to distortions in emphasis in many clinical areas, especially in relation to the etiology. . . .
>
> We have probably been insufficiently sensitive to the effects of a child's chronic asthma on family relationships, viewing reactive patterns as etiologic. . . . [They speak of] our tendency to be too ready to assume a direct link between the dynamic situation within a family and a clinical syndrome in the child.

> The cases . . . present striking examples of ways in which asthma has affected family living adversely. . . . It is evident that . . . factors of fatigue, irritability, anxiety, and financial strain all play a role in coloring the parent-child relations as they evolve through the course of the disease.
>
> Of more serious import is the high degree of negative effect of the child's illness on already existing family disturbances. . . .[34]

The critical review of often well-conceived assumptions by an expert team does not detract from the importance of psychiatric care in cases of asthma where such care is needed. It does focus on the need for more objective investigations of clinical impressions, and not only those of psychiatrists, before accepting apparently obvious associations. The need for careful epidemiologic investigation is made evident by such studies, especially so in the application of findings in community health care.

Another relevant question that needs answering concerns possible differences between the personalities of parents of asthmatic children and parents of nonasthmatic children. Fitzelle[35] found no significant differences in personality test responses of two groups of parents, nor in their attitudes towards child rearing. He also found no differences between parents of severe and mild cases of asthma.

There is need for long-term study of the incidence of asthma in order to further evaluate the relevance of personality factors in its epidemiology.

Measurement is desirable in case studies of individual patients but clinical judgment in interpretation is an important element in all such care. This is perhaps even more so in psychologic aspects of care in which unstructured interviews are fundamental to the whole process of diagnosis, therapy, and evaluation. However, in epidemiologic and community health appraisal, measurement is essential. Without it there is no foundation for action or for any scientific understanding of the health relevance of different behavior and personality factors. The use of measurements in the description of personality is making personality assessment available in epidemiologic investigations. Among the structured questionnaires that are in use in health studies are such tests as the Minnesota Multiphasic Personality Inventory (MMPI),[36,37] Cattell's Personality Factor Test (16 PF),[38] Eysenck's Maudsley Personality Inventory,[39] and the Taylor Manifest Anxiety Scale.[40]

REFERENCES

1. Gesell A: The Mental Growth of the Pre-School Child. New York, MacMillan, 1925.
2. Gesell A, Amatruda CS: Developmental Diagnosis. New York and London, Hoeber, 1941.
3. Knobloch H, Pasamanick B: Distribution of intellectual potential in an infant population. In Pasamanick B (ed.): Epidemiology of Mental Dis-

order, Publication No. 60. Washington, DC, American Association for the Advancement of Science, 1959.

4. Galton F: Hereditary Genius, 2nd ed, 1892. Reprint. London, Watts, 1950, p 28.
5. Quetelet M: Letters on Probabilities, 1st ed. 1846. English translation by Downes Layton, 1849.
6. Penrose LS: The Biology of Mental Defect, 3rd ed. London, Sidgwick and Jackson, 1963.
7. Susser MW, Watson W: Sociology in Medicine, 2nd ed. London, Oxford Univ Press, 1971.
8. Clarke AM, Clarke ADB: Mental Deficiency, The Changing Outlook, 2nd ed. London, Methuen, 1965.
9. Wilkie F, Eisdorfer C: Intelligence and blood pressure in the aged. Science 172:959, 1971.
10. Cattell RB: Description and Measurement of Personality. New York, World Book, 1946, pp 1, 216.
11. Vernon PE: Personality Assessment. A Critical Survey. London, Methuen, 1964, p 6.
12. Jahoda M: Current Concepts of Positive Mental Health. New York, Basic Books, 1958, pp 51,71.
13. Steuart GW, Wilson RN: Health education and mental health. In Galdston SE (ed.): Mental Health Considerations in Public Health. Public Health Service Publication No. 1898. Washington, DC, US Department of Health, Education, and Welfare, 1969, pp 53–55.
14. Kirkpatrick P, Michael ST: Study methods. Mental health ratings. In Srole L, Langner TS, Michael ST, et al. (eds.): Mental Health in the Metropolis. The Midtown Manhattan Study, Vol. 1. New York, McGraw-Hill, 1962, Chap. 4, p 62.
15. Dunbar HF: Psychosomatic Diagnosis. New York, Hoeber, 1943.
16. Dunbar HF: Synopsis of Psychosomatic Diagnosis and Treatment. St. Louis, Mosby, 1948.
17. Dunbar HF: Emotions and Bodily Changes, 4th ed. New York, Columbia Univ Press, 1954, p 746.
18. Brodman K, Erdmann AJ Jr, Lorge I, et al.: The Cornell Medical Index—health questionnaire. J Clin Psychol 8:119, 1952.
19. Abramson JH: The Cornell Medical Index as an epidemiological tool. Am J Public Health 56:287, 1966.
20. Abramson JH, Terespolsky L, Brook JG, et al.: Cornell Medical Index as a health measure in epidemiological studies. Brit J Prev Soc Med 19:103, 1965.
21. MacMillan AM: A survey technique for estimating the prevalence of psychoneurotic and related types of disorders in communities. In Pasamanick B (ed.): Epidemiology of Mental Disorder, Publication No. 60. Washington, DC, American Association for the Advancement of Science, 1959.
22. Leighton DC, Harding JS, Macklin DB, et al.: The health opinion survey. In The Character of Danger, Vol. 3. New York, Basic Books, 1963, Chap. 7, Appendix E.
23. Hare EH, Shaw GK: Mental Health on a New Housing Estate. London, Oxford Univ Press, 1965.
24. Ferrer HP: Screening for Health. Theory and Practice. London, Butterworths, 1968.
25. Allport GW, Odbert HS: Trait-names: A psycho-lexical study. Psychol Monogr 47:171, 1936.

26. Cattell RB: The Sixteen Personality Factor Questionnaire, rev. ed. Champaign, Illinois, IPAT, 1957.
27. Caffrey B: Behavior patterns and personality characteristics related to prevalence rates of coronary heart disease in American monks. J Chronic Dis 22:93, 1969.
28. Barrow JG, Quinlan CB, Cooper GR, et al.: Studies in atherosclerosis. III. An epidemiologic study of atherosclerosis in Trappist and Benedictine monks. A preliminary report. Ann Intern Med 52:368, 1960, p 375.
29. Barrow JG, Quinlan CB, Edmands RE, et al.: Prevalence of atherosclerotic complications in Trappist and Benedictine monks. Circulation 24:881, 1961.
30. Quinlan CB, Barrow JG: Prevalence of coronary heart disease in Trappist and Benedictine monks. Circulation (Suppl 3) 33–34: 193, 1966.
31. Rogerson CH, Hardcastle D, Duguid K: A psychological approach to the problems of asthma and asthma-eczema-prurigo syndrome. Guys Hosp Rep 85:289, 1935.
32. Lipton EL, Steinschneider A, Richmond JB: Psychophysiological disorders in children. In Hoffman LW, Hoffman ML, (eds.): Review of Child Development Research, Vol. 2. New York, Russel Sage Foundation, 1966.
33. Neuhaus EC: A personality study of asthmatic and cardiac children. Psychosom Med 20:181, 1958.
34. Dubo S, McLean JA, Ching AYT, et al.: A study of relationships between family situation, bronchial asthma, and personal adjustment in children. J Pediatr 59:402, 1961.
35. Fitzelle GT: Personality factors and certain attitudes towards child rearing among parents of asthmatic children. Psychosom Med 21:209, 1959.
36. Hathaway SR, McKinley JC: A multiphasic personality schedule (Minnesota). I. Construction of the schedule. J Psychol 10:249, 1940.
37. Dahlstrom WG, Welsh GS: An MMPI Handbook. Minneapolis, Univ of Minnesota Press. 1960.
38. Cattell RB: Personality and Motivation Structure and Measurement. New York, World Book, 1957.
39. Eysenck HJ: Manual. The Maudsley Personality Inventory. London, Univ of London Press, 1959.
40. Taylor JA: A personality scale of manifest anxiety. J Abnorm Psychol 48: 285, 1953.

6
The Distribution of Health and Disease in the Community

It is usual to describe the health of a community by analyzing health indices in different groupings of the community. The health indices are those discussed in the preceding chapters—mortality, morbidity, and disability rates—as well as analyses of somatic and psychologic attributes, such as physical growth, intellectual and behavioral development, anthropometric and biochemical variables, and personality characteristics.

The characteristics used to differentiate various segments of a community will obviously vary according to the kind of community and the particular health conditions. Thus in measuring the outcome of pregnancy differences may be grouped according to parity and length of gestation, education and social class, or family and ethnic group. These are demographic characteristics of universal validity in differentiating between members of communities. They include basic biologic characteristics such as age, sex, and other genetic differences; predominantly social categories such as social status and role; and biosocial characteristics such as family and ethnic groups. The associations that may be found between these various community characteristics and health often point towards the causes of the associations. In themselves, however, such associations should not be interpreted as being causal. The causes of the differential distribution of health and disease will be reviewed in Sections 3 and 4.

DEMOGRAPHIC TRENDS AND COMMUNITY HEALTH

The membership of a community is in continual process of change through birth, death, and migration. The relationship between these changes determines the survival and continuity of the community. Indices of biologic survival include birth, death, and fertility rates, and life expectancy. When considered together and in relation to the composition of the population group, these indices may be studied as demographic trends.

The concept of demographic transition as the foundation of the theory of modern population change and population growth cycles has been developed by a number of workers.[1-5] Three different phases are usually referred to. The demographic trend over a period of time may be one of stability in age and sex composition, or stability related to a high death rate and a high birth rate. This stability may be disturbed by modification of one or another of these rates. Thus in many developing countries today we can observe a second demographic phase, where there has been a reduction of the death rate without a corresponding reduction in the birth rate. This demographic trend has been one of rapid growth of population known to demographers as the "demographic gap." The third phase is seen in many of the more developed countries where the demographic gap is being closed by a decreasing birth rate so that a low mortality rate and a low birth rate reintroduce a more stable demographic picture.[1]

The health implications of each of these three demographic phases are highly relevant to community medicine. In the first phase, biologic survival is threatened by any new epidemic which might have the capacity to markedly reduce an already tenuously balanced population. Starvation, through failure of crops and the introduction of new virulent infections, has been one of the main means of limiting population growth and even interfering with biologic survival of the group.

In the second phase, that of the demographic gap, the rapidly increasing population could lead to a considerable reduction in the state of health. The imbalance between food production and population growth has posed one of the major health problems of this century and promises to tax the ingenuity of man for many years to come. Poverty, rural-urban migration, and pressure on the land available for peasant and agricultural communities are among the most demanding results of this second phase which have immediate health implications.

The third demographic phase has presented a different challenge. Standards of living and of maternal and child health care in the more developed countries are continually improving and being applied to wider and wider segments of the population, thereby reducing childhood mortality. With this decline in mortality and a reduction in the birth rate, the demographic picture has become one of an aging population. Aging in itself may not be a health problem, but when associated with chronic illness it does constitute a leading public health problem. The increasing number of older people who are disabled is a major health hazard of this particular demographic phase.

There is a reciprocal relationship between health and population change. The health of a population is on the one hand an important determinant of, and on the other hand is determined by, its demographic composition. Modern health services have considerable influence on population growth. The control of malaria is an example of this fact. The maternal and child health movement, with its pre- and postnatal clinics and its infant and preschool child clinics, is of equal importance. Another example is the use of sulfa and antibiotic drugs in the mass treatment of many illnesses. The successful treatment of pneumonia by antibiotics is an outstanding example of the impact of medicinal treatment in lowering mortality rates. Health services may also affect birth rates through prescription of various forms of contraception. Prevention of unwanted births is as much a responsibility of health services as is the reduction of premature mortality rates.

It is mistaken to infer from their present effects, potential and actual, that health services were always a major factor in the demographic trends that took place in European communities. The decline in various infectious diseases as causes of death and the reasons for this decline are discussed below.

One of the main causes of the rapid increase in population in Europe during the 19th century was a marked decrease in mortality. In England and Wales, for which national statistics have been available since 1838, "five diseases or groups of diseases accounted for the decline of mortality in the nineteenth century after 1838: tuberculosis for a little less than a half; typhus, typhoid and continued fever for about a fifth; scarlet fever for a fifth; cholera, dysentery and diarrhea for nearly a tenth; and smallpox for a twentieth." (Table 6-1).[6,7]

Reviewing the available historic evidence, McKeown summarizes the relative importance of various factors responsible for the decline in mortality in the second half of the 19th century. They included the rise in the standard of living, more especially improvement in the diet; sanitary improvement, following the sanitary revolution; and a favorable trend in the relations between infecting agents and the human host, e.g., in scarlet fever, in which the change has been considered to be a result of a genetic variation in the virulence of the hemolytic streptococcus. Genetic selection of population through survival probably had a role in decline of mortality from tuberculosis, but this was less important than improvements in diet and standard of living. It will be noted that specific personal preventive or curative medical action is not included among the important causes of decline in mortality during the 19th century. The effects of therapy were negligible, being restricted to vaccination against smallpox, which had a small part in the decline in overall mortality.

The decline in mortality is regarded by many as the starting point of the subsequent decline in fertility. On the other hand it has been suggested that both the decline in mortality and in reproduction is explained

TABLE 6-1. Mean Annual Mortality Rates per 1,000,000* Due to Certain Communicable Diseases 1851–1860 and 1891–1900

CAUSE	1851–1860 *a*	1891–1900 *b*	DIFFERENCE *a* − *b*	PERCENT OF TOTAL DIFFERENCE [(*a* − *b*)100]/ 3,085	
Tuberculosis—respiratory	2,772	1,418	1,354	43.9	47.2
Tuberculosis—other forms	706	603	103	3.3	
Typhus, enteric fever, simple continued fever	891	184	707	22.9	
Scarlet fever	779	152	627	20.3	
Diarrhea, dysentery, cholera	990	715	275	8.9	
Smallpox	202	13	189	6.1	
Whooping cough	433	363	70	2.3	
Measles	357	398	− 41	− 1.3	
Diphtheria	99	254	− 155	− 5.0	
Other causes	13,980	14,024	− 44	− 1.4	
Total	21,209	18,124	3,085	100	

**Standardized to age and sex distribution of 1901 population.*
(From McKeown.[6])

mainly by the improvement in standards of living.[2] The changes in population of western countries may not be a model on which to predict world changes. We cannot assume that the decline in mortality which is taking place in many developing countries will be automatically followed by a decline in fertility. The decline in mortality in many of these countries has been the direct result of major health action such as the control of malaria, rather than being a result of a rise in the standard of living. Not only has change occurred with very limited, if any, real participation by local communities, but it has not been associated with economic and educational advance.

The Pare-Taveta Malaria Scheme in East Africa offered an opportunity to measure the demographic effects of an experimental program of malaria control. The aim of the experiment was to test the effects of residual spraying of huts on malaria transmission. The spraying eliminated *Anopheles funestus* and reduced *Anopheles gambiae* to less than one-fifth of their original densities, and malaria transmission was almost completely eliminated.[8–10] The first cycle of spraying began in 1955, and the last cycle, the sixth, in 1959. Reports on malaria transmission and population are available for the 7-year period after this program (until 1966).[11,12]

There was a marked drop in general mortality rates in the experimental malaria-control areas. The crude mortality rate dropped from 23.5 per 1,000 at commencement of the experiment to an average of 14.6 in one such area and to 16.4 in another in the 5-year period 1962–1966. Like the crude mortality rate, infant mortality rates declined sharply from 212 to 105 per 1,000 live births. This change in mortality was accompanied by a marked increase in fertility, malaria control resulting in both decrease in mortality and increase in live birth rates. In this way a relatively static population increased at an average annual rate of over 2.50 percent in these areas. A decline in fertility may yet take place, but the immediate effect of malaria control differed from the demographic trends which have been described in Western Europe.

In what will surely become a classic among epidemiologic investigations of a community health problem, Wyon and Gordon[13] review the factors influencing population growth in the villages they investigated. The Khanna Study of population problems in the rural Punjab involved 11 study villages, with a total population of over 12,000. The age-sex pyramid indicates a young population which was the result of consistently high birth rates over a long period of time and of high death rates. The death rate among females, from age 5 months to 50 years, was higher than that of males. A summary of their findings indicates a multiplicity of influences originating from within the population itself as distinct from those originating from without. These various influences determine rates of births, deaths, and out-migration (Table 6-2). The implications of population growth for community health care and its role in helping communities towards population control are evident from the items which Wyon and Gordon found to be important factors in such population growth. Many of the items are not only integral parts of the daily practice of community health centers but are factors which are influenced by well-planned services. Thus the high risk of losing children, which is rated as the most important determinant of increasing births, is not only amenable to change by direct health care but can be modified through a broad program of health and community development.

The waxing and waning of epidemic diseases and the severity of their expression have not only been influenced by social factors, but infectious disease has had considerable effects on society. This impact has been most obvious during epidemics of severe disease when depopulation and social disorganization result.

Whatever the causes of the appearance and rapid spread of plague

TABLE 6-2. Factors Influencing Population Growth in the Punjab Villages Studied by Wyon and Gordon, 1956–1960*

INFLUENCES TENDING TO INCREASE BIRTHS	INFLUENCES TENDING TO DECREASE BIRTHS
1. High risk of losing children	1. Long breast feeding
2. Need for sons	2. Delayed cohabitation of women
3. Readiness to endure a low standard of living	3. Knowledge of and practice of birth control
4. Women start cohabitation at early age	4. Ambition for higher standard of life
5. All women marry	5. Cost of marrying daughters
6. Ignorance of birth control	6. Increasing sense of ability to control own future
7. Low status of women	7. Separation of husband and wife
8. Low frequency of sterility	8. 20 percent of males remain single
9. No occupations for women other than marriage	9. Lower fecundity with increasing age
10. Democracy means counting of heads	10. Low rate of coitus at older ages
11. Fashion for shorter breast feeding	11. Improved health services, less fear of losing children
12. Improved health services for mothers, less pregancy wastage	12. Improved survival of children
13. Possibility of civil unrest	13. Improved methods of birth control
	14. High cost of rearing children and preparing them for adult life
	15. Occupations for women as an alternative to marriage
	16. Higher status of women
	17. Difficulties in finding jobs outside the village
INFLUENCES TENDING TO INCREASE DEATHS	**INFLUENCES TENDING TO DECREASE DEATHS**
1. Low status of females	1. Increased willingness to strive to keep children
2. Low status of children	2. Improved health services
3. Low status of aged	3. Improved ability to feed children
4. Low status of low castes	
5. Infections	
6. Failure of rains	
7. Lack of materials for farming and industry	
INFLUENCES TENDING TO INCREASE OUT-MIGRATION	**INFLUENCES TENDING TO DECREASE OUT-MIGRATION**
1. Poor chances of livelihood in home village	1. Desire to stay in village
2. Good chances of employment in other parts of India and beyond	2. Improved chances for livelihood in own village
	3. Unemployment outside home village

**The influences are numbered according to their order of importance as considered by Wyon and Gordon on the basis of their study.*
(Adapted from Wyon and Gordon.[13])

into Europe in the 14th century following a succession of famine years, 1333–1334, 1337–1342, and 1345–1347, it spread rapidly from Sicily and Italy in 1348 through many European communities and caused extensive disorganization.[14] The immediate extensive disorganization is conveyed in Boccaccio's *The Decameron*, in his poignant description of the plague in Florence.[15]

The depopulation that resulted from the epidemics of plague over the next 300 years in different parts of Western Europe and Britain caused a profound change in the social structure.[16,17] Peasants and laborers in the towns became scarce. The feudal serf system was dependent on a relative abundance of men and a scarcity of available land. The high mortality changed this and men who were serfs found themselves in demand and were able to escape their serfdom. However, the plague epidemics may themselves not have been the primary cause of breakdown of feudalism within the feudal manor and village. There had already been changes in the system, by which the strong position of the manor in England was being weakened, in the period before the Black Death of 1348–1349. The effects of the disaster have been analyzed by Trevelyan in his study of English social history, but the changes outlined were not confined to England.

> When a third or possibly a half of the inhabitants of the Kingdom died of plague in less than two years, what was the effect on the social and economic position in the average English village? Obviously the survivors among the peasantry had the whip-hand of the lord and his bailiff. Instead of the recent hunger for land there was a shortage of men to till it. The value of farms fell and the price of labour went up at a bound.[17]

AGE AND SEX

Age and sex are two universal categories which determine the nature of individual life experience in all societies. They are perhaps the two most basic biologic characteristics in their influence on health and on social structure and culture. All societies expect role differentiation between the two sexes at different ages; they direct their ways of rearing boys and girls accordingly, and thereby initiate life-long differences in experience. There are sex differences in the play of children and adults, in the division of labor at home and in occupations, in political and religious activities, and, of course, in family functioning. Apart from reproduction and infant care, which are universal functions of women, role differences between the sexes are not the same in different cultures. Differences in health and disease between the sexes are therefore to be expected and may be related to biologic and sociocultural factors.

A Comparison of Mortality Rates in Two Countries

Change in age-sex growth rates, morbidity, and mortality has been a striking feature of the history of many peoples. Variation in the age-sex differentials of health indices are evident in comparisons of various population groups. Comparison between different countries, or in the same country at different times, is a common starting point for epidemiologic investigation. Age-sex mortality differences between communities are among the most striking features of demographic studies. These differences may not be consistent for different ages nor for the sexes, as illustrated in a comparison of the mortality rates of two Eastern Mediterranean countries: Greece and Israel.[18] Taking the average of the age-sex Israel rates for 1965, 1966, and 1967 as 100, the relative mortality ratio for each sex at different ages in Greece for the same period is shown in Table 6-3 and in Figure 6-1.

In both sexes there is a marked difference in infant mortality between the two countries. The average male and female rates in Greece for the 3-year period were 36 and 33 compared with the respective average rates in Israel of 24 and 19. The favorable trend in Israel persists through childhood for both boys and girls, after which the trend differs for males and females. Among males the difference between the two countries disappears by the age 15 to 24. The difference remains small through adulthood to the age group 45 to 54, after which there is a lower mortality rate in Greece. The differences between the women of the two countries is more marked. The mortality rate of Greek women is progressively lower in each age group from 35 to 64.

While the death rates in females were lower than those in males in all age-groups in both Greece and Israel, the sex differences in Greece are more marked than those in Israel from the age of 35 through 64. Taking the female mortality rates at each age as 100, the relative mortality rates for males in each country (Table 6-4) illustrate these facts.

Analysis of the reported causes of death in the two countries may be helpful in understanding these age and sex differences but has obvious problems. Different ways of reporting causes of death are among the most obvious of these. In a community in which coronary heart disease is known to be common and to be an important cause of death from cardiac ischemia, it is probable that when in doubt doctors will tend to certify this as a cause of death more commonly than they would when in doubt in communities where the condition is not so common.

Problems inherent in the use of mortality data have been summarized by Newell and Waggoner.[19]

TABLE 6-3. Comparison of Mortality Rates in Greece and Israel by Age and Sex for the Period 1965 to 1967*

SEX \ AGE	0	1–4	5–14	15–24	25–34	35–44	45–54	55–64	65–74	75 +
Male	150	116	131	97	108	95	97	91	84	102
Female	171	128	125	98	101	86	74	69	76	97

The rates for Greece are expressed as a ratio of the Israeli rates taken as 100.

TABLE 6-4. Comparison of Male and Female Mortality Rates in Greece and Israel for the Period 1965 to 1967*

COUNTRY \ AGE	0	1–4	5–14	15–24	25–34	35–44	45–54	55–64	65–74	75 +
Greece	112	102	157	215	171	149	167	171	139	109
Israel	127	113	150	213	161	134	127	131	127	106

The rates are expressed as a ratio of male to female, taking the female rates in each country as 100.

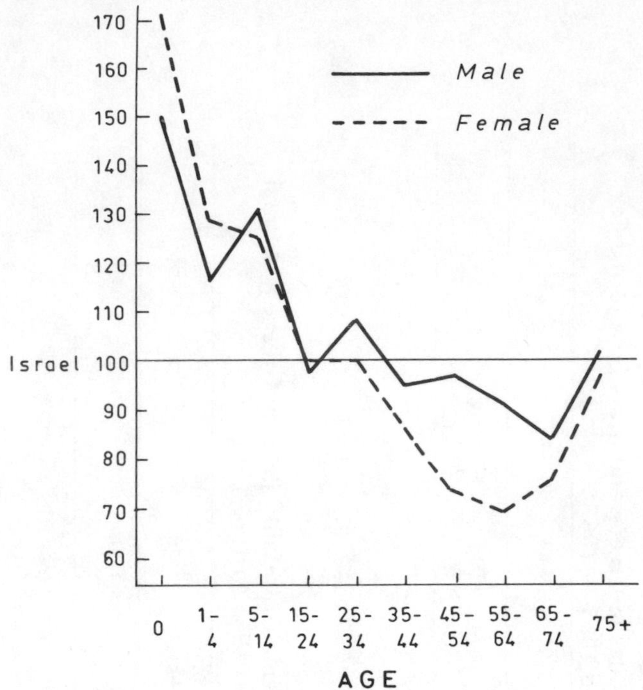

FIG. 6-1. A comparison of death rates for the years 1965–1967 in Greece and Israel, by age and sex. (The Greek rates are expressed as a ratio of the corresponding Israeli rates taken as 100). (Adapted from WHO.[18])

1. Differences in accuracy and completeness of medical information on death certificates.
2. Availability of physicians and specialized diagnostic services within different areas.
3. Accuracy of the population estimates.
4. Small numbers of deaths resulting in greater sampling variability.
5. Lack of certification of cause of death with pathologic confirmation.
6. Use of different classification systems in different locations.
7. Changing classification systems with time.

Bearing these reservations in mind and yet for the moment comparing reported causes of death of adults in Greece and Israel, the main similarities and differences are shown in Figures 6-2 to 6-4.

Figure 6-2 concerns arteriosclerotic cardiovascular disease, cerebral vascular accidents, hypertension, and diseases of the arteries. Among the outstanding differences are the very much higher mortality rates reported as due to arteriosclerotic cardiovascular disease (A81) in both

Israeli men and women. The rates for Israeli women are not only higher than those of Greek women, but are also higher than the rates for men in Greece in the age groups 55 to 64 and older.

While the differences between the two countries with respect to cerebral vascular accidents (A70) are not as marked as for those recorded as due to A81, Israel rates are consistently higher than those of Greece after the age group of 45 to 54 in women and 55 to 64 in men. In both countries this condition tends to be more commonly reported as the cause of death in women than in men.

Diseases of arteries (A85) are very much more commonly stated to be the cause of death in men and women in Israel in the older age groups than in Greece.

Figure 6-3 concerns malignant neoplasms. The difference between the women of the two countries is more marked than that between the men. Israeli women have very much higher mortality rates from various cancers than do those of Greece, the most striking difference being that of breast cancer mortality. Greek men have a higher mortality rate from cancer of the lung (A50) than do Israelis. Israeli women, on the other hand, have a higher rate than the women of Greece. Israeli men and women have consistently higher mortality rates, especially at ages 65 and over, from most other malignant neoplasms. That the differences are consistently higher and most marked in the oldest age group of men and women suggests the need for caution in acceptance of the data. Accuracy of diagnosis of cancer of specific sites such as these is difficult without autopsy examinations.

Figure 6-4 concerns various other selected differences of interest. Tuberculosis (A1 to A5) mortality is higher in Greece than in Israel, the difference being especially marked in men.

Cirrhosis of the liver (A105) is more commonly reported as a cause of death in Greek men and women than in their Israeli counterparts, the difference widening with age.

Death from rheumatic fever and rheumatic heart disease (A79 and A80) is not commonly reported in adult Greeks. It is only in older age groups that the rates in Greece approach those of Israel. The reported Israeli mortality rates show an increase with age being generally higher in women than men.

Death rates from motor accidents (A138 and A139) have a strikingly different age distribution in the two countries. The most marked difference is in older men, the Israeli rate being much higher than that of Greece. This difference is especially notable when contrasted to that of younger men, the mortality in Greece being somewhat higher. Among women, the picture is similar. Young and middle-aged women of both countries have very low mortality from this cause, with a rise in the rate among

ARTERIOSCLEROTIC CARDIOVASCULAR DISEASE

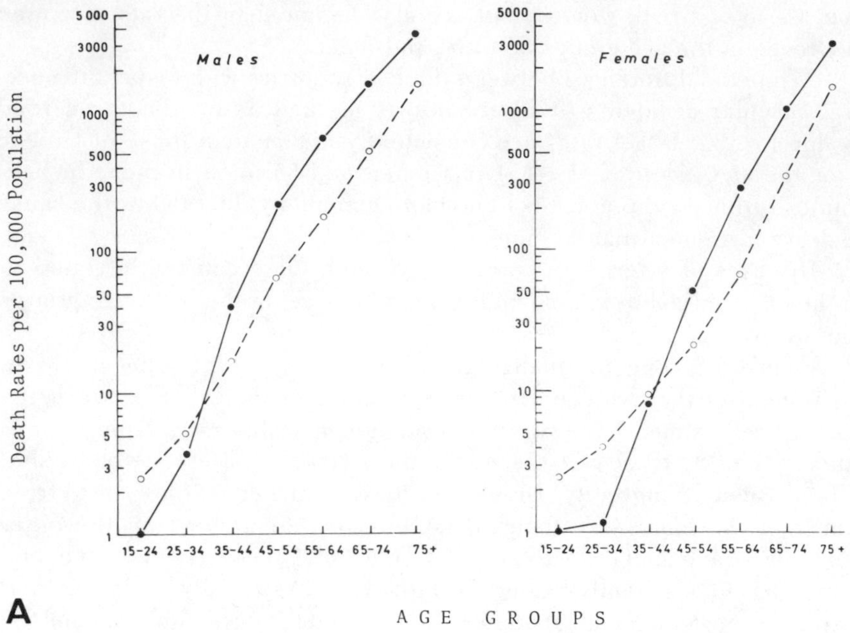

CEREBRAL VASCULAR ACCIDENTS

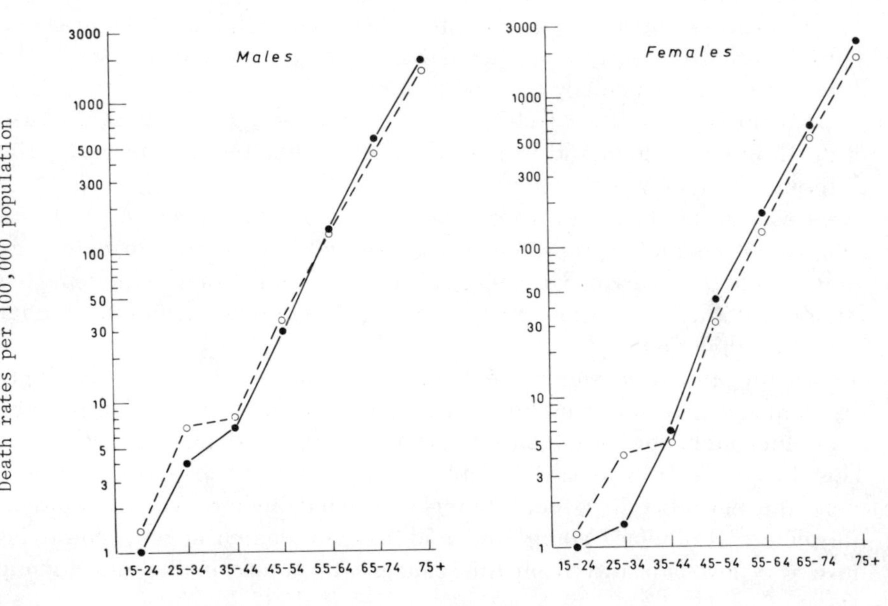

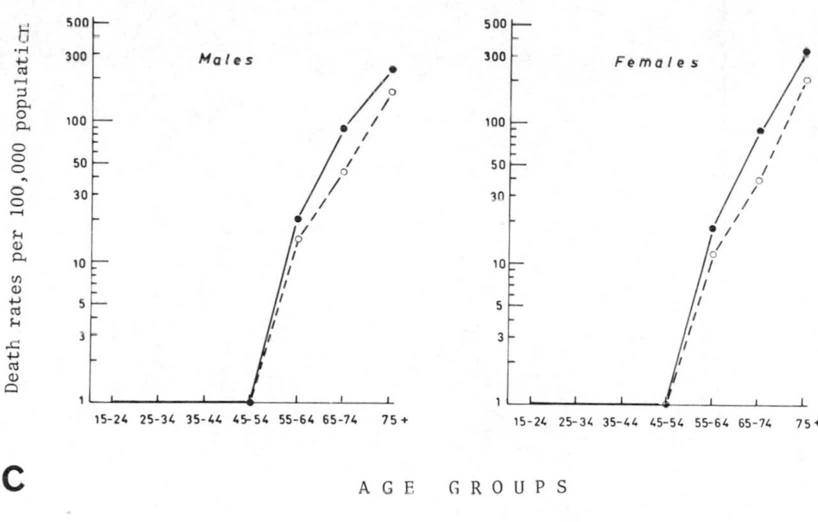

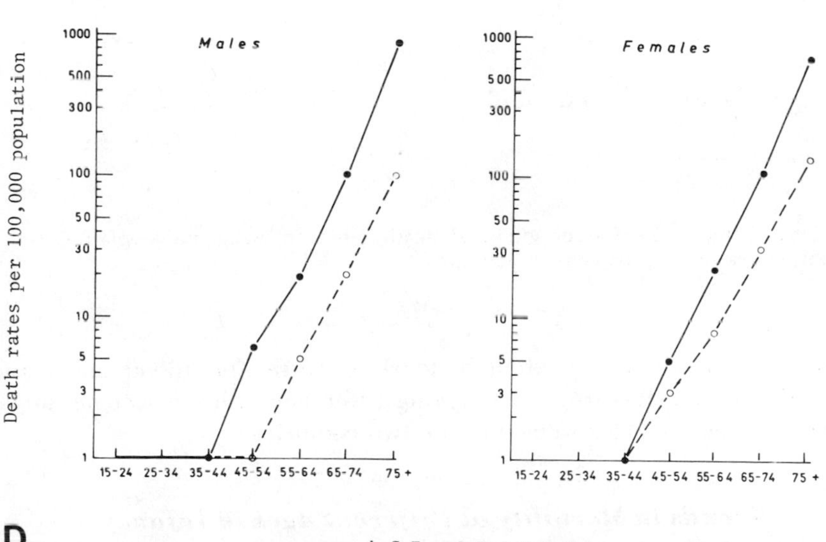

FIG. 6-2A-D. Comparison of Greek and Israeli mortality rates from some diseases of the circulatory system. Broken lines, Greek rates; solid lines, Israeli rates.

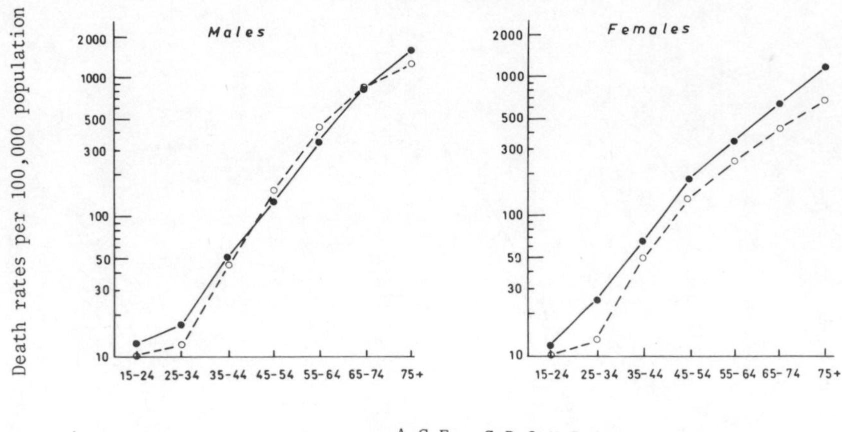

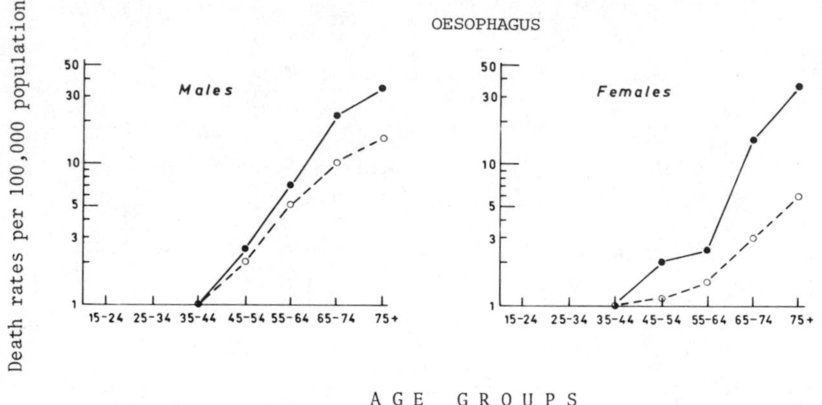

FIG. 6-3. Comparison of Greek and Israeli death rates from malignant neoplasms. Broken lines, Greek rates; solid lines, Israeli rates.

Israeli women in the age group 55 to 64 in contrast to little change among Greek women in this group. A widening difference with age becomes apparent between the older women of the two countries.

Trends in Mortality at Different Ages in Infancy

Historic change in particular countries presents a comparative picture of epidemiologic interest. Among the striking changes that have taken

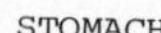

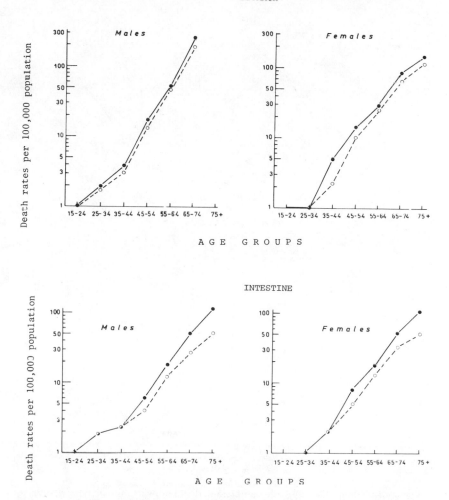

FIG. 6-3 (cont.). Comparison of Greek and Israeli death rates from malignant neoplasms. Broken lines, Greek rates; solid lines, Israeli rates.

place in the past century is that in infant mortality. There are several features of the decline in infant mortality that are pertinent to this discussion. The decline is not universal and even at the present time there are large populations for whom adequate data are not yet available. It is especially in European, North American, and other countries settled by immigrant European populations that the decrease has been such an outstanding feature. However, the rate of decline has been different in

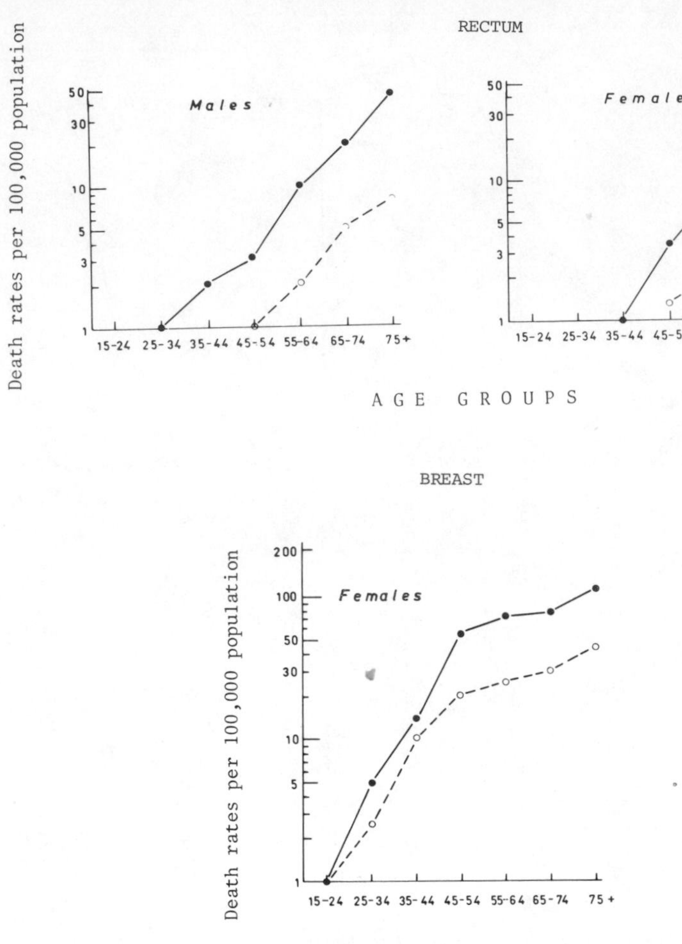

FIG. 6-3 (cont.). Comparison of Greek and Israeli death rates from malignant neoplasms. Broken lines, Greek rates; solid lines, Israeli rates.

these countries. Even when comparing countries which have had relatively low mortality rates for many years, the rate of decline has been different in the past 30 years.[20,21] In the 30-year period 1936 to 1966, the Swedish infant mortality rate declined from 44 per 1,000 live births (average for 1936 to 1938) to 12.6 in 1966, and that of New Zealand (excluding their Maori population) from 33 to 16.1 per 1,000 live births. In the same period of time the contrast was marked between two countries which formerly had very high rates; i.e., Japan, in which the rate declined from 113 to 19.3, and the Philippines, which only changed from 137 to 72.0.

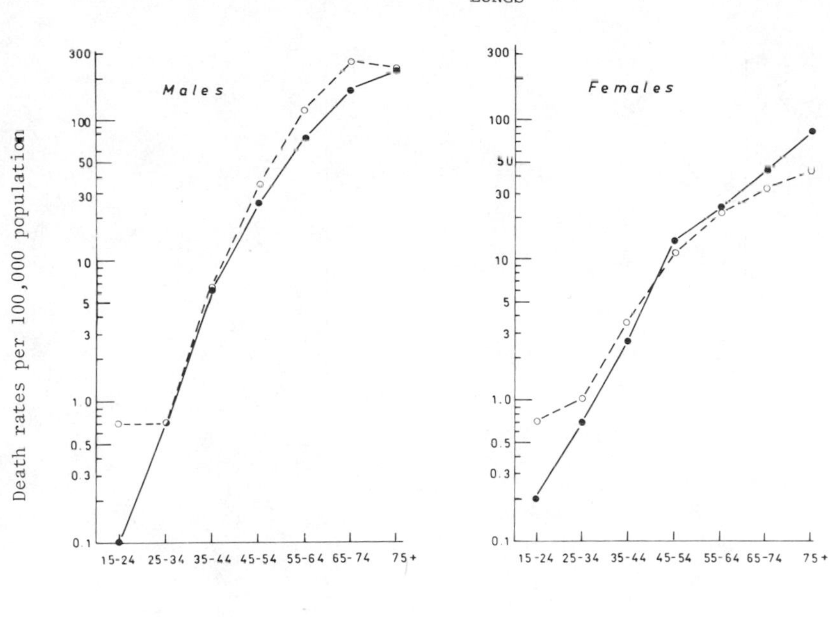

FIG. 6-3 (cont.). Comparison of Greek and Israeli death rates from malignant neoplasms. Broken lines, Greek rates; solid lines, Israeli rates.

A striking feature has been the differing rates of decrease in infant mortality at different ages in the first year and, to a lesser extent, the differential between the sexes. A more detailed analysis of the data for the Jewish population of Israel, since 1950, illustrates these age differences (Figs. 6-5 to 6-7). Additional data on causes of death at different ages in infancy are analyzed in Chapter 30.

The decline in infant mortality has been considerable in both males and females, with the female rates being consistently lower than the male rates. Charts of age specific death rates indicate clearly that the decline has occurred at all ages after the first week. It will also be noted that the sex differences are negligible at these ages, except for a higher rate in female babies aged 6 to 11 months during the years 1950 to 1955. This was at the time of mass migration of Eastern Jewish communities to Israel and may reflect a sex preference in these immigrants at that time. First week death rates have not changed in the past 20 years, and here it will be noted that there has been a marked sex difference throughout the period, especially in first day deaths.

While the relationship between fertility and mortality is the biologic

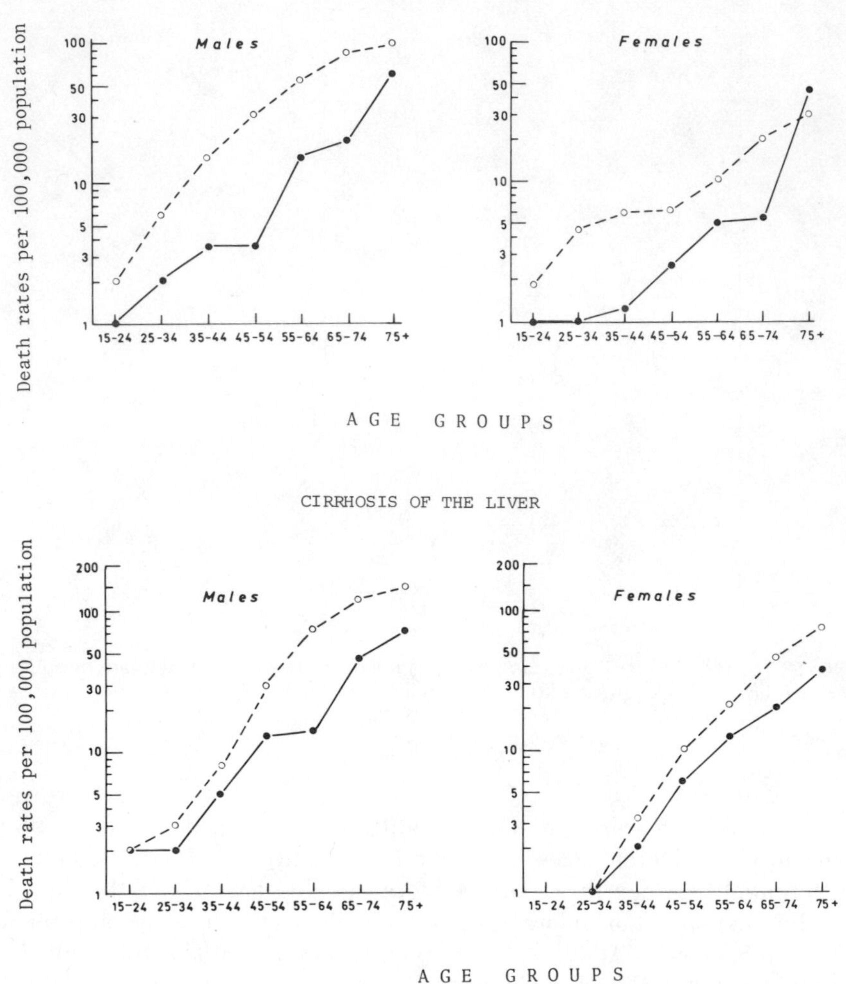

FIG. 6-4. Comparison of Greek and Israeli mortality rates from other selected causes. Broken lines, Greek rates; solid lines, Israeli rates.

foundation of demographic trends, migration is a major cause of the decline of some communities and the growth of others. It is also a most important determinant of social structure and includes international mobility and urban-rural migration, as well as internal movements in a city or other region. The relation between migration and health is reviewed in Chapter 10 in the context of the epidemiologic implications of culture change.

RHEUMATIC FEVER AND RHEUMATIC HEART DISEASE

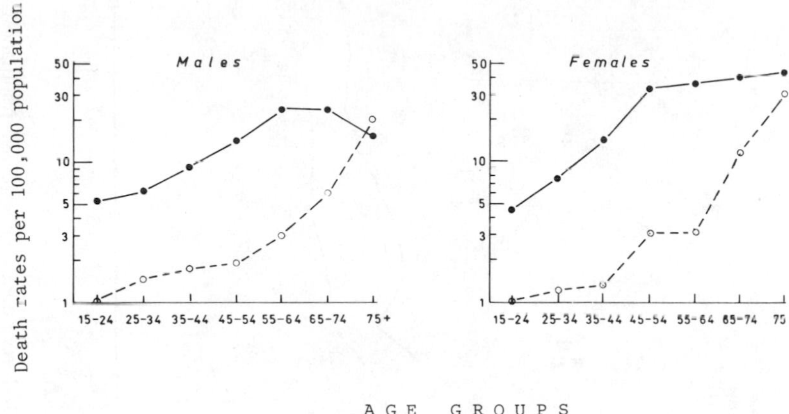

MOTOR ACCIDENTS

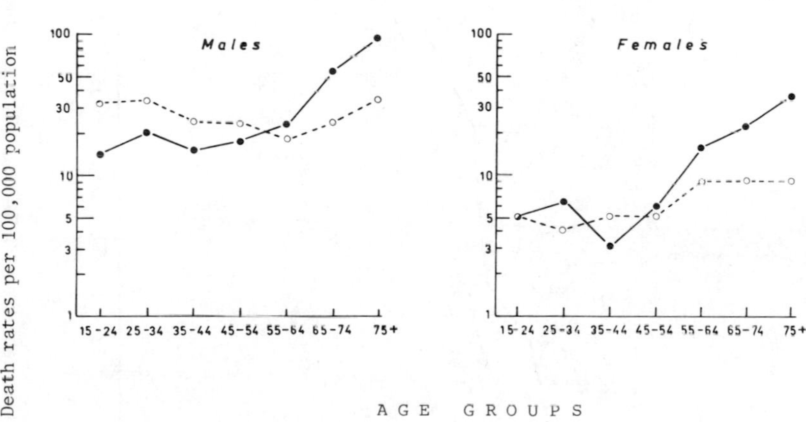

FIG. 6-4 (cont.). Comparison of Greek and Israeli mortality rates from other selected causes. Broken lines, Greek rates; solid lines, Israeli rates.

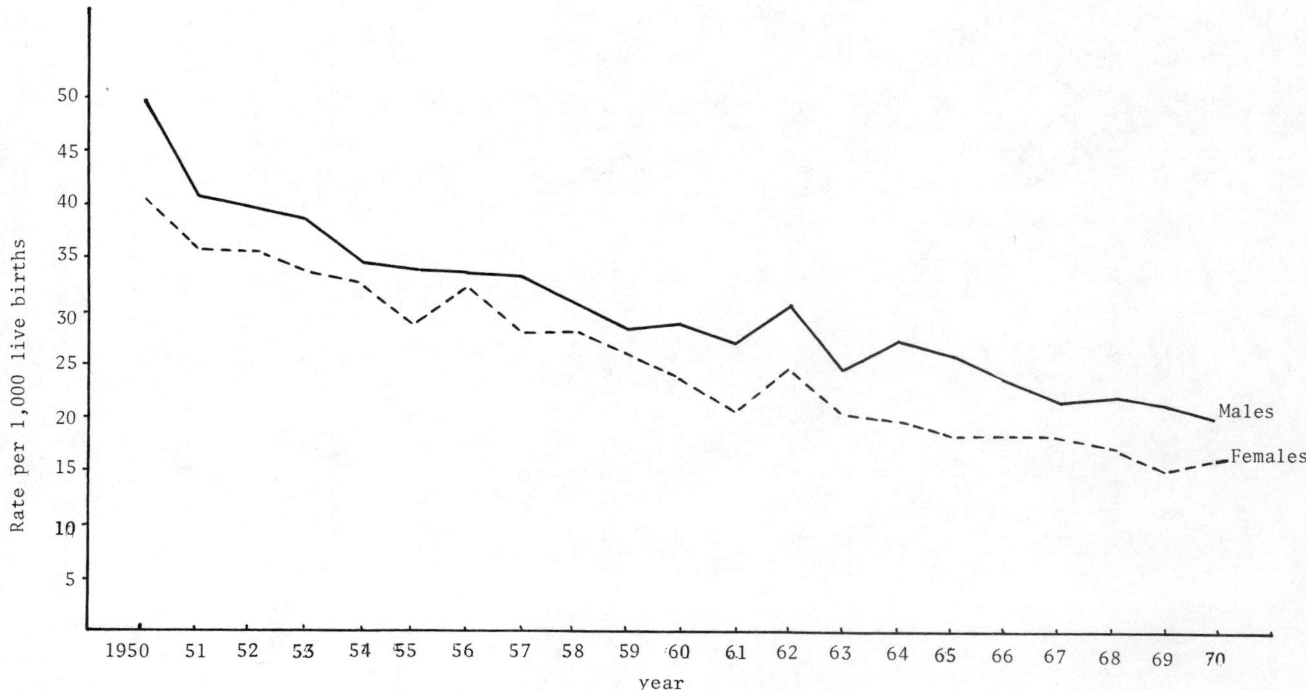

FIG. 6-5. Total Israel infant mortality rates, 1950–1970, all causes, by sex. (Adapted from data for the Jewish population from Israel Bureau of Statistics.)

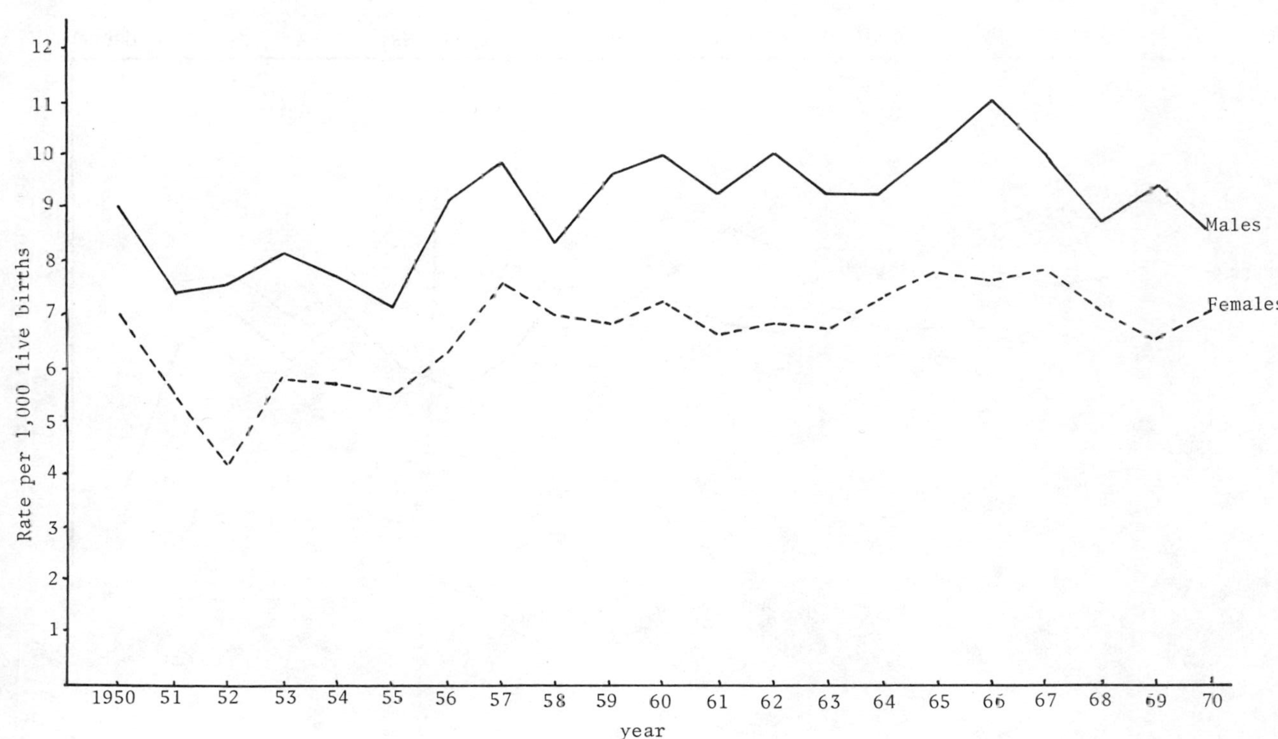

FIG. 6-6. Israel infant mortality rates, 1950–1970, all causes, by sex and age.

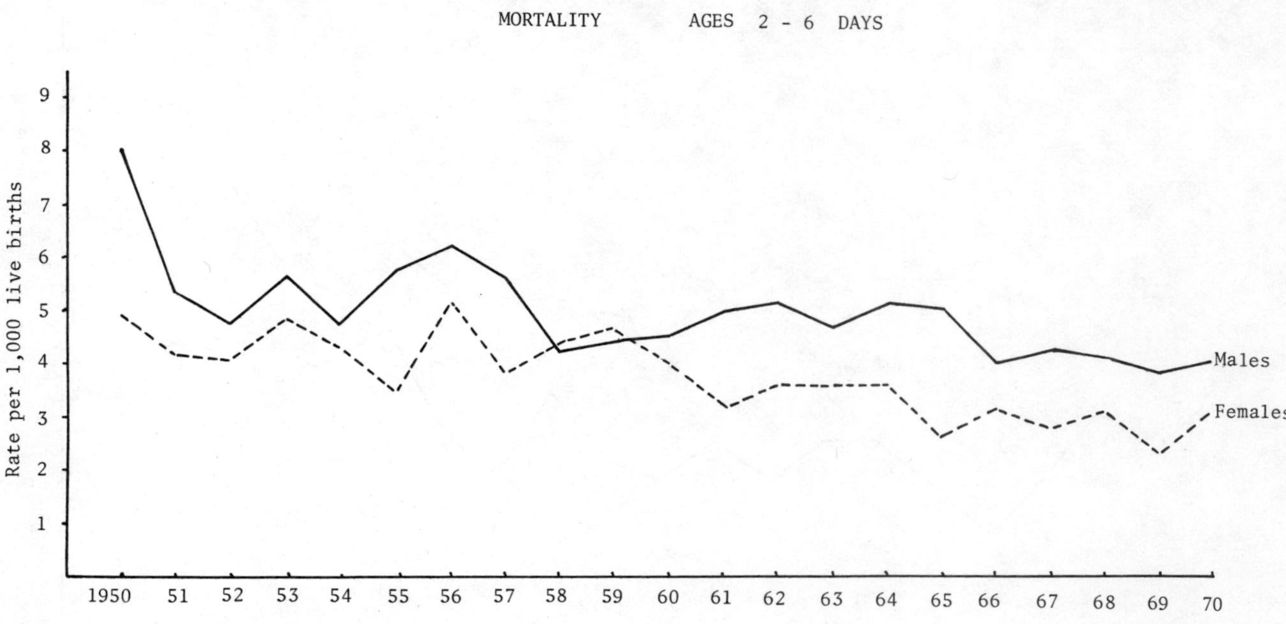

FIG. 6-6 (cont.). Israel infant mortality rates, 1950–1970, all causes, by sex and age.

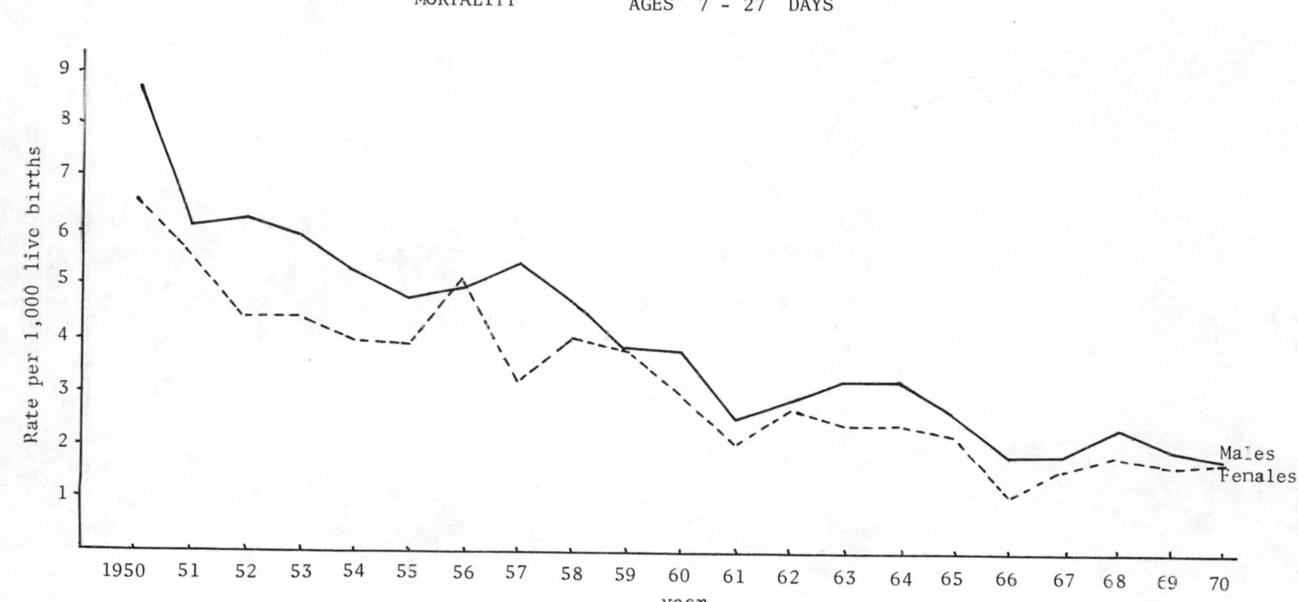

FIG. 6-6 (cont.). Israel infant mortality rates, 1950–1970, all causes, by sex and age. (Entire figure adapted from data for the Jewish population from Israel Bureau of Statistics.)

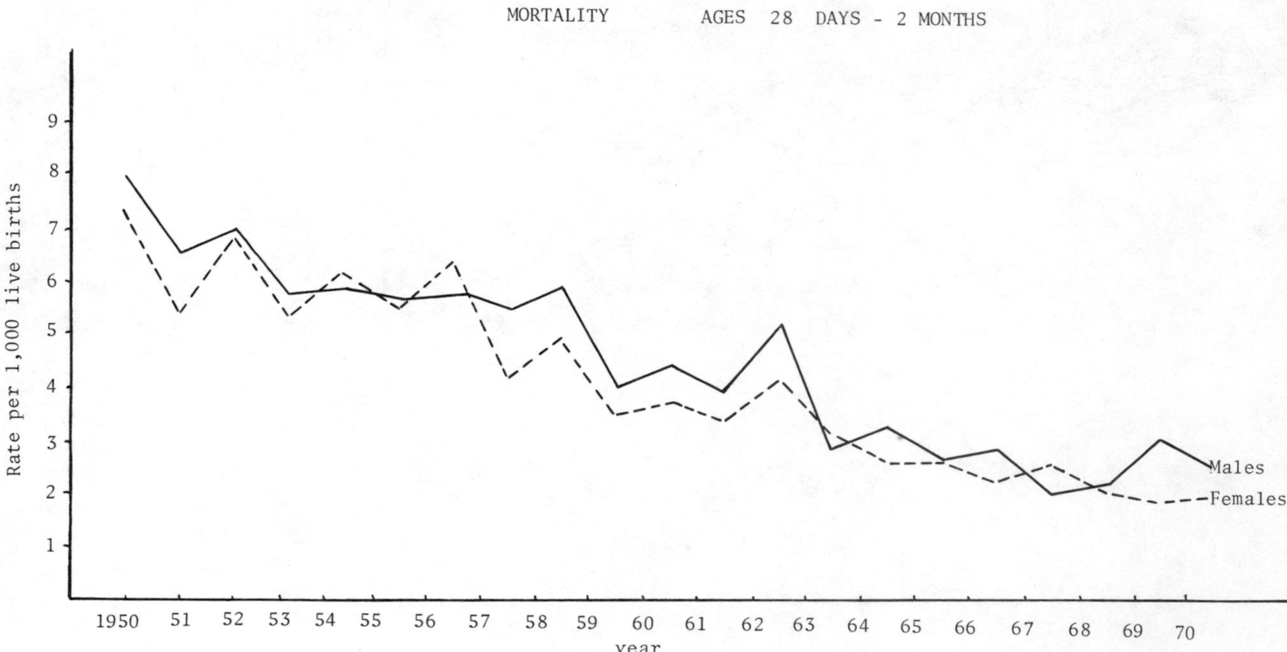

FIG. 6-7. Israel infant mortality rates, 1950–1970, all causes, by sex and age.

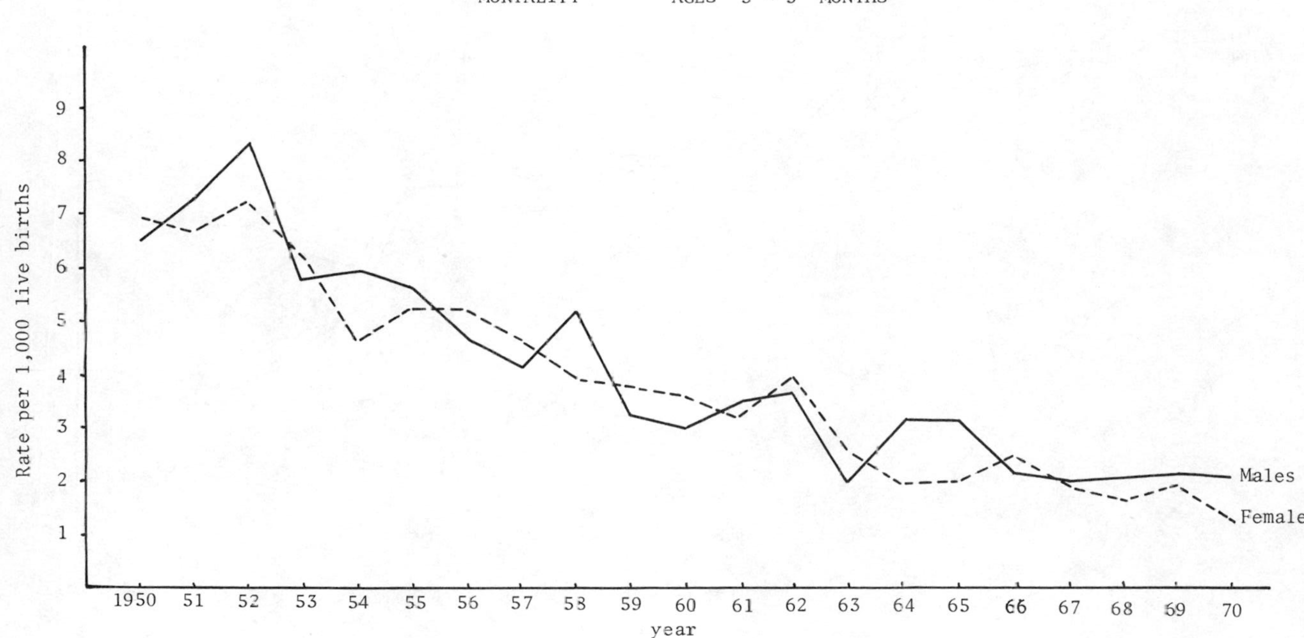

FIG. 6-7 (cont.). Israel infant mortality rates, 1950–1970, all causes, by sex and age.

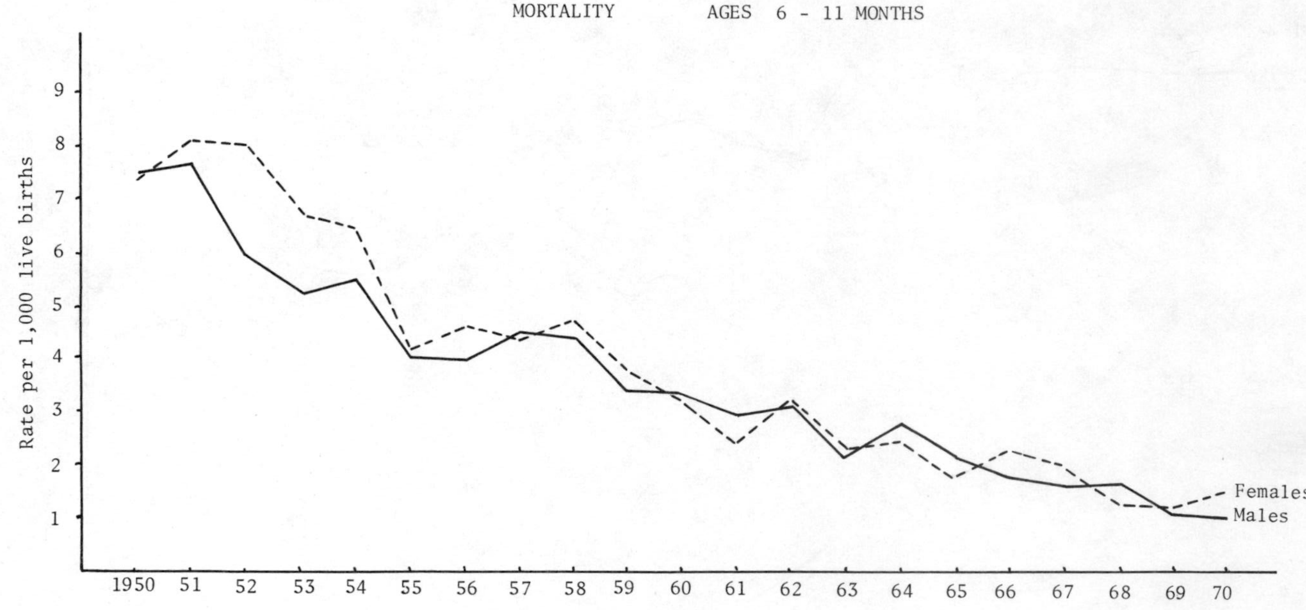

FIG. 6-7 (cont.). Israel infant mortality rates, 1950–1970, all causes, by sex and age. (Entire figure adapted from data for the Jewish population from Israel Bureau of Statistics.)

ETHNIC GROUP

In many places, especially in growing cities and countries of immigration, ethnicity is a most striking feature of social differentiation. In addition to social class it is a highly relevant determinant of difference in health and health behavior. In fact, social class differences are often associated with ethnic group differences (Fig. 6-8).[22] Study of ethnic groups is therefore useful in epidemiology and in the practice of community medicine. This usefulness obviously depends on the ethnic heterogeneity of the community or region being studied. An ethnic group is believed to have a common place of origin, a shared heritage, and distinctive features in its way of life. Thus different ethnic groups should reflect their differences in their somatic and psychologic health characteristics, and in their diseases. The community syndromes will differ according to the combinations and interactions of these constituents of health. Immigrating ethnic groups may differ from the native population in many ways. The outstanding differences may be in religion and religious practices, in race, family living and family size, or in any of the myriad ways in which cultures reveal their differences. In the course of time different ethnic groups may assimilate to become a new entity. This presupposes a sociocultural mobility different from that of socioeconomic mobility. It also entails a process of change in individuals themselves and has significance for intergenerational relationships.

The characteristics of ethnic groups which are of health-relevance are those related to the social and genetic features and the common place of origin of the group. Ethnic differences may be investigated in various ways: through cross-cultural health studies of larger populations; through

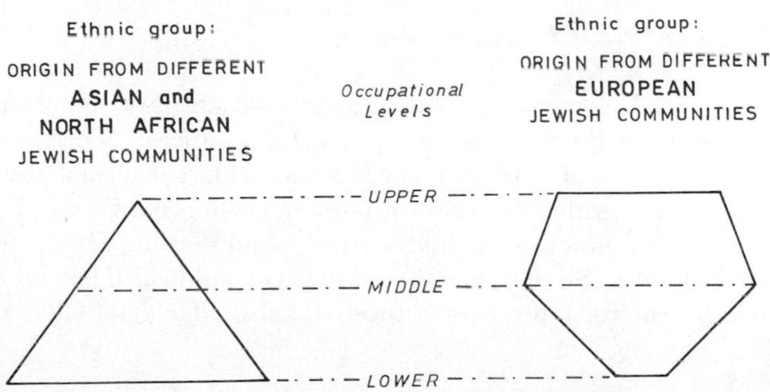

FIG. 6-8. The distribution of women of different ethnic groups according to the occupational status of their husbands. The women were maternity cases delivered in Jerusalem in 1958–1959. (From Kark et al.[22])

studies of local communities living in different places and having no contact with one another; and through studies of groups that have migrated from their original homes to a new country or new city where they have varying degrees of contact with other newcomers and people who are part of the mainstream of the new society. Differences in health of ethnic groups may be related to genetic, environmental, and sociocultural features.

Genetic Features

While not necessarily a criterion for definition of an ethnic unit, genetic constitution may be an outstanding feature of the health picture of an ethnic group, e.g., the different frequencies of genetically transmitted traits and diseases such as sickling and sickle cell disease, glucose-6-phosphate dehydrogenase (G6PD) deficiency and hemolytic anemia, thalassemia, and common diseases such as diabetes and hypertension. The elements of special relevance to the genetic aspects of the group's health include (1) the ethnic group as a breeding population or an endogamous genetic isolate; (2) natural selection and genetic features which emerge in one setting and continue thereafter when a group emigrates from an old to a new setting; and (3) assortative and preferential mate selection within the ethnic group.

Environmental Origins

In addition to the adaptation by natural selection and culture to particular environments, there are health hazards peculiar to some environments which express themselves in various communities. Some of these are strikingly manifested as ethnic health characteristics when groups of such communities migrate to other societies (e.g., multiple sclerosis, goitre, and fluorosis).

Sociocultural Features

The sociocultural elements of ethnic groups which have importance for health are seen in their social structures and cultures. Social structure includes the family and other primary groups and larger formal groupings; social stratification within the ethnic group; and solidarity. Cultural aspects include customary practice in childbearing, child rearing, family spacing, and sanitation; perception of health and disease and health behavior (e.g., diet and care sought); and values, attitudes, knowledge and beliefs relating to health.

Ethnic Group and Cancer at Various Sites

Geographic variation in the occurrence of cancer at various sites is well known. This variation between different countries is reflected in ethnic variation of cancer sites, a variation which may be due to genetic, behavioral, or environmental differences. Ethnic differences in the incidence of each particular cancer need independent study since there is no consistency in the differences and they are not likely to be related to the same determinant factors.[23–26]

The differences between ethnic groups are not always consistent for both sexes. Thus it has been noted that Swedish women in the United States have a relatively high risk for cancer of the mouth, pharynx, and esophagus, but Swedish men do not.[23,24] A similar striking inconsistency in the relative rates of lung cancer in Jewish men and women has been noted in comparisons of Jews with other ethnic and religious groups in various places in the United States and Canada.[27–29] While Jewish men have a relatively low rate of the condition, Jewish women have a higher rate than do women of other groups. This inconsistency was found even in a Jewish community, in which the women as well as the men had a higher proportion of nonsmokers than did other ethnic groups.[29] Also to be noted is the relatively high mortality rate from lung cancer among British men relative to their proportion of current cigarette smokers (Fig. 6-9).

Ethnic Group and Behavior in Illness

Doctors and nurses are aware of differences in response to pain by people of different ethnic groups. In many heterogeneous ethnic communities there are striking differences in behavior of women during labor, the more desired and valued response usually being that of the women who are more controlled and less expressive as opposed to those who are very expressive with uncontrolled crying out and screaming. Zborowski investigated response to pain by patients (all of whom were men) belonging to four American ethnic groups who were admitted to a hospital for army veterans.[30,31] The group included "old American" (Anglo-Saxon origin, usually Protestants whose ancestors had lived in the United States for more than three generations), Irish, Italian, and Jewish patients. Their responses varied not only according to the nature of the disease causing the pain, which was a major influence on response, but they differed also according to their ethnic background. The ethnic differences were

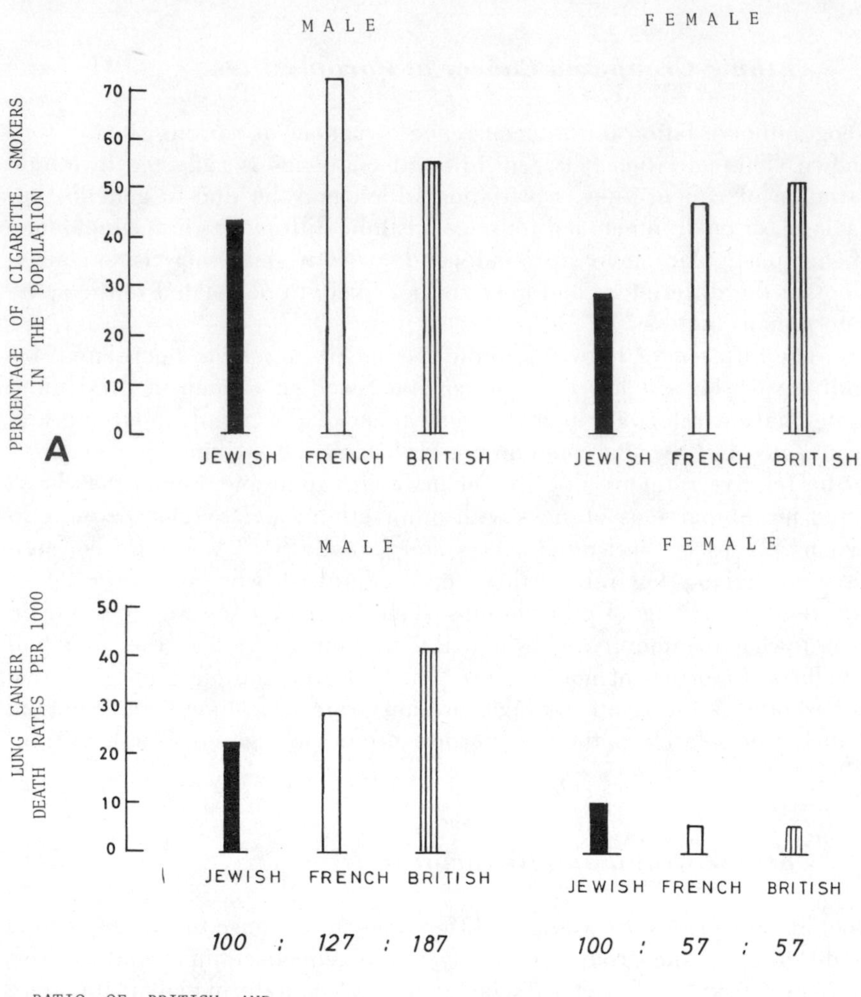

FIG. 6-9. A: Ethnic differences between the sexes in current smoking habits, in 28 census tracts in Montreal, 1967. (Adapted from Horowitz and Enterline.[29]) B: Ethnic differences in mortality from lung cancer per 100,000 population in 28 census tracts in Montreal, 1956–1966. (Adapted from Horowitz and Enterline.[29])

found when he compared patients with the same condition—herniated discs and backache.

The overt behavior of old American and Irish resembled one another in many ways and were in marked contrast to that of the Italian and

Jewish patients. The former were both nonexpressive, "playing-down" and hiding pain, while both the latter groups were highly expressive and emotional, "playing-up" and showing pain. And yet each overall behavioral pattern was distinctive. Thus in contrast to the old American patients whose manifest behavior was similar to their own, the Irish did not share the old American capacity for explicit description of pain and in attributing the pain and illness to external causes. The Irish patients' major concern with pain was its interference with work and physical activity and they would fight it by continuing to work, often until they could no longer do so. This suppression or denial of pain was evident even in hospital where they were overtly model patients in that they were nonexpressive. They also evidenced little concern for the pathology that caused the pain. The Jewish patient on the other hand was much concerned with the signifi-

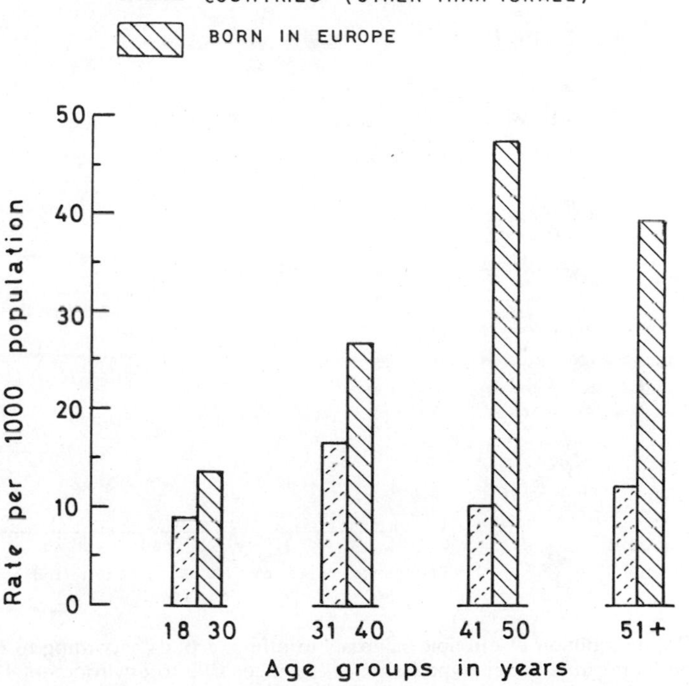

FIG. 6-10. The distribution of urolithiasis according to ethnic origin of immigrants. Hypothesis: Differences due mainly to differences in drinking habits. European groups drink less than North African and Middle Eastern ones. Partial support from experimental epidemiologic investigation in the community of Arad, compared with control population living in Beersheba. (Adapted from Frank et al.[33])

cance of the pain as symptomatic of pathology and consulted a physician immediately. While the differences are of interest and some importance for medical care, Zborowski's analysis of response to pain in its cultural context is a major contribution to understanding of health-relevant behavior. As with other patterns of behavior, "cultural traditions dictate to members of a given society not only whether they should expect and tolerate pain in a given situation, but also the correct conduct during the pain experience. . . . These traditions contain rules and norms for appropriate behavior

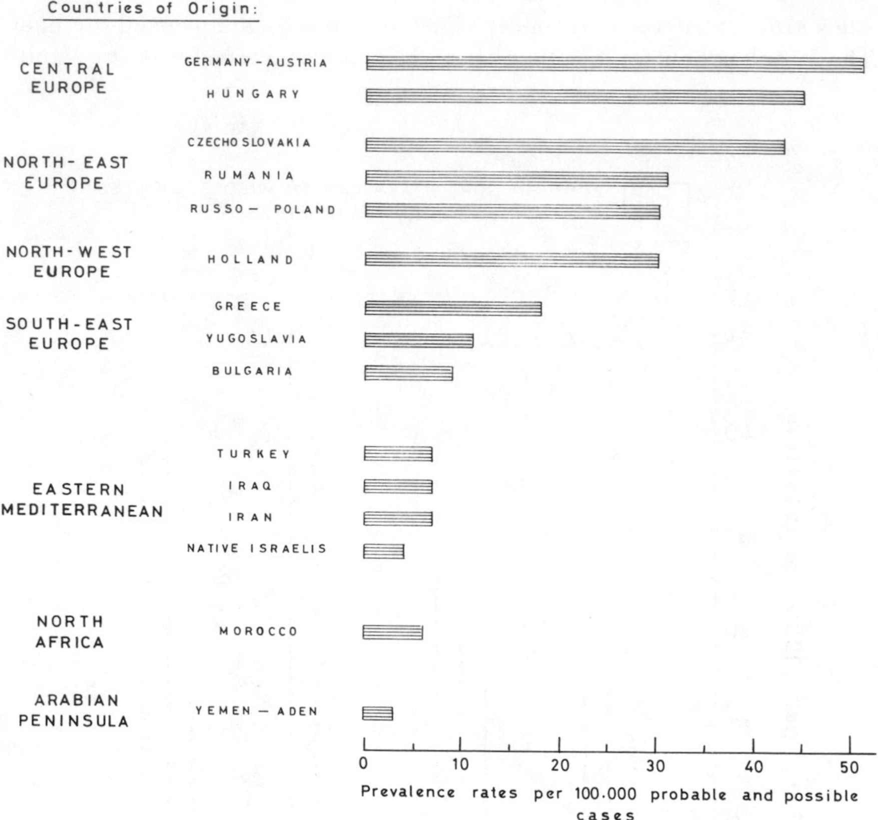

FIG. 6-11. The distribution of multiple sclerosis in ethnic groups according to country of origin and its mean latitude. Hypothesis: Differences due to environmental factors which vary with latitude, rather than ethnicity as such. This conforms to considerable epidemiologic survey evidence elsewhere. Alter and associates considered that the prevalence rate 4/100,000 for native Israelis might have been an underestimate. In Israeli natives of Jewish origin the rate was estimated as 6/100,000 and for Arabs, 1/100,000, which may be a reflection of differential use of health services at the time of the survey. (Adapted from Alter et al.[37])

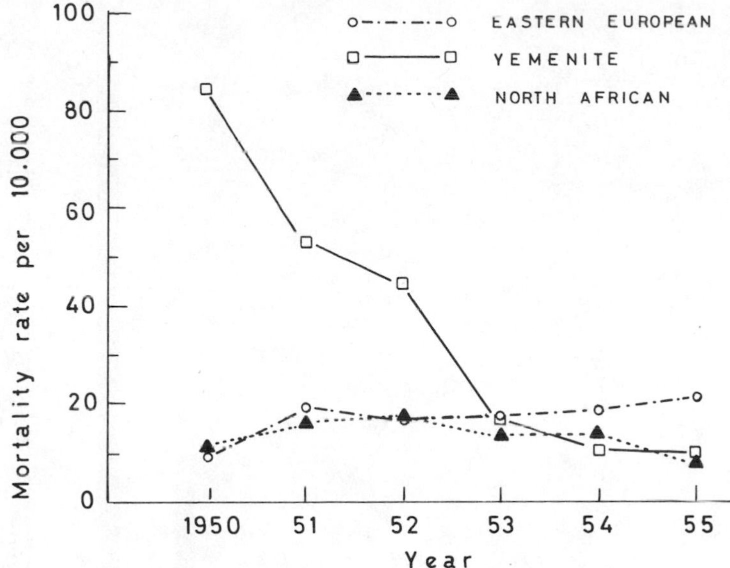

FIG. 6-12. Mortality rates from tuberculosis among Yemenite Jews who have immigrated to Israel, compared with tuberculosis rates among other immigrant groups. Summary hypothesis: High proportions of tuberculin negative on arrival in Israel and other evidence suggests tuberculous infection among Yemenite Jews in most areas of Yemen was almost unknown. Conditions under which they migrated to Israel from Yemen were very difficult, shown in exhaustion, hunger, malnutrition and various infections, trachoma, scabies, tropical ulcer, and malaria. Exposure of a "virgin" population in poor health and nutritional status to tubercle infection in Israel produced acute forms of tuberculosis—"massive exudative forms, giant cavity with bronchogenic spread, primary progressive tuberculosis . . . and miliary spread"—all of which were rare in other Jewish groups.[39] (Adapted from Gruschka.[38])

in the process of suffering. . . . These rules may vary according to age, sex, status or any other social criterion."[31]

Some Epidemiologic Implications of Ethnic Group in Israel

In 1969 the population of Israel was estimated to be 2,919,200 of which 2,496,000 were listed as Jews, 314,500 as Moslems, 73,500 as Christians, and 34,600 as Druze and other smaller groups.[32] The Jewish population is itself polyethnic. Over the 50-year period from 1919 to 1969 more than 1,700,000 Jews came from various parts of the world to settle in their ancient homeland, including some 740,000 from North African and Asian

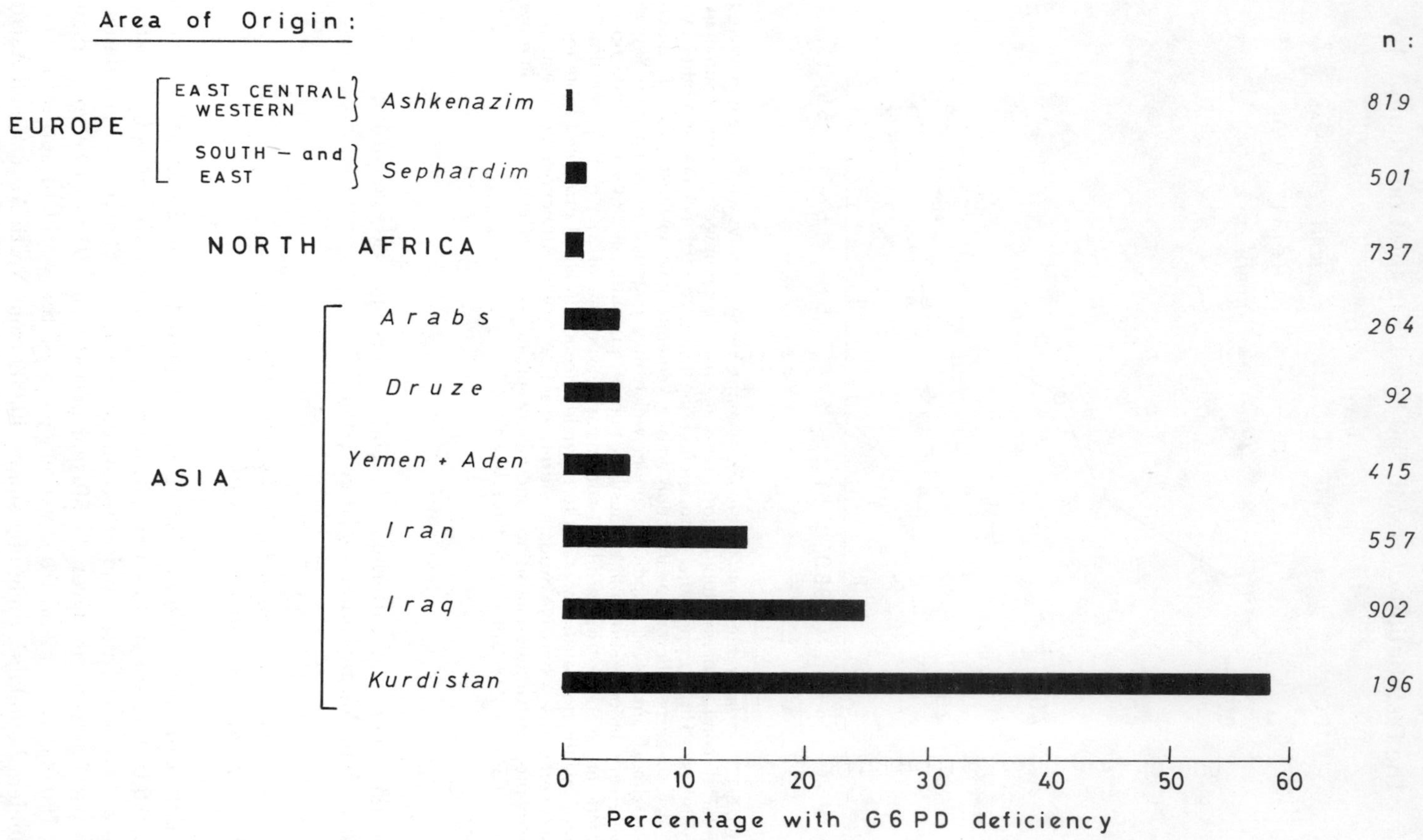

FIG. 6-13. Frequency of G6PD deficiency among males of various ethnic groups (all Jewish, except where otherwise stated) in Israel. (Adapted from Sheba et al.[40])

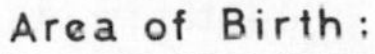

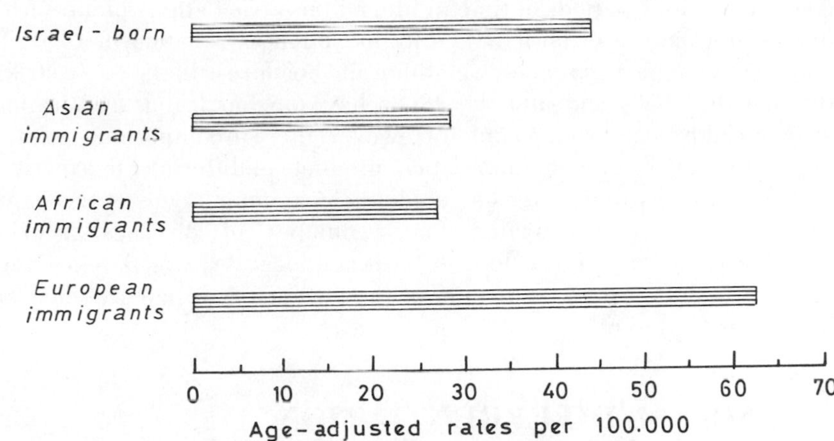

FIG. 6-14. Age-adjusted incidence breast cancer in Jewish women of Israel, 1961–1963, by area of birth. (Adapted from Shani et al.[41])

countries and over 960,000 from Europe and the Americas. In some cases this involved the mass migration of almost the total Jewish population from countries in which they had been settled for 2,000 and more years, as in the case of the Jews from Iraq and Yemen. Whole communities which have come to Israel include many relatively small and well-defined

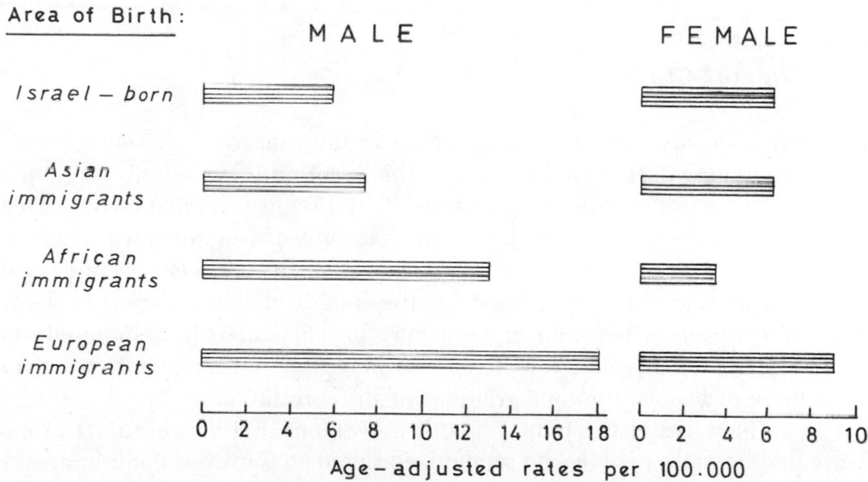

FIG. 6-15. Age-adjusted incidence of gastric cancer in Israel, 1961–1963, according to continent of origin. (Adapted from Tulchinsky and Modan.[42])

groups, such as the Cochin Indian, Kurdish, and Atlas mountain communities. The coming together of many populations who had little if any contact over long periods of time produced the varied ethnic picture which has been a feature of Israel since its inception as a nation in 1948. The more picturesque differences in clothing and headdress that were so striking through the 1950s and into the 1960s have declined and are no longer seen in children and young adults. However, there are important variations in genetic and cultural characteristics, products of differing life experience in distinctive environments. The epidemiologic implications of these qualities have been investigated for a number of diseases, such as urolithiasis,[33–36] multiple sclerosis,[37] tuberculosis,[38,39] G6PD deficiency,[40] cancer of the breast,[41] and cancer of the stomach,[42] which are illustrated in Figures 6-10 to 6-15.

SOCIAL DIFFERENTIATION

Social difference may be defined in a hierarchy of ranks or classes. Social classes, occupational grades, educational and income levels, prestige and power positions are examples of this kind of ranking of families or individuals. However, people may be separated into different groups without necessarily grading them into higher or lower levels. Ethnic and national groups, religious affiliations, urban and rural residents, and differing marital status are examples of this kind of social differentiation. The different types of groups are often more meaningful variables in health studies when investigated in relation to one another, especially when there is interdependence in their distribution. Figure 6-8 is an example of the interdependence of ethnic group and occupational gradings.

Social Class

Every person has a position or standing in the hierarchy of social status of his community. He usually inherits this position by virtue of the family into which he is born but may change it by his own achievements. This change, or vertical social mobility, may be upward or downward in the social scale. Social stratification means inequality between people and these inequalities have relevance for the health of the different classes. The differentiation between classes may be very sharply delineated, as in feudal societies; relatively fixed, as in caste systems; or there may be a more or less continuous gradient of differentiation.

The pioneers of the public health movement of 19th century Europe were middle-class people who recognized the need for reform and improvement in the living conditions of the laboring classes. The importance of class as a determinant of health was clearly stated in the Chadwick report of 1842.[43]

The differences in the average age at death in different social classes in the cities of England at that time is illustrated in Table 6-5. During the same period the social reform movement also focused on the neglected condition of children of the "low neighborhoods" and emphasized the influence of these neighborhoods on the prevailing high rate of child delinquency and crime.

Social class differences in health have been reported in many investigations.[43-47] They include differences in mortality rates,[48-56] physical and mental morbidity,[57-62] physical growth and maturation,[63-66] intelligence,[67] outcome of pregnancy,[55,56] and delinquency.[68] These social class differences in health have been related to differences in behavior, in the environment, and in material resources. The behavioral differences of relevance to health have been described in many practices, such as diet, cigarette smoking, behavior in illness and the use of medical care facilities, infant and child rearing, and assortative mating.[69-76] The differences in environment and material resources of various social classes include the physical and social condition of the neighborhood of living, income, housing, and clothing. The behavioral factors which may be responsible for the association between social class and health are discussed further in Chapter 8.

The impact of social class permeates so many facets of daily living that it is not surprising that class has such widespread associations with different somatic and psychologic conditions of health and disease. Thus the variation in physique in different social classes is not only an effect of health and nutritional differences between the classes, but is also a predictor of variation in biologic performance. This is well demonstrated in the findings of the British Perinatal Mortality Study.[55,56] Perinatal mortal-

TABLE 6-5. Social Class: Age at Mortality in Different Cities of England, 1839–1840

SOCIAL CLASS	CITIES		
	Manchester	Liverpool	London (average of three areas)
Gentlemen, professional persons, and their families	38	35	43
Tradesmen and their families	20	22	30
Laborers, mechanics, servants and their families	17	15	24

(Adapted from Chadwick.[43])

TABLE 6-6. Mortality in Males from Duodenal Ulcers in England and Wales by Age and Social Class*

AGE	SOCIAL CLASS			
	I & II	III	IV	V
45–54 in 1921–1923	10	7	8	8
in 1949–1953	11	13	12	16
55–64 in 1921–1923	12	9	8	9
in 1949–1953	20	26	21	29
65–69 in 1921–1923	18	11	10	6
in 1949–1953	40	44	37	40
70 and over				
in 1921–1923	15	7	7	6
in 1949–1953	62	48	46	46

**The death rate is expressed per 100,000 in each population group.*
(From Susser.[77])

ity rates were significantly lower in the offspring of tall women (162.5 cm and over) than in short women (under 155 cm), and tallness was directly related to social class. Similarly the outcome of pregnancy was related to cigarette smoking, there being a higher stillbirth plus neonatal mortality rate in children born to mothers who smoked during pregnancy. This habit was more common in lower social classes. Associated with these variations in mortality is the social class variation in birth weight and period of gestation. The relationship between these different health conditions, each of which is associated with social class, is not necessarily causal. The nature of the relationship needs further exploration than the social class distribution alone can provide and is discussed further in Section 2.

Secular Changes in the Association Between Mortality Rates and Social Class. Health differences between social classes change over time. These changes may be reflected in a differing frequency of the condition at different ages, as indicated for 1921 to 1923 and 1949 to 1953 in Table 6-6, presented by Susser.[77]

In the 30-year period between the two sets of data there was a general increase in the mortality rate from duodenal ulcer, but the rate of increase differed for various social classes and age groups. The result of these different rates of change was a reversal of social class differentials in some age groups, such as the 45 to 54 and 55 to 64 groups, wherein the death rate in the upper social classes was higher than in the lower social classes in the earlier period, but relatively less than the latter 30 years later. The fact that social class differences are not fixed and change over short periods of time adds to the meaning these differences have for epidemiology. At one time the variations in health of different social classes may be a reflection of wide differences in income and material possessions. After some time the economic factor may not be the outstanding feature of the class differences, which may rather be related to the spread of a particular habit from the upper to the lower social classes. Changes in dietary habits often follow these lines and therefore we may expect nutritional changes which will be reflected in growth, physique, and disease patterns.

The relation between social class and morbidity is not necessarily the same in different places nor even consistent for different demographic groups of the population in the same place. Thus in England and Wales, during the years 1949 to 1953, cancer of the lung was more common in lower social class men yet more common in upper class women.[48] Similarly, obesity has been reported to be much more common in lower social class women in some places whereas there was not such a marked social class difference in obesity in men.[61]

Change in the association between social class and mortality from various causes takes place in even shorter periods of time. Table 6-7

TABLE 6-7. The Change in Relationship Between Social Class and Health in a 10-year Period in England and Wales

Lower social class with higher mortality in 1949–1953 and 1959–1963	Pulmonary tuberculosis Bronchitis Pneumonia Ulcer of stomach Malignant neoplasm of stomach
Higher social class with higher mortality in 1949–1953 with change to Lower social class with higher mortality in 1959–1963	Coronary disease, angina Diabetes Cirrhosis of the liver Vascular lesions of central nervous system Suicide
Higher social class with higher mortality in 1949–1953 with change to No appreciable class differences in mortality in 1959–1963	Leukemia
No appreciable class difference in mortality in 1949–1953 with change to Lower social class with higher mortality in 1959–1963	Nephritis and nephrosis

(Adapted from Registrar General's Decennial Supplements for England and Wales 1951–1961. Occupational Mortality Data for 1949–1953 and 1959–1963.[48])

and Figure 6-16 summarize some of the changes in a 10-year period in England and Wales, when diseases which had been more common causes of death in higher social classes became more common in the lower social classes. These diseases included coronary disease and angina, diabetes, vascular lesions of the central nervous system, cirrhosis of the liver, as well as suicide. The lowest social class (class V) differs strikingly from the other social classes, the standardized mortality ratio in 1959 to 1963

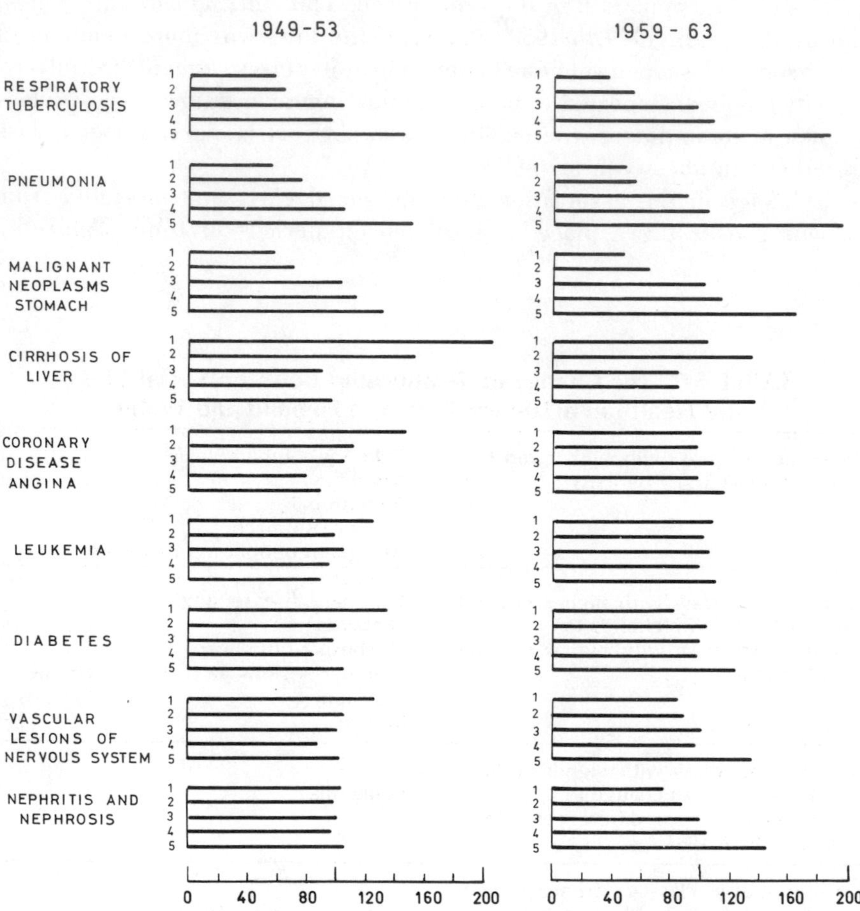

FIG. 6-16. Illustration of the change in social class distribution of various diseases in England and Wales in the periods 1951–1961. The social classes range from 1 (highest) through to 5 (lowest). (Adapted from the Registrar General's Decennial Supplements for England and Wales 1951–1961. Occupational Mortality Data for 1949–1953 and 1959–1963.[48])

being strikingly high with respect to many diseases in this class (Table 6-8).

TABLE 6-8. Standardized Mortality Ratios (SMR) for Certain Causes by Social Class for All Men and Married Women at Ages 15–64, 1959–1963

	MEN					MARRIED WOMEN				
SMR	I	II	III	IV	V	I	II	III	IV	V
Tuberculosis (001–019)	40	54	96	108	185	41	61	102	112	178
Bronchitis (500–502)	28	50	97	116	194	33	51	102	118	196
Pneumonia (490–493)	48	54	88	102	196	64	69	95	114	172
Malignant neoplasm stomach (151)	49	63	101	114	163	50	76	103	110	153
Ulcer of stomach (540)	46	58	94	106	199	81	62	101	109	172
Leukemia (204)	106	100	103	97	108	110	101	104	93	114
Coronary disease angina (420)	98	95	106	96	112	69	81	103	107	143
Cirrhosis of the liver (581)	106	136	86	85	137	94	132	92	92	115
Diabetes (260)	81	103	100	98	122	43	67	95	121	183
Vascular lesions of nervous system (330–334)	86	89	101	98	135	68	80	104	108	140
Suicide (E963, E970–E979)	91	94	87	103	184	110	98	101	84	109

(From the Registrar General's Decennial Supplement for England and Wales 1961.[48]).

Indices Defining Social Class

If the concept of social stratification is to be used for investigation of the differential distribution of health conditions, measurable indices must be devised. These include classifications by occupation, education, locality of residence, and various combinations of factors.

Occupational Classifications. In Britain a classification of all occupations into 5 social classes has been in common use for many years. It was first introduced by the Registrar-General, the information on occupation being obtained from the general population census and from mortality reports. This has resulted in a record of social class differentials in mortality rates since 1910 to 1912. The classification is based on three qualitatively different occupational groupings, and two intermediate ones.[44–46]

Social class I: Higher professions, i.e., engineers, physicians; scientists; directors and owners of big business,

insurance houses, banks, and industry
"The generally well-to-do section of the population."

Social class II: (Intermediate between I and III) Lesser professions, i.e., teachers, pharmacists, smaller business men and managers, farmers

Social class III: Skilled manual workers, artisans and craftsmen, road transport workers, motor drivers, white collar workers, clerks typists

Social class IV: (Intermediate between III and V) Semi-skilled workers in agriculture, mines, and factories

Social class V: Unskilled workers, i.e., general laborers, dock workers, porters, domestic workers

Many years later a similar index, based on the subjective judgment of the classifier, was introduced for official use in the United States census.[78] While such classifications have been widely used, more objective indices have been sought. An example of these was the study carried out by the National Opinion Research Center (NORC) in the United States in 1947.[79–81] A nationwide representative sample of almost 3,000 adult Americans was interviewed to evaluate 90 occupations according to five ratings: excellent, good, average, somewhat below average, and poor. There was a considerable degree of agreement on evaluation of the various occupations by people in different regions of the country, in small or large communities, and of different age and sex.

In a comparative opinion poll study on the prestige of various occupations in six countries, a high degree of concordance was also found.[82] The countries were the United States, the Soviet Union, Japan, Germany, Britain, and New Zealand. These are industrial countries, suggesting that, at least in industrial societies, occupation is a definitive indicator of social class.

Occupational stratification is usually correlated with other forms of class differentiation, including political, economic, and educational stratification. Occupation, education, and neighborhood of residence have been found to be interrelated. Such a correlation of factors has been used by Hollingshead in an index of social position.[83]

A problem arising in the use of these systems of occupational classification is that they bring together different kinds of activities and arbitrarily allocate them to a class. Thus, the population involved in agricultural activities is graded in various social classes along with those in industrial or professional occupations. This problem has been partially met by a system of classification which has been described by Brichler.[84] This system of classification is based entirely on the economic aspects of social functioning and does not group people into upper and lower classes.

Educational Stratification. Education is a key to understanding the association of social differences and health. Regarding culture as learned behavior, the process of education is central to any concept of the relation between culture and health. Firstly, kind of education and amount of training determines occupational position. Secondly, education through rearing at home, among peers, and in neighborhoods, determines behavior, values, and frameworks of knowledge and beliefs.

The close relationship which education often has with occupation, and hence with social class, has led to its being one of the factors by which social class is measured, e.g., in the Hollingshead Index of Social Position.[83] In one index Hollingshead uses three factors by which the head of the family is ranked: occupation, education, and residential area. An even simpler method is a two-factor index of social position in which only occupation and education are considered and in which the occupational rank is weighted more heavily than the educational rank.

In assessing the usefulness of such compound indices we must consider the purpose of delineating social differences between people and of classifying them into various categories. In epidemiology and community medicine there are several good reasons for making a separate analysis of education. Both the general standard and the kind of education are probably among the most important factors determining health-relevant behavior. Differences in child-rearing practices, such as diet, immunization, and social stimulation, may be more related to an economic factor in some situations and an educational factor in others. Thus poor growth and nutritional status of children in some segments of the community may be a direct result of not having enough money to buy food, but it may also be due to faulty concepts of the nutritional values of different foods. While economic status and educational level may be highly associated and together are important factors in differential health status ratings, they also have independent effects on behavior and hence on health. The education of girls and the final standard of education attained by mothers is probably in itself a most important social factor determining child health. Study of the standard of education of women in different social classes, and especially of girls and mothers in developing countries, in relation to outcome of pregnancy, family spacing, and child health, could be a most important foundation for community medicine and for governmental health and welfare policy in general.

Another reason for using education as an independent index is that it does not necessarily have a consistent relation with income and occupation. A discrepancy between these different elements of social status in Israel has been reviewed by Eisenstadt.[85] While investigations have revealed that the main criterion for social stratification in Israeli society is the economic factor, it seems that the high social status of those with political power, education, and occupation of the highest grades does not necessarily coincide with income level. Furthermore, these criteria for success are of relatively recent origin.

Whatever the reasons for the incongruity between different elements of importance in prestige and social status, this lack of congruity makes it undesirable to combine these variables when defining social categories for purposes of epidemiologic investigation. Furthermore, the inconsistency itself may be relevant for health and therefore worthy of investigation. Abramson reported significant differences in the Cornell Medical Index (CMI) Scores in age groups 30 and over among foreign-born Israelis in whom there were discrepancies between occupational and educational ranks compared with those in whom there was little or no discrepancy.[86] High CMI scores, which may be regarded as indicating emotional disorder, were associated with a discrepancy in either direction between educational and occupational status.

Locality. Differences in the health of people living in different localities is well known and has been recorded with respect to such widely differing disorders as delinquency and crime on the one hand and infectious diseases on the other. Locality of residence in cities is determined by several variables, of which social class is a central feature. The social class structure of a city tends to express itself in distinctive areas of the city.

In the course of an epidemiologic investigation in Jerusalem, a very clear correlation was found between occupational rating and neighborhoods of residence, when the latter were grouped according to the municipal rating for taxation purposes (Table 6-9).[22] The occupational rating system which was used was that of the Registrar-General of Britain adapted to local occupations. The municipal rating of a particular neighborhood is based on a combination of the following neighborhood attributes.

1. The nature and extent of development of roads, municipal services, transport services, and schools.
2. Type of housing construction.
3. The distance of the neighborhood from the business center of the city.
4. The composition of the population.

The differentiation between areas is often most evident in growing major industrial cities and was revealed in the pioneer ecologic studies of the American city by Park and Burgess.[87,88] The pattern of development of cities in the United States involved the emergence of concentric zones, each with its distinctive characteristics.

Zone I: The center of the city, the central business and light industry district, with a very small number of resi-

TABLE 6-9. The Relationship Between Occupational Rating of Men and the Municipal Grading of Their Neighborhood of Residence in Jerusalem 1958–1959

MUNICIPAL RATING OF NEIGHBORHOODS	OCCUPATIONAL RATING				
Groups	Highest I & II	III	Lowest IV & V	Other (not rated)	Total (%)
Highest 1	34	51	2	13	100
2	22	50	10	18	100
3	12	53	24	11	100
4	5	48	32	15	100
5	4	39	49	8	100
Lowest 6	0	35	55	10	100

(From Kark et al.[22])

dents, mainly transients living in large hotels, and homeless men.

Zone II: "Zone in transition" where the growing industrial area was encroaching on what had formerly been residential. It was an undesirable area for residence. These slum areas housed families in poverty among whom were many foreigners.

Zone III: "Zone of working men's houses"—more stable population than Zone II, with higher proportion of skilled workers and less foreign born.

Zone IV: "Residential zone," with single family dwellings, upper-middle class families.

Zone V: "Commuter's zone," still further from the central city area than Zone IV but with a similar class distribution.

A feature of the growing city was that each zone was in the process of expansion and thus encroaching on that beyond it. This expansion was itself a cause of neglect of property and environment in the expectation of replacement by business or industry, or by a lower social class.

This zonal development is not characteristic of cities in all parts of the world. Zonal distribution of different social classes may not radiate from the city center outwards. However, neighborhoods, streets, or wider localities of residence are often associated with a particular social class or with other social characteristics of the residents.

The health-relevant characteristics which differentiate residential areas of industrial cities include the following:

1. Physical appearance: maintenance and development of housing, public

buildings, roads and sidewalks, water supplies, and systems of disposal of excreta and refuse.
2. The people in the area: economic status, occupation and education, ethnic and religious groups, nativity (native to the country, city or locality, and length of residence (transitional migrant, recent migrant, or older migrant).

Differences in the health of people in various neighborhoods are often an expression of social class, but this association is not always the sole one and is often an oversimplification.

The study of Faris and Dunham focused attention on the striking association between residential zone and mental disorders,[89] and led to much speculation and some study as to causation. The highest rates for mental disorders, as assessed from the 35,000 cases committed to mental hospitals in Chicago during the years 1922 to 1934, were for persons living in the central city zone. The rates declined with increasing distance from the center towards the peripheral zones. The general pattern for cases diagnosed as schizophrenia was the same, the highest rates being in the central communities and the rooming-house areas, with declining rates according to the ecologically defined zones.

The distribution of cases diagnosed as manic-depressive psychosis was in marked contrast to the distribution of schizophrenia. The differences in the rates of manic-depressive psychosis between various neighborhoods was not consistent with any social characteristics of the ecologic type defined by the different zones of the city.

Delinquency in boys was also found to vary according to the ecologic pattern outlined by the classification of zones of the city. Shaw and McKay noted that the map of distribution of mental disorders in the city of Chicago as outlined by Faris and Dunham corresponded quite closely to their delin-

TABLE 6-10. A Comparison of Various Health Indices in Different Areas of Chicago

	Zone I	Zone II	Zone III	Zone IV	Zone V
Rates of infant mortality 1928–1933 (per 1,000 live births)	86.7	67.5	54.7	45.9	41.3
Rates of tuberculosis 1931–1937 (per 100,000 population as in 1934)	33.5	25.0	18.4	12.5	9.2
Rates of mental disorder 1922–1934 (per 100,000 population over 15 years of age)	32.0	18.8	13.2	10.1	8.4
Rates of male juvenile delinquency 1927–1933	9.8	6.7	4.5	2.5	1.8

(Adapted from Shaw and McKay.[90])

TABLE 6-11. Incidence Rate of Schizophrenia in Two Subcommunities of Detroit in 1958, by Social Class (per 1,000 population)

SOCIAL CLASS	MEASURED BY FATHER'S OCCUPATION	MEASURED BY PATIENT'S OCCUPATION & EDUCATION
I	0.87	0.0
II	0.79	0.32
III	0.44	0.35
IV	0.43	0.21
V	0.69	1.45

(Data from Dunham.[91])

quency map. They also found a significant relationship in various neighborhoods between rates of delinquency and other health characteristics, i.e., infant mortality and tuberculosis. The covariance of these variables lead them to conclude that ". . . delinquency is not an isolated phenomenon. Instead, it is found to be closely associated, area by area, with rates of truancy, adult crime, infant mortality, tuberculosis, and mental disorder, as representative community problems."[90] Table 6-10 is based on Shaw and McKay's more detailed analysis of the important elements of different pictures of health presented by various communities.

Some years later Dunham carried out another, more thorough, epidemiologic study of the social distribution of schizophrenia in a different city, Detroit.[91] Among the important findings of relevance to our present discussion are those regarding social class and residential area in epidemiologic investigation.

As pointed out by Dunham the association between social class and schizophrenia, and the concentration of schizophrenics in lower social class neighborhoods, may be a result of the developmental process of the disease itself which may adversely affect their education and occupation and hence place them in a lower social class.

When Dunham compared the incidence rates of schizophrenia according to social class of father of patient and of patient himself, the results were different (Table 6-11).

This shows that the association between social class and schizophrenia is only marked when social class is measured by the occupation and education of the patient himself. When father's occupation is used as the indicator the rates for classes I and II combined are higher than for classes III, IV, and even V. This finding is in accord with that of Goldberg and Morrison[92] in a study of male patients in England.

At this point it should be emphasized that epidemiologic investigation of the social class factor requires as much attention to the criteria of social class as is usually given to the health condition under study. It involves the following:

1. Definition of the criteria by which social class is to be measured, such as occupation, income, and education or residential area, with clear indication of how these items are to be classified.
2. Validation of these indicators of social class is especially important when the classification used in one country (e.g., the Registrar General's classification in Britain), is to be used in a different setting.
3. Family social class is often measured only by the social position of the husband and father, whether measured by his occupation, education, or other indicators. This may be generally useful but as we have seen it excludes important factors. In particular studies it may be vital to add information which will measure other aspects of social class.
4. Social Mobility.
   a. Social mobility of the family as a whole, as measured by changes over time in its areas of residence.
   b. Social mobility of the father and husband, as measured by changes over time in type of occupation, more especially vertical change as contrasted to horizontal, i.e., change in job but not in status of the occupation.
   c. Inter-generational change, as measured by the following.
      1. Comparison of fathers and sons.
      2. Movement by marriage of daughters.
5. Concordance in factors that are intrinsic to social class.
   a. Congruence in social class of wives and husbands, as measured by the social class of their respective homes of origin (families of orientation) and also by specific indicators of social class, such as their respective standard of education, and levels of occupation.
   b. Concordance of factors in the individual himself, such as consistency between his levels of education and occupation, his income or occupational position in relation to his education, and home of origin.

REFERENCES

1. Davis K: The world demographic transition. Ann Am Polit Soc Sci 237:1, 1945.
2. Glass DV: Population growth and population policy. In Sheps MC, Ridley JC (eds.): Public Health and Population Change. Pittsburgh, Univ of Pittsburgh Press, 1965.
3. Cowgill DO: The theory of population growth cycles. Am J Sociol 55: 163, 1949.
4. Notestein FW: Population—the long view. In Schultz TW (ed.): Food for the World. Chicago, Univ of Chicago Press, 1945.
5. Omran AR: The epidemiologic transition: A theory of the epidemiology

of population change. New York, Milbank Mem Fund Q 49:509, 1971.
6. McKeown T: Medicine and world population. In Sheps MC, Ridley JC (eds.): Public Health and Population Change. Univ of Pittsburgh Press, 1965, p 32.
7. McKeown T, Record RG: Reasons for the decline of mortality in England and Wales during the Nineteenth Century. Population Stud 16:94, 1962.
8. Draper CC, Smith A: Malaria in the Pare area of N.E. Tanganyika. I. Epidemiology. Trans R Soc Trop Med Hyg 51:137, 1957.
9. Draper CC, Smith A: Malaria in the Pare area of N.E. Tanganyika. II. Effects of three years' spraying of huts with dieldrin. Trans R Soc Trop Med Hyg 54:342, 1960.
10. Wilson DB: Report on the Pare-Taveta Malaria Scheme 1954–1959. Dar-Es-Salaam, Government Printer, 1960.
11. Pringle G: Malaria in the Pare area of Tanzania. III. The course of malaria transmission since the suspension of an experimental programme of residual insecticide spraying. Trans R Soc Trop Med Hyg 61:69, 1967.
12. Pringle G, Matola YG: Report on the Pare-Taveta Vital Statistics Survey 1962–1966. Amani, Tanzania, East African Institute of Malaria and Vector-borne Diseases, 1967.
13. Wyon JB, Gordon JE: The Khanna Study. Population Problems in the Rural Punjab. Cambridge, Harvard Univ Press, 1971.
14. Durant W: The Renaissance. New York, Simon and Schuster, 1953.
15. Boccaccio G: The Decameron. Translated by John Payne. New York, Liveright, 1943.
16. Nohl J: The Black Death. English translation by CH Clarke, George Allen and Unwin, London, 1926.
17. Trevelyan GM: English Social History. London, Longmans, Green, 1944, p 8.
18. WHO: World Health Statistics Annual 1965, 1966, and 1967. Geneva, WHO, 1968, 1969, 1970.
19. Newell GR, Waggoner DE: Cancer mortality and environmental temperature in the United States. Lancet 1:766, 1970.
20. WHO: Annual Epidemiological and Vital Statistics 1947–1949. I. Vital Statistics and Causes of Death. Geneva, WHO, 1952.
21. WHO: World Health Statistics Annual, Vol. 1. Vital Statistics and Causes of Death. Geneva, WHO, 1969.
22. Kark SL, Peritz E, Shiloh A, et al.: Epidemiological analysis of the hemoglobin picture in parturient women of Jerusalem. Am J Public Health, 54:947, 1964.
23. Kmet J: The role of migrant population in studies of selected cancer sites. A review. J Chronic Dis 23:305, 1970.
24. Haenszel W: Cancer mortality among the foreign-born in the United States. J Nat Cancer Inst 26:37, 1961.
25. Staszewski J, Haenszel W: Cancer mortality among Polish-born in the United States. J Nat Cancer Inst 35:291, 1965.
26. Haenszel W, Kurihura M: Studies of Japanese migrants. I. Mortality from cancer and other diseases among Japanese in the United States. J Nat Cancer Inst 40:43, 1968.
27. Newill VA: Distribution of cancer mortality among ethnic subgroups of the white population of New York City, 1953–1958. J Nat Cancer Inst 26:405, 1961.
28. King H, Diamond E, Bailar JC: III. Cancer mortality and religious pref-

erences. A suggested method in research. Milbank Mem Fund Q 43:349, 1965.
29. Horowitz I, Enterline PE: Lung cancer among the Jews. Am J Public Health 60:275, 1970.
30. Zborowski M: Cultural components in response to pain. J Soc Issues, 8: 16, 1952.
31. Zborowski M: People in Pain. San Francisco, Jossey-Bass, 1969, p 32.
32. Central Bureau of Statistics: Statistical Abstract of Israel, 1970, No. 21. Jerusalem, Government Press, 1970.
33. Frank M, De Vries A, Atsmon A, et al.: Epidemiological investigations of urolithiasis in Israel. J Urol 81:497, 1959.
34. Frank M, Atsmon A, De Vries A, et al.: Urolithiasis. In Goldschmidt E (ed.): The Genetics of Migrant and Isolate Populations. New York, Williams and Wilkins, 1963.
35. Frank M, Atsmon A, Sugar P, et al.: Epidemiological investigation of urolithiasis in the hot arid southern region of Israel. Urol Int 15:65, 1963.
36. Frank M, de Vries A: Prevention of urolithiasis. Arch Environ Health 13: 625, 1966.
37. Alter M, Halpern L, Kurland LT, et al.: Multiple sclerosis in Israel. Arch Neurol 7:253, 1962.
38. Gruschka T: Health Services in Israel. A Ten Year Survey 1948–1958. Jerusalem, Israel Ministry of Health, 1959.
39. Rakower J: Tuberculosis among Yemenite Jews. Volume of Reports. The Israel Tuberculosis Convention, Tel Aviv, 1959.
40. Sheba C, Szeinberg A, Ramot B, et al.: Epidemiologic surveys of deleterious genes in different population groups in Israel. Am J Public Health 52:1101, 1962.
41. Shani M, Modan B, Steinitz R, et al.: The incidence of breast cancer in Jewish females in Israel. Harefuah 71:337, 1966.
42. Tulchinsky D, Modan B: Epidemiological aspects of cancer of the stomach in Israel. Cancer 20:1311, 1967.
43. Chadwick E: Report on the Sanitary Condition of the Labouring Population of Great Britain, 1842. Republished and edited by MW Flinn. Edinburgh, Edinburgh Univ Press, 1965.
44. Stevenson AC: Recent Advances in Social Medicine. London, J & A Churchill, 1950.
45. Morris JN: Uses of Epidemiology. Edinburgh, E & S Livingstone, 1964.
46. Susser MW, Watson W: Sociology in Medicine, 2nd ed. London, Oxford Univ Press, 1971.
47. Kosa J, Antonovsky A, Zola IK (eds.): Poverty and Health. A Sociological Analysis. Cambridge, Harvard Univ Press, 1969.
48. Registrar General's Decennial Supplements, England and Wales, 1951 and 1961. Occupational Mortality. London, Her Majesty's Stationery Office, 1958 and 1971.
49. Benjamin B: Social and Economic Factors Affecting Mortality. The Hague, Mouton, 1965.
50. Moriyama IM, Guralnick L: Occupational and social class differences in mortality. In Trends and Differentials in Mortality. New York, Milbank Mem Fund Q, 1956.
51. Heady JA, Heasman MA: Social and Biological Factors in Infant Mortality. London, Her Majesty's Stationery Office, 1958.

52. Illsley R: Social class selection and class differences in relation to stillbirths and infant deaths. Brit Med J 2:1520, 1955.
53. Douglas JWB: Health and survival of infants in different social classes. A national survey. Lancet 2:440, 1951.
54. Daly C, Heady JA, Morris JN et al.: The independent effects of social class, region, the mother's age and her parity on infant mortality. Lancet 1:499, 1955.
55. Butler NR, Bonham DG (eds.): Perinatal Mortality. The First Report of the 1958 British Perinatal Mortality Study. Edinburgh and London, E & S Livingstone, 1963.
56. Butler NR, Alberman ED (eds.): Perinatal Problems. The Second Report of the 1958 British Perinatal Mortality Study. Edinburgh and London, E & S Livingstone, 1969.
57. Hare E: Mental illness—social class in Bristol. Brit J Prev Soc Med 9: 191, 1955.
58. Antonovsky A: Social class and the major cardiovascular diseases. J Chronic Dis 21:65, 1968.
59. Marcial VA: Socioeconomic aspects of the incidence of cancer in Puerto Rico. Ann NY Acad Sci 84:981, 1960.
60. Graham SM, Levin M, Lilienfeld AM: The socioeconomic distribution of cancer of various sites in Buffalo, NY, 1948–1952. Cancer 13:180, 1960.
61. Moore ME, Stunkard A, Srole L: Obesity, social class, and mental illness. JAMA 181:962, 1962.
62. Hollingshead AB, Redlich FC: Social Class and Mental Illness. A Community Study. New York, Wiley, 1958.
63. Acheson RM: Sex, socioeconomic status, and secular increase in stature. A family study. Brit J Prev Soc Med 18:25, 1964.
64. Tanner JM: Growth at Adolescence, 2nd ed. Oxford, Blackwell Scientific, 1962, Chap 5.
65. Michelson N: Studies in physical development of Negroes. IV. Onset of puberty. Am J Phys Anthropol NS 2:151, 1944.
66. Kark E: The menarche in African and Indian girls. In Kark SL, Steuart GW (eds.): A Practice of Social Medicine. Edinburgh, E & S Livingstone, 1962.
67. Susser M: Mental subnormality in the community. In Community Psychiatry, Part 4. New York, Random House, 1968.
68. Morris T: The Criminal Area. Study in Social Ecology. London, Routledge and Kegan Paul, 1957.
69. Warner WL, Lunt PS: The Social Life of a Modern Community. New Haven, Yale Univ Press, 1941.
70. Mechanic D: Medical Sociology. New York, Free Press, 1968.
71. Johnson AL, Jenkins CD, Patrick R, et al.: Epidemiology of Polio Vaccine Acceptance, Monograph No. 3. Jacksonville, Florida State Board of Health, 1962.
72. Northcutt TJ, Jenkins CD, Johnson AL: Factors influencing vaccine acceptance. In Neill JS, Bond JO (eds.): Hillsborough County Oral Polio Vaccine Program, Monograph No. 6. Jacksonville, Florida State Board of Health, 1964.
73. Breslow L, Hochstim JR: Sociocultural aspects of cervical cytology in Alameda County, California. Public Health Rep 79:107, 1964.

74. Kedward HB: Social class habits of consulting. Brit J Prev Soc Med 16: 147, 1962.
75. Simmons OG: Social Status and Public Health, New York, Social Science Research Council, 1958.
76. Newson J, Newson E: Infant Care in an Urban Community. London, George Allen and Unwin, 1963.
77. Susser MW: Social medicine in Britain. Studies in social class. In Welford AT, Argyle M, Glass DV, et al. (eds.): Society, Problems, and Methods of Study. London, Routledge and Kegan Paul, 1962.
78. Edwards AE: Comparative Occupational Statistics for the United States, 16th Census, 1940. Washington, DC, US Government Printing Office, 1943.
79. North CC, Hatt PK: Jobs and occupations. A popular evaluation. Public Opinion News 9:3, 1947. Reprinted in Bendix R, Lipset JM (eds.): Class, Status, and Power. Glencoe, Ill, Free Press, 1953.
80. Hatt PK: Stratification in the mass society. Am Sociol Rev 55:533, 1950.
81. Kahl JA: The American Class Structure. New York, Rinehart, 1959.
82. Inkeles A, Rossi PH: National comparisons of occupational prestige. Am J Sociol 61:329, 1956.
83. Hollingshead AB: The index of social position. In Hollingshead AB, Redlich FC (eds.): Social Class and Mental Illness. A Community Study. New York, Wiley, 1958, Part 5.
84. Brichler M: Classification of the population by social and economic characteristics. The French experience and international recommendations. J R Stat Soc A 121(2):161, 1958.
85. Eisenstadt SN: Israeli Society. London, Weidenfeld and Nicolson, 1967.
86. Abramson JH: Emotional disorder, status inconsistancy, and migration. Milbank Mem Fund Q 44:23, 1966.
87. Park RE, Burgess EW: The City. Chicago, Univ of Chicago Press, 1925.
88. Burgess EW (ed.): The Urban Community. Chicago, Univ of Chicago Press 1926.
89. Faris REL, Dunham HW: Mental Disorders in Urban Areas. Chicago, Univ of Chicago Press, 1939.
90. Shaw CR, McKay HD: Juvenile Delinquency and Urban Areas. Chicago, Univ of Chicago Press, 1942. Revised ed. 1969, p 106.
91. Dunham HW: Community and Schizophrenia. Detroit, Wayne State Univ Press, 1965.
92. Goldberg EM, Morrison SL: Schizophrenia and social class. Brit J Psychiatry 109:785, 1963.

SECTION 2

Community Determinants of Health and Disease

In all human societies people live in social groups functioning in relation with one another in the fulfillment of their respective roles. In its most elementary form the survival of a people depends on its reproduction and its ability to sustain its members at least to their reproductive life span. Measures of reproductive efficiency and survival after birth are a reflection of the functioning of a society to meet these basic needs for its continued existence. Measures of the quality of health are more refined indicators of its social and ecologic equilibrium.

The characteristics of a population group which are of health relevance may be viewed as an interacting system of its biologic, social, and cultural qualities. Study of these features of a population group is the keystone to epidemiologic understanding of cause of disease and determinants of well-being. It is not merely the unit of study that distinguishes epidemiology, but also its interest in the group processes which determine the distribution, the biologic gradient, and the varied expressions of disease. Like other medical sciences, epidemiology is interested in cause and it is especially in its concern with the group that it can further develop its distinctiveness.

Focus on community processes which are of relevance to the community's health is the feature of epidemiology in community medicine. The questions asked are oriented towards explaining the ways by which society determines the differential distribution of the state of health of its constituent groups.

How do these groups, families, and communities influence the state of health of their members? What are the various factors in community living which initiate disease and determine the severity of its expression and its outcome? What are the processes which promote or improve the health of a community?

To understand the way society influences genetic and environmental determinants of health we must understand the relative importance of these determinants in specific conditions. Results of social action have been most evident with respect to environment, for good or ill. This will not always be so. Genetic engineering will be possible and will require social action, depending on the value system, at least as much as does environmental engineering. Atmospheric pollution by industry and soil erosion by agriculture are due to ignorance of their epidemiologic implications for health and of their wider ecologic relevance to life. Pollution and erosion are indicators of what may be in store for society when genetic engineering becomes possible. They point to the need for an epidemiology which is oriented towards understanding the impact of social process on health and hence towards the health effects of social action.

The various community processes which affect the community's health may be classified as follows:

1. Processes of transmission and social interaction between members of the community and their human environment.
2. Shared experience of the community as a whole or its subgroups.
3. Processes of change which are an outstanding feature of present-day societies.

The main elements of these processes are summarized in Tables 7-1—7-3.

In examining these various processes, it is obvious but nevertheless pertinent to stress the importance of the community's past and present. Both contemporary and historical processes are involved in determining the present and future health status of a population group.

TABLE 7-1. Processes of Transmission and Interaction Between Members of a Community and Their Human Environment

THE PROCESSES	BIOLOGIC AND PSYCHOLOGIC ASPECTS	SOCIAL ASPECTS
Genetic transmission	Natural selection and fertility Health status of parents	Assortative mating Population control
Transmission of infection	Host reactions Immunologic processes Intrauterine transmission from mother to fetus	Structure and functioning of groups that determine rate and direction of transmission of microorganisms among its members Sanitation and pollution control
Transmission of culture	Learning ways of thinking, believing, and behaving Internalization	Socialization patterns in family and other groups
Interaction	Homeostatic regulating mechanisms Mother-fetus-infant interaction Personality development	Network of relationships Role structure

TABLE 7-2. The Shared Experience of Members of a Community or Its Subgroups

Genetic
Exposure to a common environment: physical, chemical, biologic
Material resources: housing, means of communication, wealth-poverty
Social structure: leadership, status system, informal and formal social groupings
Culture: customary practices, knowledge, beliefs, values, and socialization system
Health service system and other services and facilities

TABLE 7-3. Processes of Change

CHANGE IN THE LIFE EXPERIENCE OF INDIVIDUALS IN THE COMMUNITY
Change associated with phases of growth, development, maturation and age
Change in life situation, including stressful experiences, bereavement, deprivations
Migration
Social mobility
CHANGE AFFECTING THE COMMUNITY OR SUBGROUP AS A WHOLE
Biologic change:
in the genetic make-up
in biologic survival and age-sex distributions
in patterns of health and disease.
Social and cultural change:
in social structure and size
in customary practices
in the value-system
in the health care system
Environmental, technologic, and economic change:
in the natural environment
in man-made changes

7
Health-Relevant Community Characteristics

Community characteristics which are of relevance to epidemiologic studies include its various groupings, the customary practices of its members, the cultural background of its value-attitudes, and its knowledge and beliefs (Fig. 7-1). The following material is based on the approach of Arensberg and Kimball,[1] who delineate three components of the social system of a group, i.e., the "structure of interaction termed a relational system, a system of customary behavior, and a system of values."

Groups in the Community

In epidemiologic studies the term "group" has been used somewhat loosely to refer to various groupings of people. These may be differentiated into at least two distinct types of groups,[1] one in which the individuals concerned relate with one another, and another in which the groups are of a categorical nature and in which the individuals do not necessarily relate.

Categorical Groups. These may be defined by both biologic and social characteristics such as sex, age, and blood groups and other genetic markers, as well as by occupation, education, social class, religion, and ethnic characteristics. These categorical groups are among the most frequently used in epidemiologic studies. Their importance is well established and their epidemiologic relevance is more sharply delineated if studied together with the relational system of the community and its customary practices.

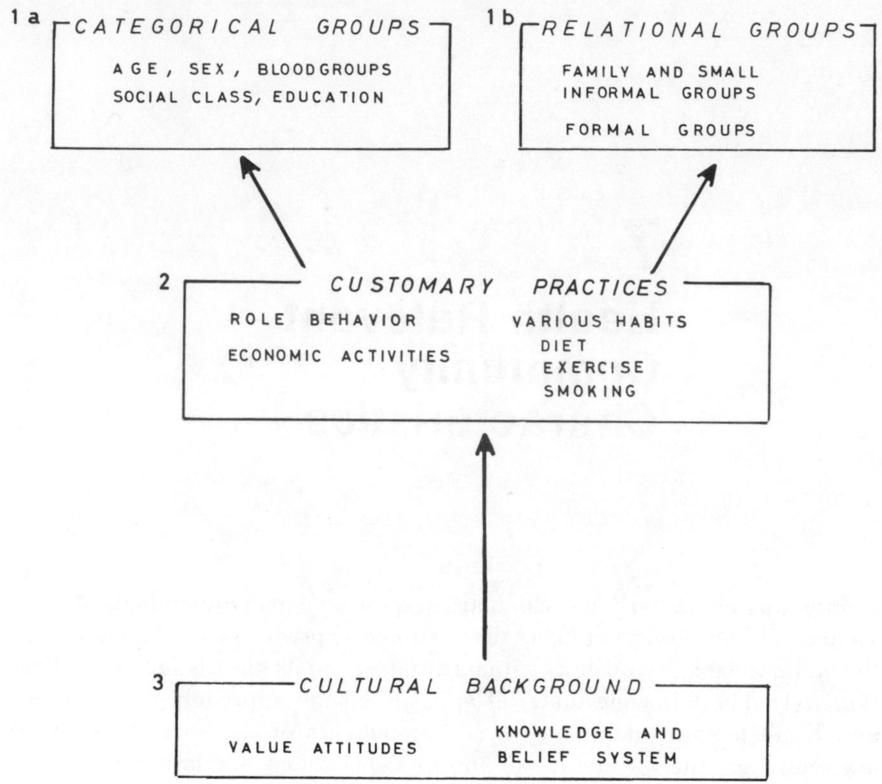

FIG. 7-1. Health relevant characteristics of a community.

Relational Groups. These include small groups such as the family, informal friendship, and other primary groups, as well as more formal groups.

Cooley introduced the term "primary" to describe groups "characterized by intimate face-to-face association and cooperation. They are primary in several senses, but chiefly in that they are fundamental in forming the social nature and ideals of the individual."[2] They are usually relatively small, the relationships between the individuals are informal, contacts are frequent and continue over a long period of time. The "family, playgroup of children, and the neighborhood or community group of elders"[2] were seen by Cooley as the most important primary groups. In countries and cities where immigration is common, the primary groups of immigrants coming from the same "home country," town, or village become important in the perpetuation of their traditions, and in their degree of integration into the new community. In reviewing much research on the role of the small group, Berelson and Steiner conclude that it "strongly influences the behavior of its members by setting and/or enforcing standards (norms) for proper behavior by its members," and further "the more stable and cohesive the group is, and the more attached the members are to it, the more influential it is in setting standards for their behavior."[3]

Epidemiologically, these groupings are of considerable interest and should be an important focus of community health research. Their role in infection and infectious disease is well established, but as fields of social interaction and other processes determining health much research remains to be done.

In contrast to the primary group and small informal groups generally, are the more structured and less personal larger associations which have been described as "secondary groups." They include governmental organizations, trade-unions, and much of the health service system in more developed countries. Understanding their structure and function in different social systems is essential to successful planning and development of public health services, hospitals and health centers, health and medical care in general, and the effective utilization of facilities by the community.

Customary Practices

There are customary practices which are expressly concerned with some aspect of health. They may be protective of the group as a whole, as in ensuring the sanitary standards of its water supply or its air, or promotive of the health and nutrition of certain groups, e.g., expectant mothers or infants, or in ensuring care of the sick or aged. Important and varied as these practices may be, most patterns of behavior of communities are not purposefully directed to their health implications. Nevertheless their influence on health is often more profound and more pervasive than are the effects of those practices more specifically directed to health. They include family living, work and play, education of children and adults, religious practices, and other community activities.

The Environment and Health. The relationship between community and environment, which is unstable and changeable over time, is often one of disequilibrium rather than of balance. The components of the physical environment (natural, man-modified, or man-made) and the human environment itself constitute an interdependent system (Fig. 7-2). Small hunting communities may have been integral elements of their environment with little destructive impact on their ecologic setting and they might have lived in relative plenty. Studies of surviving hunting communities suggest this to be true[4] yet the cost in health may be very much higher than we are nowadays ready to accept. Along with man's increasing ability to use and modify his environment grows the need to do so for rapidly

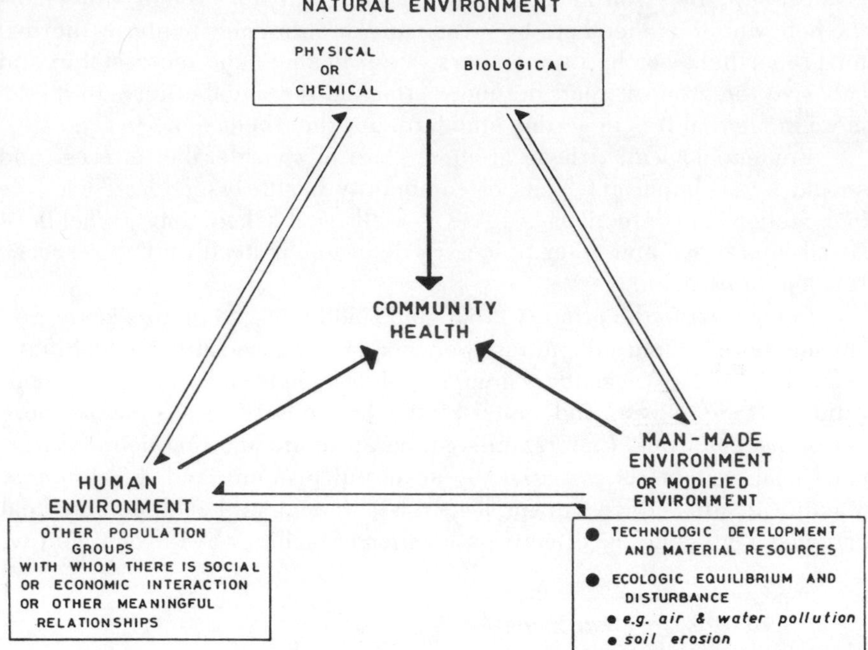

FIG. 7-2. The components of the physical environment and the human environment: an interdependent system.

increasing populations living in larger and more densely crowded communities. While the aim may be for an ecologically balanced process the facts are usually different, and major technologic advance is often accompanied by disturbance or destruction. Awareness of the need to promote ecologic balance has been acutely stirred by the development of smog in and around the world's widening industrial centers, the destruction of the fertile layers of the soil through erosion, and the undermining of life by pollution of land, air, rivers, and the seas. While the scientific evidence of the effects of insult and neglect of the environment accumulates, the human anguish and struggle for mere survival has been told in great sagas, such as John Steinbeck's classic story of migration from a land that had been made into a dustbowl,[5] or in the compelling indictment by Rachel Carson against the poisoning and destruction of life by the widespread use of insecticides.[6]

Pollution of the Environment. Pollution of the environment in the crowded cities that developed with the industrial revolution stimulated the 19th century public health movement of Europe which was spearheaded by

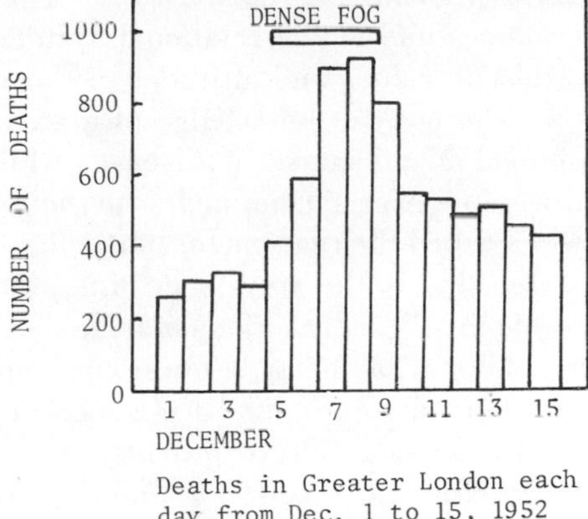

FIG. 7-3. The increase in deaths during the London smog of December 1952. (From Logan.[9])

a revolution in environmental sanitation.[7,8] The focus was on pollution of streets and water by the indiscriminate disposal of organic refuse such as human excreta, and on overcrowding within houses, housing density, poor housing, and neglect of personal hygiene.

The esthetic effects of air pollution by smoke and its effects on vegetation and buildings have been known for many centuries. Acute episodes of increased mortality and morbidity associated with fog led to more systematic study of the effects of air pollutants and control measures. The dramatic effects on community health of envelopment by fog have been noted in a number of areas following the episodes in 1930 and in the Meuse River Valley in Belgium; in Donora, a city near Pittsburgh, in 1948; and the intensively studied effects of the London smog of December 1952. The increase in deaths in this London episode was marked and was more especially a result of an increased mortality from chronic bronchitis and other lung diseases, as demonstrated in Logan's analysis (Fig. 7-3).[9]

Cultural Background

Expected behavior which has its roots in the value-system regulates such fundamental requirements for social functioning as reciprocal role behavior. A social unit functions when its members perform their roles in the expectation that others will fulfill theirs. Marriage and the family, schools and universities, student bodies, and industry and work groups all depend on this mutual fulfillment of expected behavior. Without such reciprocal role behavior there is disequilibrium and disorganization, and eventually no shared goals.

Culture, Behavior, and Health. The cultural background of customary practices and of the relational system of different social groups involves the basic values and attitudes of these groups.

The body of knowledge of a group, involving concepts of the nature of health and cause of disease, while not shared by all individuals of the group, exerts its influence on their daily practices. Thus many mothers, when asked the reasons for particular infant rearing practices, may merely state "this is the way to do this," or more tolerantly, "this is the way we do this." Their actions may be determined by a specialist, a traditional practitioner, a doctor, a nurse, perhaps even more often an older woman, their own mothers, husband's mother, or a wise older lady of the village. In this way, a culture provides a ready answer as to what to do, what to eat and the way to eat, how to dress and maintain cleanliness, and how to perform all manners of activities of daily living. The individual does them because that is what is done and he does not need to explore or rediscover ways of acting that will meet certain needs.

INHERITANCE AND LIFE EXPERIENCE

A community's health reflects the interaction between the genetic constitution and life experience of its members. Differences in inheritance, in behavior, and in environment are expressed in the differential distribution of health and disease among various segments of the community.

At conception a newly-formed zygote inherits a constitution, "*G*," and immediately begins active behavior as a new individual interacting with his environment. This is the beginning of a continuing life experience within his environment.

The meaningful element of life experience is that which has been internalized and is an integral part of the individual. It is these internalized experiences which modify the developing organism. This process continues with succeeding experiences in a continuum of constitutional development and change (Fig. 7-4). The state of health may be viewed as a product of the integration between genetic qualities (*G*), internalized past experiences (*Ex*), and present life situation.

Inheritance

Genetic diversity between populations is associated with differences in health status and genetic determinants of disease are an obvious area of epidemiologic relevance. So too is the role of genetic determinants in the variation of health-related characteristics within a population. Related to this central interest of community medicine in genetics are the

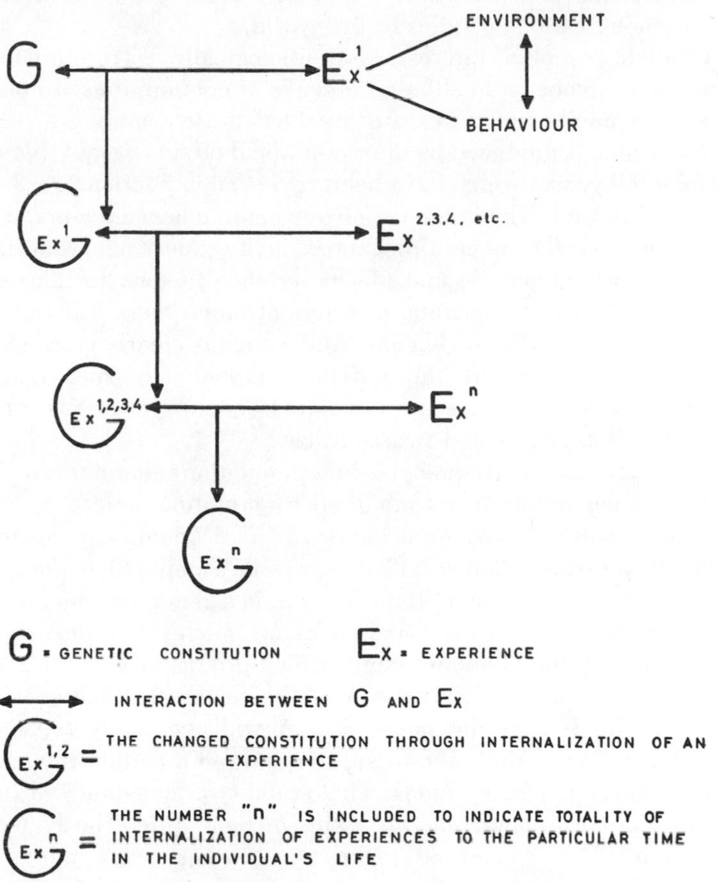

FIG. 7-4. Illustrating the change in constitution through internalization of experience.

findings of population geneticists concerning the genetic diversity of population groups and the causes of these variations, including the influence of disease on the biologic fitness of the group.

There are a number of diseases in which the main cause is readily determined to be genetic. These are the conditions recognized to be caused by a single gene, genes at a single locus, or by chromosomal abnormalities. They are relatively uncommon when viewed against the overall prevalence of disease in most communities, but because of their clear genetic mode of transmission and their clinical relevance they have been of major interest in medical genetics. They are classified as disorders of autosomal dominant, recessive, or intermediate inheritance; sex-linked (X-linked) inheritance;

and chromosomal abnormalities.[10-12] The disorders have different frequencies among various peoples of the world.

Of much potential interest epidemiologically is the influence of polygenic inheritance on health and disease of communities. In polygenic inheritance a number of genes are involved in determining a particular character, which is produced by their combined effect. Height, blood pressure, and intelligence, which have been reviewed in Section 1, are characteristics of this kind. The influence of polygenic inheritance is not always readily distinguished from multiple factors in life experience. Multifactorial causation, in which genetic and life experience factors are closely knit, makes delineation of the genetic component much more difficult than in those disorders in which single gene inheritance is clearly marked. Investigations aimed to measure the genetic component in such health and disease attributes may involve study of gene frequency in various population groups, as well as family and twin studies.

Gene Frequency. Gene frequencies in a population remain the same from generation to generation if not modified by mutation, selection, or other factors which will be considered below. Thus a "dominant" gene is not dominant in the sense that it will increase in a population group at the expense of a "recessive" gene. It means that in a genotype which is heterozygous, consisting of dominant and recessive alleles, the phenotype will be determined by the dominant gene. Blood groups of genotype AO and AA will both appear as phenotype A, A being the dominant and O the recessive allele. It does not mean that A will eventually replace O in the population group. Both genes will continue to maintain the same frequency in succeeding generations. This stability or constancy of the gene frequency in a population is known as the Hardy-Weinberg phenomenon,[11,13,14] named after the two workers who independently described it. Stability or constancy of genetic frequency in a community may be interfered with by several processes.

Assortative Mating. This is a selective mating process wherein like tends to mate with like. The likeness may range through a number of social, physical, and psychologic attributes. Here, we are especially concerned with mating between family-related individuals, i.e., with consanguineous marriages. While this in itself will not affect the overall gene frequency, it will affect the frequency of homozygous recessive individuals in relation to heterozygous individuals. It does this by increasing the chances of mating between persons with similar genes because the more closely individuals are related, the more they have certain genes in common.

As a general principle it may be stated that "the rarer a recessive gene, the higher will be the chance of encountering the affected homozygotes among the offspring of consanguineous marriages. Also, the higher the frequency of cousin marriages in the population, the larger will be their contribution to the total of affected homozygotes."[15]

Gene Flow. Gene flow represents the opposite process from consanguineous mating or mating within a small isolate. It is a change in genetic constitution of a group due to new genes being introduced by mating between members of different population groups. Examples of this are intermarriage between a migrant population and a host community, or mating during invasion and conquest.

Genetic Drift. By genetic drift is meant the chance occurrence of a gene in a particular group for reasons unrelated to mutation or selection. A small group of migrants may readily differ from the larger population which it leaves: "some genes from the original population may not be included. . . . while others may be over-represented.[14] Thus, the migration of a small group of people from one country to another may by chance have included one or several persons with a particular gene which is rare in the community from which they came and may even not have been noted. The gene may become common in the descendents of the pioneer group of migrants, and accordingly this type of genetic drift is known as the "founder effect."

Examples of such "founder effects" are Dean's description of porphyria variegata[11,16,17] in some 9,000 descendants of a couple who married in 1688 in South Africa, McKusick's report of dwarfism-polydactyly among the Old Order Amish of Pennsylvania,[13] and possibly Tay-Sachs disease among those Ashkenazy Jews whose ancestors came mainly from villages of southern Lithuania and north-east Poland.[18,19]

Fertility and Gene Frequency. Another aspect of the chance occurrence of genes in a population is related to differences in fertility which are not a function of the genetic constitution itself. There are considerable differences in fertility between individual married couples, between social classes and ethnic or religious groups, and between different communities and nations. Social factors are the main causes of differential fertility and hence of differences in growth of various segments of a population. The increasing facility to control reproduction is perhaps the most important single factor differentiating reproduction rates. The differential population growth may well affect the gene frequency of succeeding generations. Thus it has been estimated that only 12 percent of Frenchmen living at the time of the French revolution in 1789 were represented by their progeny in the generation living in 1880.[15] In prognostic studies of the frequency of genes which are of epidemiologic interest demographic investigations of reproductive rates, family size, and mating are therefore important.

Mutation and Selection. Characteristic of genes is their capacity to replicate themselves identically. Gene mutation, i.e., change in a gene, occurs spontaneously and at a low rate in relation to the genetic totality. Thus, while replication is a characteristic of genes, so too are mutations. Replication of such mutant genes is uncommon. They are usually disadvantageous to the individual inheriting them and may discontinue in the group if their detrimental effects result in death before maturity or otherwise prevent reproduction. However, they may be biologically advantageous, and under such circumstances, even though rare, they may be perpetuated in the population.

Natural selection does not only determine survival of a species in the broad sense of the term, but it is also involved in survival or disappearance of particular genetic traits. Two common health problems of recent times have resulted from advances in medical treatment and environmental sanitation. The development of mutant strains of organisms resistant to the effects of particular antibiotics results in selective survival of the resistant population. These mutations are chance events, not stimulated by the drug itself, but the drug then acts as a selective agent of the resistant strains.[20,21] Similarly, insecticide resistance of arthropods[21] is a world health problem both in the direct impact of insecticides on the spread of infections by arthropod vectors, and on the disturbance in the ecology of the habitat due to change in the dosage of the insecticide to meet the challenge of resistance. Another commonly quoted example of natural selection in modern times has been the increase of the dark-colored moth in England since the industrial revolution.[22–24]

The genetic implications of attempts at biologic control have been illustrated by the epidemiologic observations of Fenner and his associates in Australia.[25–27] The European rabbit, which was originally introduced to Australia by settlers from Europe, bred to the extent that it became a pest. All attempts failed until the myxoma virus was introduced. This virus occurs naturally in wild rabbits of Brazil, causing them relatively mild disease. When introduced to Australia it caused severe disease which spread through the rabbit-infested area of Australia between 1950 and 1957, reducing the rabbit population to between 1 to 2 percent of its premyxoma infection level. The infection is spread by mosquitos acting as mechanical transmitters; there is no evidence of virus multiplication in the mosquito. By 1955 the disease was becoming less severe due to changes in the rabbits and in the virus. The more resistant rabbits which survived the rapidly fatal early epidemics bred and thus produced a more resistant rabbit population. In addition, the virus became less virulent, a fact which was confirmed when the virus was tested against rabbits which had not been exposed to the early epidemics. Dobzhansky[14] has summarized the results of this "natural" experiment.

> Death of the host means death of the parasite: the longer an infected rabbit remains alive the greater the chance that a mosquito will transfer the virus it contains to another rabbit. Natural selection favored a mutual accommodation between the virus and the Australian rabbit; the situation observed in the Brazilian rabbit is perhaps a result of such an accommodation.

Natural selection and mutation may maintain a balance when the rate of mutation corresponds with the rate at which the trait is eliminated. This is what is thought to occur with a number of mutants, as in achondroplastic dwarfism where a low rate of mutation is accompanied by a low rate of survival and the condition is maintained as a relatively infrequent occurrence.

There may be a condition in which genes may be both advantageous and disadvantageous: they may be disadvantageous in the homozygote, but may be advantageous in the heterozygote. Thus a mutant gene may be lethal in the homozygote genotype but, when present with an alternate allele on the same locus, the heterozygote may be advantageous to survival. Not only may the heterozygote be superior to the mutant homozygote, but also to the normal homozygote. The maintenance of the heterozygote is thus of advantage to the population. There may be many examples of this but at the present there are only a very limited number in which a definitive epidemiologic relation with a health condition has been found, such as sickling and plasmodium falciparum malaria. The subject is further discussed in Chapter 16 regarding some genetic consideration of the epidemiology of infection and disease.

The similarity in genetic structure of members of various groups is estimated by the proportion of genes they are likely to have in common. This varies according to the closeness of the relationship, from the near-identical structure of monozygous twins to that of immediate family and to more distant kin and ethnically-related groups.

In small isolated communities in which varying degrees of inbreeding have been common for generations, the members will have a relatively high proportion of genes in common. There are often characteristic features in the genetic structure of such a community which distinguish it from others. The Kalahari Bushmen of Botswana differ from other Africans in their physique and in the distribution of a number of blood genetic markers; this is evidence of the long period of their history over which they lived in isolation from other African peoples.[28] These characteristics often emerge as distinct for different ethnic groups when they leave their relatively isolated living and migrate to other countries or to the cities. Kurdish Jews now living in Israel have a relatively high frequency of thalassemia and of G6PD deficiency.[29] Study of those who migrated from Eastern Turkey and from Northern Iraq indicate that they ". . . share certain features which set them apart from all other ethnic groups studied so far."[30,31] In contrast to the relative homogeneity of isolated communities is the heterogeneity of modern industrial metropolitan communities, which were originally formed through mass migrations of people from different rural communities and often from different countries. Between these extremes there are many communities which have distinct genetic characteristics and yet resemble other communities of the region, suggesting common ancestral genes or varying degrees of gene flow between groups that may at some time have been markedly different.

Life Experience

In the present context, the term experience extends beyond its more usual connotation of knowledge based on previous observation or on feelings arising from earlier incidents in life. It also involves diverse experiences such as the following.

Feeding practices and dietary habits determining nutritional status, metabolism and growth
Experiences conditioning the nervous system which determine subsequent behavior
Learning by experience from exposure to antigens in development of immunity.

Life experience is determined by the social and environmental settings in which it takes place. One of the central epidemiologic questions in community medicine concerns the role of the social group as a determinant of the health of its members. Epidemiologically, does the social group have meaning beyond the aggregate of health and personal characteristics of its individuals? The health of a group is usually described in quantitative measurements of various aggregates of individuals: mortality rates, incidence and prevalence rates of diseases, or distributions of health-relevant characteristics—anthropometric, biochemical, or psychologic. Analysis of associations between these health variables and those describing the personal characteristics of the individuals may indicate causal relationships. However, the association may only be found in certain settings and even if a causal association is established it may only be valid in a particular social situation. Thus when the social factors determining a health state in a population group are sought, it is not only the personal characteristics of individuals that will need examination, but also qualities of the group as a whole. While there is a unique quality to the life experience of all individuals, there is much that is shared with others. As in genetic constitution, shared experience involving both personal behavior and similar environmental exposure varies from the intensely close resemblance in the life experience of identical twins, through that between members of the same family, to the similarities within an ethnic group. Ethnic groups may be viewed as "an aggregate of kinship units, the members of which either trace their origin in terms of descent from a common ancestor or in terms of descent from ancestors who all belonged to the same categorized ethnic group."[32] There is also the shared life experience of schoolmates and other peer groups, and that of religious groups or other special-interest groups, as well as those of various social strata definable as social classes or as educational and occupational categories.

Members of a community with a relatively homogeneous culture will share much of their life experience. Such culture groups include traditional, relatively isolated rural communities with little or slow culture change. They will obviously have similar customary practices and will relate with one another in a relatively stable framework of well-established roles. There will be a high degree of reciprocity in role behavior and in concordance between expected and actual behavior. Members of such a community will tend to rear their children in similar ways, thereby transmitting their culture as a homogeneous social heritage to the next generation. This rearing will be in marked contrast to that of other communities, and will express itself in the distinctive culture of each particular group. The early life experience of children is a foundation of their physical and personality development. Thus, even though there are individual differences, it may be expected that there will be a pattern of health in a relatively homogeneous group which distinguishes it from other groups which have different cultures.

When both the cultural and genetic factors of a population group are distinct it may be expected that the patterns of health of its various segments will resemble one another, and wide differences in its subgroups will not be a feature of the overall picture of health. On the other hand, in heterogeneous, changing communities the picture will be very different, not only from that of smaller homogeneous communities, but also between subgroups of the total heterogeneous community. It may be expected that there will be marked differences in the health status of different segments of the community, and these differences will probably extend to the pattern of disease, as well as to their somatic and psychologic characteristics.

Genetic and cultural processes guide the life experiences of all members of a community, setting limits to expectation of life, to responses to the environment, and to their behavior. In turn, internalization of life experience continually modifies the constitution of the members (Fig. 7-4) which, in its interaction with their changing personal life situation and the environment, determines their health.

REFERENCES

1. Arensberg CM, Kimball ST: Culture and Community. New York, Harcourt, 1965, p 268.
2. Cooley CH: Social Organization. New York, Scribner's, 1909. Republished: New York, Schocken Books, 1962, pp 23, 24.
3. Berelson B, Steiner GA: Human Behavior. New York, Harcourt, 1964, pp 331, 332.

4. Lee RB, Devore I (eds.): Man the Hunter. Chicago, Aldine, 1968.
5. Steinbeck J: The Grapes of Wrath. London, Heinemann, 1939.
6. Carson R: The Silent Spring. New York, Houghton Mifflin, 1962.
7. Chadwick E: Report on the Sanitary Condition of the Labouring Population of Great Britain, 1842. Republished by Flinn MW (ed.). Edinburgh, Edinburgh Univ Press, 1964.
8. von Pettenkoffer M: The Value of Health to a City, 1873. Translated and presented by HE Sigerist. Baltimore, The Johns Hopkins University Press, 1941.
9. Logan WPD: Mortality in the London fog incident, 1952. Lancet 1:336, 1953.
10. Carter CO: An ABC of Medical Genetics. London, Lancet, 1965.
11. Fraser Roberts JA: An Introduction to Medical Genetics, 5th ed. London, Oxford Univ Press, 1970.
12. McKusick VA: Medical genetics. In Harvey AM, Cluff LE, Johns RJ, et al. (eds.): The Principles and Practice of Medicine, 17th ed. New York, Appleton, 1968.
13. McKusick VA: Human Genetics. Englewood Cliffs, New Jersey, Prentice-Hall, 1964.
14. Dobzhansky T: Mankind Evolving: The Evolution of the Human Species. New Haven, Yale Univ Press, 1962, pp 282, 303.
15. Sutter J: The relationship between human population genetics and demography. In Goldschmidt E (ed.): The Genetics of Migrant and Isolate Populations. New York, Williams and Wilkins, 1963, p 160.
16. Dean G: The Porphyrias: A Story of Inheritance and Environment. London, Pitman Medical, 1963.
17. Dean G: The porphyrias. Brit Med Bull 25:48, 1969.
18. Livingstone FB: The founder effect and deleterious genes. Am J Phys Anthropol 30:55, 1969.
19. Chase GA, McKusick VA: Founder effect in Tay-Sachs disease. Am J Hum Genet 24:339, 1972.
20. Tepper BS: Microbial resistance to drugs. In Sladen BK, Bang FB (eds.): Biology of Populations. New York, American Elsevier, 1969.
21. Brown AWA: Insecticide Resistance in Arthropods. WHO Monogr Ser 38: 1, 1958.
22. Kettlewell HBD: The phenomenon of industrial melanism in the Lipidoptera. Ann Rev Entomol 6:245, 1961.
23. Kettlewell HBD: Selection experiments on industrial melanism in the Lipidoptera. Heredity 9:323, 1955.
24. Kettlewell HBD: Further selection experiments on industrial melanism in the Lipidoptera. Heredity 10:287, 1956.
25. Fenner F, Day MF, Woodroofe GM: Epidemiologic consequences of the mechanical transmission of myxomatosis by mosquitos. J Hyg 54:284, 1956.
26. Fenner F, Marshall ID: A comparison of the virulence for European rabbit (oryctolagus cuniculus) of strains of myxoma virus recovered in the field in Australia, Europe, and America. J Hyg 55:149, 1957.
27. Fenner F: Myxomatosis in the Australian Wild Rabbit—Evolutionary changes in an Infectious Disease. Harvey Lectures 1957–1958. New York, New York Academy, 1959.
28. Tobias PV: The peoples of Africa south of the Sahara. In Baker PT, Weiner JS (eds.): The Biology of Human Adaptability. Oxford, Clarendon, 1966.
29. Cohen T, Bloch N, Goldschmidt E, et al.: G6PD deficiency and thalassemia

in Jews from Kurdistan. In Goldschmidt E (ed.): The Genetics of Migrant and Isolatc Populations. New York, Williams and Wilkins, 1963.
30. Steinberg AG, Levene C, Goldschmidt E, et al.: The Gm and Inv allotypes in kindreds of Kurdish Jews. Am J Hum Genet 22:652, 1970.
31. Horowitz A, Cohen T, Goldschmidt E, et al.: Thalassemia types among Kurdish Jews in Israel. Brit J Haematol 12:555, 1966.
32. Parsons T: The Social System. Glencoe, Ill, Free Press, 1951, p 172.

8
Culture and Health

The epidemiologic relevance of culture for health involves methodical study of the causal role of culture, or specific elements of culture, on health and disease distribution. Comparative studies of health in different culture groups are the foundations of geography of disease. Similar kinds of thinking stimulate historical studies of change in the health and disease pattern in relation to culture change over time. Geographic and historic comparison are thus often starting-points for investigation of disease. There is the more difficult task of studying the cultural impact on health within a relatively homogeneous culture group, especially when the investigator is part of the group and regards his life experience and the culture of his community as "normal." Perception and recognition of culture as a determinant of health of one's own community came late in the health services, more especially since it pertains to change in personal behavior in order to improve the community's health.

MEANING OF CULTURE

Society and culture describe closely related social characteristics of man. "Society is grouping; culture is the patterning of behavior in groups,"[1] or, even more simply stated by Stuart Chase, "A *society* refers to a group of people who have learned to work together. A *culture* refers to the way of life which the group follows."[2]

The essential characteristics of culture have been concisely outlined by Parsons: ". . . Culture is *transmitted,* it constitutes a heritage or a social tradition; secondly, . . . it is *learned,* it is not a manifestation, in particular content, of man's genetic constitution; and third, . . . it is *shared.*"[3]

Its meaning for the individuals of a community is clearly conveyed by the following extract from Ruth Benedict's *Patterns of Culture:*

> The life history of the individual is first and foremost an accommodation to the patterns and standards traditionally handed down in his community. From the moment of his birth the customs into which he is born shape his experience and behavior. By the time he can talk, he is the little creature of his culture, and by the time he is grown and able to take part in its activities, its habits are his habits, its beliefs his beliefs, its impossibilities his impossibilities.[4]

> Culture provides the rules, that define the roles that make the relationships that constitute the group.[5]

As such, culture is perhaps the most relevant social determinant of community health. Its influence on health penetrates through prevailing concepts about the nature and cause of health and disease; these concepts are then translated into action in the health care system as a whole, and in personal and group health practices. The pervasive effects of culture are evident in the ways in which communities promote health and prevent disease, and in the provisions they make for care of the sick and disabled. Use of these facilities and health-relevant behavior in the family, at school and at work, or in love and play are intrinsic elements of culture. Furthermore there are the many specific customs which influence health but can often only be understood through their place and meaning within a particular culture.

Families of a particular group do not share all aspects of the culture nor do parents transmit its totality to their children. Different aspects of the culture are given varying emphasis, producing what are, in effect, many family subcultures. Similarly, different social classes and religious or ethnic groups of a particular society, while sharing much of the society's culture, differ from one another sufficiently to be recognizably dissimilar in their behavior.

While social classes may cut across national boundaries, it would be wrong to assume that the subculture of such classes is the same in all nations. The subculture of an upper social class in one country may resemble that of a similar social class in another country and yet differ from it in major respects of relevance to health. Both the similarities and the differences are of epidemiologic interest. Thus in almost every industrialized society social class differences in life expectation are marked,[6,7] but this is not to state that life expectation is the same in similar social classes in different parts of the world. The association between social class and mortality rates at different ages, and hence in life expectation, may be caused by a considerable number of behavioral factors.

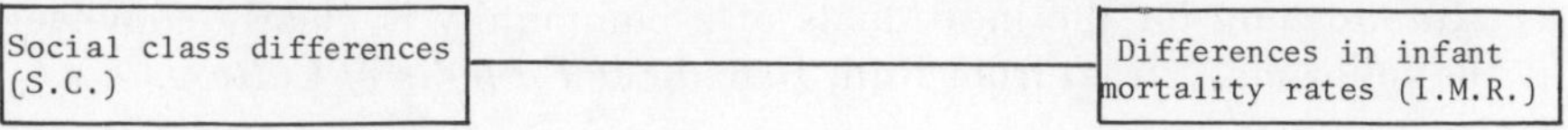

FIG. 8-1. Diagram representing the differential infant mortality rates according to social class.

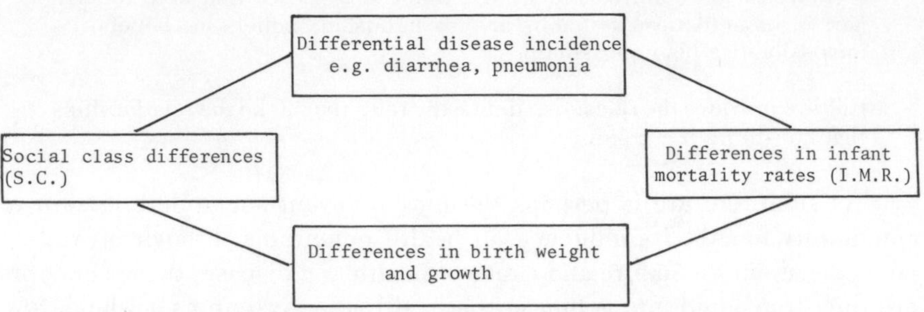

FIG. 8-2. The intervening variables, disease and somatic characteristics, which result in differential infant mortality rates according to social class.

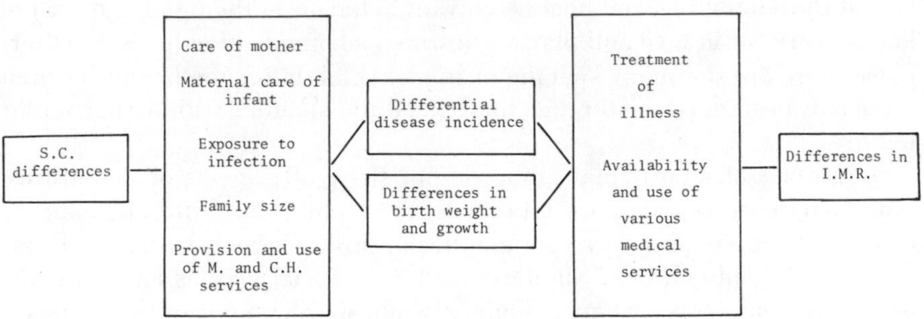

FIG. 8-3. The causal connections between the associations of Figure 8-2 shown as differences in behavior.

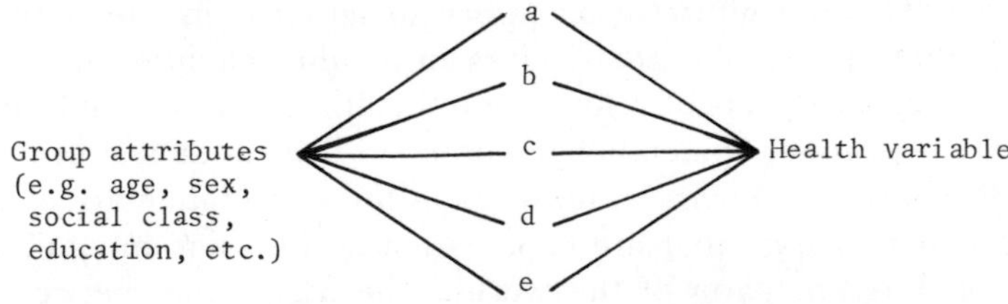

FIG. 8-4. General model of behavioral factors which determine an association between group attributes and a health variable.

The well-known association between social class and infant mortality rate may be expressed in the following model, in which the relation between the independent variable, social class, and the dependent variable, infant mortality rate, is analyzed. The analysis follows through intervening variables of health and disease (Fig. 8-1). Often the investigation is not carried further to elucidate the role of behavioral variables in the differential incidence of these conditions and in their outcome. The importance of their inclusion is shown in the second part of the model (Fig. 8-2). An association between social class or other group characteristics of a population and a particular health variable can often be causally linked by behavioral factors which are culturally determined, as shown in Figures 8-3 and 8-4.

CUSTOMARY PRACTICES AND HEALTH

There are basic biologic needs around which much of culture is developed and it is the germane customary practices surrounding these needs that are often of direct relevance to health and survival of the population group. They include:

Diet and feeding practices
Protection from injury or exposure, e.g., housing, clothing, and protection from infection
Care of sickness and prevention of disease
Sex relations and reproduction

Behavioral determinants of health are often part of a causal chain or network. In many communities survival depends on successful initiation and maintenance of breast-feeding. The ease with which lactation is established and breast-feeding maintained is a striking feature of such communities. The expected behavior of these mothers is breast-feeding, usually for considerable periods of time. There are several culturally prescribed actions which in themselves may or may not be consciously directed to ensuring adequate breast-feeding but which have this effect. In a study of a rural peasant community[8] the following relevant observations were made:

The high rate of breast-feeding in this community was shown by the fact that 99.4 percent of babies were being breast-fed at one month of age. The proportion declined very slowly during the first year, namely, 99.2 , 96.6, 96.3, and 84.4 percent of babies were breast-fed at ages of 3, 6, 9, and 12 months, respectively. Engorgement of breasts and breast abscess were very rare, and cracked nipples or complaints of tender nipples seldom noted.

When for some reason the mother could not breast-feed, which was usually due to maternal death or severe illness, the baby died unless an alternative breast-feeding arrangement was made. The reestablishment of lactation by the grandmother was sometimes successful.

Good mothering was highly valued. This involved the value of fertility and of rearing children, the basic element of which was survival. Successful lactation was essential for this. Women reached their highest status as mothers of grown-up children, especially as mothers of adult sons.

There were several interesting practices which were supportive of this highly valued role of mothering. Topless dress was traditional for young girls before marriage. Among school-goers and others who were from nontraditional homes, blouses and full dresses were worn but the brassiere and other tight binding of breasts was uncommon. Self-manipulation of nipples and breasts was commonly practiced through puberty, to ensure a well everted nipple and firm breasts. The stated objectives were cosmetic, not subsequent performance in lactation. Inverted or flattened nipples were very rarely seen in health care of mothers and infants.

Another common practice was breast massage. In this case the purpose was to initiate breast-feeding. Following birth, the baby was not put to the breast until colostrum had been replaced by milk. This lasted from 3 to 5 days and sometimes more, during which time the baby was fed other foods. The mother's breasts were massaged, warm cloths applied and the breasts milked to extract colostrum, after which feeding of the baby would start. Demand breast-feeding was the practice; time control was not a factor, and feeding times remained irregular with the mother adjusting in an easy ongoing feeding relationship.

The successful initiation of breast-feeding was seen as the foundation of a continuing function of comforting the baby, i.e., as part of a physically close mother-baby relationship. Babies slept with their mothers, who were required by custom not to have coitus with their husbands while breast-feeding. When the mother went to work, or went visiting or on various errands, she usually carried her baby tied on her back.

Table 8-1 summarizes the practices which were directly or indirectly associated with successful initiation and maintenance of breast-feeding in this community.

The extent to which the behavior is prescribed by the culture is of importance. A practice may be found to be common and yet not be deeply rooted in the value- and belief-system of the community. Another customary practice may be so rooted in the value system as to appear immutable. One may speak of these practices respectively as "soft points" of the culture, i.e., readily changeable or changing; and "hard points" of the

TABLE 8-1. Practices Which are Directly or Indirectly Associated with the Successful Initiation and Maintenance of Breast-feeding in a Rural Peasant Community

	CUSTOMARY PRACTICES	HEALTH-RELEVANT RESULTS
Puberty	Nipple and breast manipulation —everting nipple	Hardening of nipples Nipples everted, prominent
Dress	Topless or loose-fitting blouses Brassiere or other tight binding of breasts not used	Firm, everted nipples, exposed with no flattening
Postnatal days	Massage of breasts until free of colostrum before putting baby to breast	Free flow of breast milk
Breast-feeding	No time-control or time-regulation Baby fed by its "demand" and by mother's "feeling"	Breasts fill readily and milk flows with ease Breast very seldom engorged Cracked nipples very rare

culture, i.e., persistent or very slowly changing. In the rural community just referred to, the use of cereal drinks in the first week of life was a readily changeable practice; although widespread it was a recent innovation associated with decline of cows' milk production. A very much harder point to change, if one had tried to do so, would have been the introduction of time or clock-regulated feeding. Not only was the clock not yet a part of this peasant community's daily living (hence there were no clock-time norms for work and household activity), but there was rejection of the thought of denying a baby its comfort when in need. "Why should a mother want to do that?"

It is often difficult to recognize the effect on health of a custom which is deeply rooted in a community's culture. This is especially so if the custom is thought to be harmful. The history of medicine, and of thought and science in general, is replete with examples of the violent response of a society to the questioning of its basic values as expressed through its institutions and through the customary behavior of its members. Fortunately many customs are not so deeply rooted as to prevent investigation into their impact on health, and, if found harmful, for the people to conceive of their change. How can epidemiologic inferences be made regarding the role of customary practices in causing disease or in determining other psychologic and somatic characteristics of health relevance? Inferences about the causal role of custom, especially if it is the custom of groups other than that of the "judge or observer," are readily made but are difficult to prove.

There are many communities who defecate in their rivers and thereby pollute the water supplies which they themselves and others drink. There are now many communities who fill the atmosphere with smoke from industry and home fires and with the exhaust from motor vehicles, thereby polluting the air they themselves and others breathe.

When Koch's postulates, used for establishing a microorganism as the specific cause of a disease, are applied to the complex question of relating customary practices to the health of a community, they limit the scope of study to specific causal factors which are themselves products of the particular custom.

In the first case referred to above, custom has converted water into a vehicle carrying organic matter which may contain potentially pathogenic organisms. In the second case, air has been converted into a vehicle laden with physical and chemical pathogenic substances. The fact that both the water and the air are vehicles of pathogenic substances and not pathogenic in themselves does not absolve them as main causal factors of the diseases which result from exposure to them. Thus polluted water is not the only way a community may be infected with salmonella typhosi, but as one of the important vehicles of this organism it is often a cause of epidemics of typhoid fever. Similarly, the customs that produce the pollution are causal of the diseases that result from it. And it is these practices that often need change.

In considering the concept of causality, Lilienfeld felt that it was reasonable to adopt a pragmatic approach. "One major reason for determining etiological factors of human disease is to use this knowledge to prevent the disease. Therefore, a factor may be defined as a cause of a disease, if the incidence of the disease is diminished when exposure to this factor is likewise diminished."[9] Support for such a concept should not be interpreted as discounting the importance of a continuing search for specific causal networks of various health conditions. It does, however, emphasize that the whole or macroscopic elements of the network should always be investigated, not only to provide greater understanding of the circumstances under which disease occurs, but also because action at this level is often very effective in controlling the causal conditions and hence in preventing the disease.

This viewpoint is of particular help in our exploration of the determinant role of culture in community health. The factors which have played a part in secular changes in growth and maturation, outlined in Chapter 4, no doubt include important changes in customary practices: diet in its relation to nutrition, sanitation in relation to transmission of infection, and especially food hygiene. The history of cigarette smoking is an outstanding example of a habit which has become a widespread practice, increasingly accepted first among men, then women, and still more recently among adolescents and even younger children. Its relation to a number of diseases has been the subject of a large number of epidemiologic studies, on the basis of which several comprehensive reviews have been published.[10–14]

Cigarette smoking is now suspected as a cause of increase in mortality rates and of conditions such as lung cancer, chronic bronchitis, ischemic heart disease, gastric and duodenal ulcer, and low birthweight. The fact that cigarette smoking is associated with so many conditions has raised doubts about its causal role. The nonspecificity of the relationship between cigarette smoking and the various diseases, and the fact that experimental evidence is lacking, are among the questionable aspects of its causal role. The question that arises is at what point is it reasonable to accept the probability of a causal relationship between a customary practice, such as smoking, and various diseases? And as a corollary to this, at what point is it unreasonable, and even unethical, to delay taking action?

A custom and a particular health variable, or a syndrome of the variable, can be regarded as related or associated if the health variable changes according to the degree to which the custom is practiced. The relation may be direct or inverse. Such an association or correlation is not in itself evidence of a causal relationship but is a first step in the investigative process. Further consideration in attributing a causal role to customary practices involves epidemiologic investigation of the strength or degree of the association between the dependent and independent variables, and the consistency of the association. The time element is itself fundamental in determining the direction of a causal relationship. Did the customary practice precede the appearance of the particular health condition under consideration? Historical evidence based on incidence studies is of importance in answering this question, but experimental epidemiologic investigation is desirable, when practicable and ethical. The evidence may be summarized as follows.

Indirect Evidence

Communities in which the disease is common are those in which the particular custom is practiced. Historical changes and geographic differential distributions are of interest in this regard.

Direct Evidence

Retrospective Studies. The custom is more commonly practiced by persons with the condition than in comparable persons who do not have the particular condition.

Prospective Studies. Follow-up studies of cohorts of people who practice the custom compared with those who do not, demonstrate a higher incidence of the health condition in the former group. The length of time and the intensity with which the practice is carried out are also factors determining differences.

Experimental Studies. Studies of the effects of changing practices are, by their very objective of experimentally modifying a custom, dependent on the "hardness" or "softness" of the particular custom; i.e., such studies depend upon the ease with which people are prepared to change. Furthermore, some direct experiments, such as stimulating the practice of a suspected harmful habit, are unethical and not possible in human epidemiologic studies. Less direct experimental studies are those in which experimental groups are encouraged towards the potentially desired behavior, such as reduction in cigarette smoking, changing diet, and so on.

The association may not be demonstrable in all situations. Thus hypertension is associated with a high rate of ischemic heart disease in some communities, while in others where hypertension is present ischemic heart disease is rare. In this event hypertension is a *cause* of ischemic heart disease in some circumstances but not in others. The concept of a network of factors operating together is important in this regard. One factor may be neither necessary nor sufficient in itself to cause a disease but it may well be an important cause under some circumstances.

Another consideration in making inferences as to the causal role of a customary practice is that they should be in accord with scientific thought, i.e., they make "biologic sense."[9]

REFERENCES

1. Gillin JL, Gillin JP: Cultural Sociology, rev. ed. New York, Macmillan, 1948, p 140.
2. Chase S: The Proper Study of Mankind. New York, Harper & Brothers, 1948, p 61.
3. Parsons T: The Social System. Glencoe, Ill, Free Press, 1951, p 15.
4. Benedict R: Patterns of Culture. New York, Mentor, New American Library, 1934, p 2.
5. Wilson EK: Sociology: Rules, Roles, and Relationships. Homewood, Ill, Dorsey, 1966, p 45.
6. Antonovsky A: Social class, life expectancy and overall mortality. Milbank Mem Fund Q 45:31, 1967.
7. Morris JN: Uses of Epidemiology, 2nd ed. Edinburgh, E & S Livingstone 1964.
8. Kark SL: The initiation of breast-feeding. In Kark SL, Steuart GW (eds.): A Practice of Social Medicine. Edinburgh, E & S Livingstone, 1962.
9. Lilienfeld AM: Epidemiological methods and inferences in studies of noninfectious diseases. Public Health Rep 72:51, 1957.

10. US Public Health Service: Health Consequences of Smoking, Public Health Service Publication No. 1696. Washington, DC, Government Printing Office, 1967.
11. US Public Health Service: Health Consequences of Smoking, PHS Publication No. 1696, Supplements for 1968 and 1969. Washington, DC, Government Printing Office, 1968, 1969.
12. Royal College of Physicians: Smoking and Health. London, Pitman Medical & Scientific, 1962.
13. Royal College of Physicians: Smoking and Health Now. London, Pitman Medical & Scientific, 1971.
14. Fletcher CM, Horn D: Smoking and Health. WHO Chron 24:345, 1970.

9
Some Epidemiologic Considerations of Continuity in Life Experience

Meaningful associations between distributions of health and disease in demographic or social groupings are those which stimulate fruitful hypotheses regarding causal factors. These may be the foundation for further analytic or experimental epidemiologic research or they may be used in planning health services and action programs in the interests of the public's health. The causal factors with which we are presently concerned are the life experiences, past and present, of the community as a whole and of its various cohort groups.

Life experience involves attributes which are opposite and yet complementary, e.g., continuity and change, acquisition and loss. Taken together these are attributes of the life span of all individuals and of the groups which they form. Measurement of the meaning of life experience for health requires careful consideration of these qualities. The significance of past life experience in determining the present picture of health and disease is generally accepted, but epidemiologic methods of investigating the specifics of these relationships are limited.

THE COHORT PHENOMENON

An historical change in the age distribution of various diseases may be evidence of an ongoing effect of past life experiences. Thus the pandemic of encephalitis lethargica of 1917 to 1926 was followed by a considerable change in the age distribution of parkinsonism, of which the most important cause is encephalitis lethargica.

Before the epidemic the mean age of onset of parkinsonism in the

United Kingdom was in the fifties. The immediate result of the epidemic was a rise in the incidence of postencephalitic parkinsonism and the mean age of new cases dropped by some 15 years. Cases of parkinsonism continued to occur in those who were exposed to the epidemic, with the mean age of new cases rising steadily. By 1971 the mean age of onset approached that before the pandemic of encephalitis lethargica of 1917 to 1926. The age of onset of parkinsonism can be expected to rise still further as the cohort of people affected during the encephalitis epidemic of 1917 to 1926 dies off, providing there is not another epidemic of encephalitis. Cohort analysis of this kind can add much to understanding secular change in age distribution of various diseases or their prevalence at a particular time.

In his use of the cohort method in a study of tuberculosis death rates, Wade Hampton Frost made a basic contribution to the epidemiologic method of studying the continuity of effects of earlier life experience on the apparent change in age distribution of a disease.[1] Studying the age selection of mortality from tuberculosis in different decades over the period 1880 to 1930 in Massachusetts, he found the following.

> Looking at the 1930 curve, the impression given is that nowadays an individual encounters his greatest risk of death from tuberculosis between the ages of fifty and sixty. But this is not really so; the people making up the 1930 age group fifty to sixty have, in earlier life, passed through *greater* mortality risks.

He demonstrated this in a number of illustrative figures and in a table of the data. The table is reproduced here as Table 9-1.

Susser and Stein have used this method of cohort analysis in a study of the changing age occurrence of peptic ulcer in England and Wales.[2]

Positive findings in a cohort analysis are indicative of the fact that successive age cohorts have had a distinctive experience with a particular disease and probably with the determinants of the disease. When specific causes of death have their highest age specific rate in older people, this may be "a residual of higher rates in the earlier life" of that cohort.

The cohort approach, if it is to be more than a statement of the probable impact of the past on the present and future, must be supported by methods of study of factors that cause the cohort phenomenon. Longitudinal studies in which secular trends in somatic and psychologic attributes are analyzed together with a changing trend in disease occurrence would be better understood if studied in the context of the life experience of successive cohorts.

The world is now undergoing a rapid rate of change which is deeply affecting living habits and life styles in infant and child rearing, formal education of children and adults, family living, work and play, role differentiation and relationships between the sexes and between age groups, and

TABLE 9-1. Death Rates per 100,000 from Tuberculosis, All Forms, for Massachusetts, 1880 to 1930, by Age and Sex, with Rates for Cohort of 1880 Indicated

AGE	1880	1890	1900	1910	1920	1930
Males						
0–4	760	578	309	209	108	41
5–9	43	49	31	21	24	11
10–19	126	115	90	63	49	21
20–29	444	361	288	207	149	81
30–39	378	368	296	253	164	115
40–49	364	336	253	253	175	118
50–59	366	325	267	252	171	127
60–69	475	346	304	246	172	95
70 +	672	396	343	163	127	95
Females						
0–4	658	595	354	162	101	27
5–9	71	82	49	45	24	13
10–19	265	213	145	92	78	37
20–29	537	393	290	207	167	92
30–39	422	372	260	189	135	73
40–49	307	307	211	153	108	53
50–59	334	234	173	130	83	47
60–69	434	295	172	118	83	56
70 +	584	375	296	126	68	40

(From Frost.[1])

economic development and social stratification. It would be surprising if succeeding cohorts did not reflect different health problems. The resultant changes could be expected to have a continuity of effect on health and the cohort phenomenon illustrated by Frost's analysis should be found with respect to a number of diseases.

A disease will manifest the cohort phenomenon if its causes decline or cease to operate. The reappearance of the causes will change the age-cohort trend which had become apparent. Here it is important to stress that the reintroduction of one element of a causal network will not necessarily be followed by the disease being expressed as it had formerly expressed itself, unless the one element is accompanied by the other elements of the causal network.

The more a specific cause of a disease is sufficient in itself to cause the disease in question, with limited differences in gradient and expression, the more its reintroduction to a community is likely to change the age-cohort trend that had become apparent.

The investigation of change in life experience and health status is of central importance in epidemiology. It is not only of interest to ultimate understanding of historical processes affecting the health of populations, but in predicting the health outcome of current changes in life situations which, if modified, alter the prognosis for future health. Historical methods of study include examining the life history of cases, or histories of major events and changes affecting successive cohorts. The methods of study may be retrospective or prospective. Both are important and while the latter is the cohort method of choice, it is expensive, time consuming, not always practicable, and, therefore, must be used with discrimination.

CHILDHOOD EXPERIENCE, CULTURE, AND BEHAVIORAL DEVELOPMENT

The life experiences of individuals determine, and are determined by, the individuals' growth and development. Each phase of growth is succeeded by the next in a genetically ordered pattern of development characteristic for the species. The kind of development during one phase may therefore be expected to influence succeeding phases and the effects of interference with growth will depend on the phase of individual development at which it took place. The epidemiology of congenital malformations requires knowledge of fetal development in relation to events and experiences that have distinct effects at different phases of fetal life. Similarly, epidemiologic investigation of abnormal growth or behavior demands a foundation knowledge of the course which development follows, with its morphologic, physiologic, mental, and social aspects. Erikson [3–5] has formulated a concept of the healthy personality as a process of development of various personality components, the whole being dependent on a succession of phases developing at the "proper rate and the proper sequence." Theoretically, failure in development at any phase will pervade the personality structure during subsequent life. And this is no less true for a group than it is for the individual.

There are times in the life of many communities during which the family home is disrupted and members of the family are separated. Wars and natural disasters may create the demand for special residential facilities for infants and children. Even in "normal" times baby homes or residential nurseries, orphanages, and boarding schools are a feature of many communities. In their war-time observations of babies evacuated into residential nurseries Freud and Burlingham[6] noted contrasting implications of institutional rearing at different ages. From birth to 5 months of age babies in the Hampstead Nursery, London, developed better than comparable babies in their working-class homes, but the picture was reversed in the second half of the first year of life. The differences in the first 5 months of life were the more regular gain in weight among the nursery babies, their better general appearance, and less frequent intestinal disturbances. In the second half of the year the superiority of the family-reared babies was evidenced by their better social response and behavior development. During the second year they found the institutional child superior in muscular control and in feeding while the family child was superior in speech development and habit training. They conclude their observations in the following inferences.

> The institutional child in the first two years has advantages in all those spheres of his life which are independent of the emotional side of his nature; he is at a disadvantage wherever the emotional tie to the mother or to the family is the mainspring of development. Comparisons between children under these contrasting conditions serve to show that certain achievements such as speech and habit training are closely related to the child's emotions, even though this may not be apparent at first glance.[6]

The possibility of modifying behavioral development in an institutional setting and the differential response of distinctive elements of development noted by Freud and Burlingham have been demonstrated experimentally by Rheingold.[7] A group of 6-month-old babies in an institution, who were subjected to "mothering" by a single person over a period of 8 weeks, did not differ in motor skills but differed markedly in social responsiveness from a control group of babies who continued to have their routine institutional care. The difference in social responsiveness was not confined to the "mother figure" herself but extended to others as well.

The public health importance of the quality of social interaction in infancy and early childhood received widespread attention after the publication of a forceful and challenging monograph by John Bowlby, *Maternal Care and Mental Health*.[8] It is a review of the mental health aspects of homeless children which was carried out on behalf of the World Health Organization (WHO). When published by the WHO in 1951 it had an almost immediate impact on public health practice through its influence on social policy regarding the care and placement of children, and in the research it stimulated to test its main contentions. Its relevance for community health concerned its focus on the importance of a continuing, warm, mothering relationship through infancy and early childhood for healthy personality development and the converse result, i.e., the severe personality disturbance that could result from maternal deprivation.

In its severe form the syndrome has been called "psychopathic behavior disorder of childhood,"[9] "affectionless character,"[10] and "primary affect hunger."[11] "Anaclitic depression" was the term used by Spitz to describe the unfortunate children observed by him in a highly impersonal institutional setting, in which lack of expression and indifference to all that went on around them were outstanding features. "These children would lie or sit with wide open, expressionless eyes, frozen immobile face, and a faraway expression as if in a daze, apparently not perceiving what went on in their environment."[12]

In the many studies and discussions that followed the publication of Bowlby's 1951 monograph, it is clear that there are several distinctive aspects of the life experience of babies. They include the following.

Institutional care versus home care
Separation from mother versus continuity of being together with mother
Maternal deprivation versus "a warm, intimate, and continuous relationship with the mother (or permanent mother-substitute)"

It will be readily appreciated that there are many cases in which a baby's situation involves each of these elements. In fact, in the extreme types of care reviewed by Bowlby this was the situation. However, between the two extremes of care, at home by an accepting mother in a healthy, happy family setting, and that of the impersonal, isolated sterile institution, there are many potential variations in the kind of personal relationship framework within which the infant develops and is cared for.

As useful as "maternal deprivation" has been in calling attention to the importance of maternal care for subsequent mental health, it has been subject to much questioning as regards both its definition and its meaning for health.

Maternal deprivation was defined by Bowlby as ". . . . a general term covering a number of different situations. Thus, a child is deprived even though living at home if his mother (or permanent mother-substitute) is unable to give him the loving care small children need. Again, a child is deprived if for any reason he is removed from his mother's care."[8]

In discussing the reasons for the controversy which followed Bowlby's monograph, Ainsworth pointed to some of the problems resulting from a too wide or too inclusive use of the term "maternal deprivation." She suggested that ". . . distinctions should be maintained between the following: (a) insufficiency of interaction implicit in deprivation; (b) distortion in the character of the interaction, without respect to its quantity; and (c) the discontinuity of relations brought about through separation."[13]

The effects of separation in infancy will be more objectively studied in the family context in which the separation takes place, the experiences following separation, the frequency of separations, and the age at which it takes place. In a review of the meaning of separation from parents during early childhood, Yarrow[14] points to the major variables needing attention when comparing the findings of different investigations and in prognosing the outcome. He includes the age at time of the separation, duration of separation, the quality and character of the relationship with the mother before and after the separation, and the role of constitutional factors.

The cultural medium in which children are reared is highly relevant to the consideration of the life experience of children as a determinant of personality and intellectual development. The small nuclear family of mother, father, and children places considerable onus of caretaking and mothering on the one adult woman of the home. Although this type of family living is the common type in middle-class homes of industrial cities there are other common forms of household, such as the sharing between several adult women of responsibility for taking care of infants and children. This may be in the framework of households composed of extended family units,[15,16] or the type of combined family and group care that is so characteristic a feature of kibbutzim in Israel.[17] Comparative studies between various types of communities may not only contribute to basic knowledge of healthy development and different ways of attaining it, but will prevent the too ready generalization from studies in uniform and homogeneous settings.

After sifting much of the controversy that followed publication of Bowlby's monograph in 1951 there remains a high degree of consistency in the inferences that can be made from the studies performed, especially with respect to the importance of early life experience for subsequent mental health. It is true that differences have been found in studies of institutionalized children which point to the significance of the kind of caretaking in the institution and hence to the significance of the child's life experience rather than institutionalization itself.[18] This was evidenced in the comparison of babies and children in institutions with different rearing methods. In one institution children admitted from the age of less than one month and who never saw their mothers after that were kept in separate cribs, on their backs, with limited personal contact. Comparing them with children in institutions with more staff, the children being held when fed and having much more interpersonal interaction generally, Dennis found retardation very marked in the first group and considered this to be caused by the position into which children were put and to their lack of handling.[19]

Perhaps even more pertinent to our present considerations are the findings of a number of workers indicating that serious personality disturbances, often similar in kind to those described in institutionalized children, were found in children who had not been separated from their mothers or homes but who had not had sufficient affection or relatedness with parents, or who had distorted relationships, as in the case of those with mentally abnormal mothers.[20,21]

Yet another question needing further study in differing cultural settings is the permanency of the effects of unsatisfactory life experience in infancy and early childhood. The retardation in intellectual development may well be permanent and yet improvement has been reported.[22,23] Group care may be a major social instrument in promoting intellectual development in children who might otherwise be retarded by the cultural deprivation they experience in their homes. A well-balanced program of family care and group care may make an important contribution to healthy development in physique and behavior, and a number of significant studies are in progress.[24] Thus institutionalization in infancy and early childhood may under some circumstances be highly detrimental to health, but may yet be a force for the promotion of health and prevention of some of the ill-effects of unsatisfactory home care. Partial institutionalization of infants and very young children is a growing feature of societies in which an increasing proportion of women work away from home. The experience of kibbutzim in Israel is of interest in this regard.

Kibbutz Culture and Child Rearing

The importance of the whole life experience for health of a population group is illustrated in personality studies of children reared in a kibbutz. Prognosis as to the outcome of a particular system of rearing may be inaccurate if investigation is restricted to only one aspect or time-period of the system. In the early 1950s Caplan made some challenging observations about the emotional life of Israeli children reared in communal settlements. His impressions at that time are summarized here in several quotations.[25]

On infancy and young childhood, to about 6 years of age, he had this to say:

> Kibbutz children look as though they are suffering from maternal deprivation.
>
> There is a tremendous amount of thumbsucking, temper tantrums, and general lack of control over aggression—much more so than among children raised in families. Enuresis is endemic.
>
> When you observe the young children, especially the toddlers, they look like deprived children in institutions.

On children over the age of 6 years: ". . . the incidence of signs of disturbance falls, and it falls more and more rapidly as the children approach adolescence."

By the age of about 10 to 11 years: ". . . signs of emotional disturbance appear only as frequently as they do in children brought up in our culture."

From age 10, through adolescence to young adulthood:

> If we drew a graph of incidence of disturbed children in the two cultures, the kibbutz line would start higher and begin falling at about age 6. At age 10 it would cross the line of our culture, and from then on it would reveal progressively less disturbance among kibbutz children than our own. They have a much smoother adolescence . . . and as young adults they are remarkably nonneurotic.

On the young adult:

> The young adult of the kibbutz is a remarkable specimen: He is very sociable, and has excellent interpersonal relationships. He is a stable, phlegmatic individual—rather extroverted, and is prepared to sacrifice himself for his group to a notable degree. He does not make egotistical demands on the group, and he is everything the original settlers wanted their children to be.

Among the limited number of scientific psychologic studies concerning the personality of kibbutz children, Rabin's comparative study of children and young adults reared in kibbutzim and moshavim[26] supports the main impressions of Caplan. The "kibbutz" and "moshav" are different types of agricultural settlement in Israel, one of the differences being that the children of the moshav live and are reared in the family home. His selection of kibbutzim and moshavim for this study was directed to reducing other important variables which might confound the essential comparison between kibbutz- and family-reared children. The founders of the settlements resembled one another in "country of origin, educational level, idealism, and in a great many of their national and political values and attitudes." In fact there was "a good deal of similarity in the human material" in the settlements he chose; eight kibbutzim and four moshavim. A summary of his findings is presented in Table 9-2, showing that a comparatively emotionally disturbing infancy in kibbutz children is not manifested in older children and young adults, who are at least as well adjusted and as well developed intellectually and emotionally as the family-reared children, if not more so.

Kibbutz Child-rearing. The impact of the value system of a community on the ways of rearing its children and hence on their health is illustrated by the kibbutz. Despite important differences between kibbutzim, kibbutz living is a distinctive culture in the society of Israel, and is a culture which has been changing since its inception.[27–32] Developed because of economic and agricultural necessity rather than as a preplanned society based on ideology, it soon developed a pragmatic and community-oriented socialist way of life. The basic precept of personal labor with the corollary of not employing hired labor has been relaxed over time, especially after

TABLE 9-2. Personality of Kibbutz Children Compared with Family-reared Children of Moshavim

INFANCY	
10–18 months— 5 kibbutzim 4 moshavim	Griffiths Mental Development Scale (Gesell type observational study of the children): No significant differences between the two groups of children in locomotive, hearing and speech, and eye-hand coordination or manipulation areas of development. Kibbutz children significantly inferior in "personal-social" scale. Vineland Social Maturity Scale (information about the child: from metapelet for kibbutz children and from mothers of moshav children): Kibbutz children scored lower than nonkibbutz children, but neither group would be regarded as retarded. Note: ". . . the discrepancy between the low achievement in the personal-social area as compared with other areas of the developmental scale"
TEN-YEAR-OLDS	
4th and 5th schoolgrades, ages 9–11— 6 kibbutzim 4 Moshavim	Tests: Draw a Person, Rorschach, Blacky Pictures (family of dogs), Sentence Completion: "Kibbutz ten-year-olds are judged to be at least as mature, as well developed intellectually and emotionally and, generally, as well adjusted as their peers in the ordinary family setting. In most instances, the indices we have employed even point to the superiority of the kibbutz children in these areas." Note: the low achievement in personal-social area in kibbutz infants is not found in the ten-year-olds. If anything the trend is towards their superiority over the nonkibbutz children at this age.
ADOLESCENTS	
Mainly 17-year- olds; 12th schoolgrade— 4 kibbutzim 3 moshavim	Tests: Rorschach, TAT (Thematic Apperception Test) and Sentence Completion: "Intellectually, kibbutz adolescents function at least as well and perhaps somewhat better than the controls. . . . with respect to overall "adjustment," no marked differences between the groups were noted. . . . Kibbutz adolescents are less intensely involved affectively with members of their family and evidence less conflict with them. . . . There is evidence of less strong personal amibition in terms of vocational or professional advancement in the kibbutz group; yet, ambition in the direction of personal, cultural, and intellectual growth seems to be present to a higher extent than in the controls."
YOUNG MANHOOD	
Army	Comparison of kibbutz and nonkibbutz soldiers from rural settlements. Tests: Some of the Incomplete Sentence and the TAT Army tests used among soldiers referred to the officers selection unit. More of kibbutz group of soliders are accepted for training as officers. If such selection is a measure of "adjustment," it "supports the trend stated previously for kibbutz children and adolescents that subsequent to the period of infancy the kibbutz subjects make an adequate adjustment."

TABLE 9-2. (cont.)

SELECTED FINDINGS	
	"Less aggression and hostility is generally projected in the materials obtained from kibbutz subjects. The more militant vigilant attitude to the environment is maintained. Personal autonomy and early withdrawal from parental control are also noted. . . . Additional trends for the kibbutz man are his greater comfort in, and dependency upon, the group and his more frequent ambivalence about independent functioning. . . . Kibbutz young men do not rebel against their society; on the contrary, they feel rooted in it, expect to return to it following military service, and perpetuate its collective values in preference to individual plans and ambitions."

(Adapted from Rabin.[26])

the mass immigration following the formation of Israel as an independent state. Its ideology of economic and social equality, with emphasis on the liberation of women and children to enable them to fully develop their abilities, has faced challenges in the differential distribution of sex roles. Men have the key productive functions and women have the domestic or service functions. The economic importance of production may often result in those involved in its direction having a greater say in decision making.

Specialization, demanded by increased knowledge, technology, and skills, may preclude rotation of duties. The composition of committees may even reflect this in the knowledge needed before individual members can make important contributions to decision making. While rotation may continue it may in effect be restricted to small groups of persons, each becoming more expert in particular fields. This may well be reflected in the weekly kibbutz meeting of all members, and free discussion and participation in decision making by everybody may be reduced by the presence of experts in each field. The trend to family homes in some kibbutzim and the living together of parents and children may lead to an increase in domestic responsibility of women and their increasing concern with rearing their own children. The processes of change constitute challenges to basic kibbutz ideology and are reflected in child-rearing and education. Appreciation of these changes and of the variation between different kibbutzim warns against too facile generalization about kibbutz living and personality development of the kibbutz child. The limitations of the summary tabulations (Tables 9-3–9-5) must be stressed, and yet

TABLE 9-3. Some Features of the Value-system and Practices of Kibbutzim

VALUE-SYSTEM	PRACTICES
Personal work with emphasis on agriculture	Cooperative work—in productive, domestic service, and educational aspects
Economic and social equality	Communal ownership of land and buildings, including housing
Collective responsibility	Communal responsibility
	Democratic decision making through regular meetings of all members and rotational membership of committees by election
	Meeting needs of members—feeding, clothing, housing, health promotion and medical care, entertainment, annual vacations
	Child rearing and education*
	Specific training of members for their roles
	Care of dependent parents of members and retired members
Communal living	Communal activities
	Central dining room and recreation center
	Gardens and lawns
	Sports, e.g., swimming pools

*Table 9-4.

they do present a picture of what is, despite its internal variations, a distinctive culture undergoing change.

In the traditional kibbutz the child belongs to at least two highly significant groups at any one time from his arrival at the infants' home after birth in hospital to the end of his childhood. One group is his family (parents and siblings) and the other his peer group of children (cohort group) with its changing metapelet (one who cares). As he graduates from one children's house to the next during his infancy and young childhood, the child is involved with several mothering adults. These include the mother herself and the metapelet, and the different metapelet he gets when he graduates from infants' house to the toddlers' house. This may have the effect of partial deprivation and might help explain the comparative personal-social retardation of kibbutz infants studied by Rabin. However, the need for careful and detailed observation of the reality is illustrated by the findings of Gewirtz and Gewirtz.[34] During the first 8 months of life the kibbutz infant had contact with his mother for much more time each day than with the metapelet. This fact supports consistent observations of other workers of the close attachment of the kibbutz child with his parents and siblings.[30–35] In elaborating his concept of attachment behavior Bowlby makes such observations on kibbutz children. The development of attachment behavior in infants is related to two variables:

TABLE 9-4. Traditional Kibbutz Children's Rearing and Education—The System of Living in Children's Houses

	AGE OF CHILDREN	SIZE OF COHORT/ PEER GROUP	SIGNIFICANT RELATIONSHIPS	
		Living group	Nonfamily	Family
Infants' Home‡	Birth to 12 or 15 months	5 to 6 babies in a room of the home which houses 12 to 20 babies After return from maternity hospital baby goes to infants' home	Metapelet* and assistant increasing role in direct care after early period in which mother much involved	In early period care by mother including feeding, social stimulation, and response to various needs of baby; in later period infant remains with parents' and sibs in parents' room and garden at fixed times of day
Toddlers' Home‡	About 1 to 4 years	5 to 6 children	Change to new home involves change of metapelet	With family at fixed times of the day, usually late after-afternoon
Kindergarten	4 to 6 years	15 to 20 children, arranged by bringing together some three of the groups graduating from toddlers' home	Ganenet† New metapelet	As above
"Elementary School" Home	7 to 12 or 14 years	The same cohort as above, but several cohorts are in the various standards that constitute an elementary school	The children's group itself—Child Society; "Matron" of the home; teachers; various members of the kibbutz	As above
"High School" Home	12 or 14 to 18 years	Same cohort from kindergarten through high school; many kibbutzim, not having their own high school, travel together to the nearest kibbutz high school	The group itself; teachers; members of the kibbutz; youth guide concerned with extracurricular activities	With family at fixed times of the day, usually late afternoon

**A metapelet (plural: metaplot) is a specially trained member of the kibbutz, has responsibility for care of infants and children in their groups. The word literally means "carer."*

†A ganenet is a specially trained kindergarten supervisor (from the word "gan," meaning garden).

‡In some kibbutzim the infants' and toddlers' homes are not separate houses–the group of children continues from infancy to four years of age without necessarily changing its metapelet.

TABLE 9-5. The Difference Between Traditional Kibbutz Rearing and Rearing in a Kibbutz Which Has Changed*

TRADITIONAL

Pattern which has persisted in most kibbutzim for many years:

- Children living in children's houses (Table 9-4), i.e., sleeping, eating, and various day activities
- Parents: Living in rooms provided for couples
  - Eating in communal dining room and various activities in communal dining room or other communal facilities
- Parents and children have at least a daily contact—usually fixed times

THE CHANGE

Encouraging more family living:

- Family home with several rooms and "kitchenette" facility (refrigerator, hot plate)
  - Parents and children sleeping in family home
- Mother returns from maternity hospital with baby to family home
- Children's "homes" become increasingly day-care and day activity centers rather than homes, except for later "high school" age children who may move away from parents' home to their own special house
- Dining: Increasing joint participation of children (especially older children) with members in communal dining room, and of whole family in minor meals and occasional evening meal at home with food from the communal kitchen

**Family living has been a feature of some kibbutzim since their inception. In fact in the first kibbutz established in the country children have slept with their parents since its founding. In this respect it differed from what became the main, "traditional," pattern, outlined in Table 9-5.*

"(1) sensitivity of mother in responding to her baby's signals; and (2) the amount and nature of interaction between mother and baby."[36]

The metapelet has a number of children to care for and therefore has limited time to initiate interaction herself, such as talking, smiling, and otherwise "communicating" with each baby. Nor can the metapelet always respond immediately to each baby's signal. In contrast, the kibbutz mother, when in the infants' home, is usually engaged with her own baby and may well spend more effective time in personal interaction with her baby.

Perhaps the distinguishing feature of kibbutz child-rearing, whether traditional or more family-centered, is its emphasis on the children as a group towards whom the community as a whole has the responsibility of ensuring equality of opportunity for full development.

All material needs, health and medical care, and formal education are ensured by the community and are not dependent on the economic situation of the family or educational status of the mother and father. Important elements of social development are similarly provided in the children's groups themselves. Growing up as a member of a group to which each child belongs, a group which has continuity for the child throughout his childhood has been stressed as a positive process in personality development.

> A common goal, collective striving, and group action give a sense of belongingness. The very structure of the kibbutz society does not permit the isolation of the individual and existential vacuum to become major phenomena . . . (which are such prominent features) . . . in the life of the individual in present-day industrialized Western society.[26]

Insistence on group-rearing in infancy may well be a cause of the difficult beginning that many traditionally-managed kibbutz babies appear to have, but later the group life would appear to promote healthy personality development and even correct or reverse its earlier effects. It would be important to compare personality and physique of children and adults reared along traditional kibbutz lines with those whose upbringing is in kibbutzim emphasizing family- and group-rearing.

The impact of the value-system of a community on its ways of rearing its children and hence on their health is illustrated by the kibbutz. The problem of subjecting the processes involved to epidemiologic study and analysis is not readily solved. The importance of culture as a determinant of health is not in question; rather what is in question is the ability of epidemiology to investigate cultural processes in a way that makes it possible to be more specific about the causal relationships between a community's value-system, its behavior pattern, and its state of health.

REFERENCES

1. Frost WH: The age selection of mortality from tuberculosis in successive decades. Am J Hyg 30:91, 1939. Republished in Maxcy KF (ed.): Papers of Wade Hampton Frost, M.D. New York, Commonwealth Fund, 1941, pp 593, 596.
2. Susser M, Stein Z: Civilization and peptic ulcer. Lancet 1:115, 1962.
3. Erikson EH: Childhood and Society. New York, Norton, 1950.
4. Erikson EH: Growth and crises of the "healthy personality." In Kluckholm C, Murray HA (eds.): Personality in Nature, Society, and Culture. New York, Knopf, 1953.
5. Erikson EH: Identity: Youth and Crisis. New York, Norton, 1968.
6. Freud A, Burlingham DT: Infants without Families. New York, Medical War Books, International Univ Press, 1944, p 26.
7. Rheingold HL: The Modification of Social Responsiveness in Institutional Babies. Monogr Soc Res Child Dev 21:63, 1956.
8. Bowlby J: Maternal Care and Mental Health. WHO Monogr Ser, No. 2, 1951.
9. Bender L: Psychopathic behavior disorders in children. In Lindner RM, Seliger RV (eds.): Handbook of Correctional Psychology. New York, Philosophical Library, 1947.
10. Bowlby J: Forty-four juvenile thieves, their characters and homelife. Int J Psychoanal 25:19, 1944.
11. Levy DM: Primary affect hunger. Am J Psychiatry 94:643, 1937.
12. Spitz RA, Wolf KM: Anaclitic depression. An inquiry into the genesis of psychiatric conditions in early childhood. In Freud A, Hartmann H, Kris E (eds.): The Psychoanalytic Study of the Child, Vol. 2. New York, International Univ Press, 1947, p 314.
13. Ainsworth MD: The effects of maternal deprivation: A review of findings and controversy in the context of research strategy. In Deprivation of Maternal Care: A Reassessment of its Effects. WHO, Public Health Pap 14:1, 1962.
14. Yarrow LJ: Separation from parents during early childhood. In Hoffman ML, Hoffman LW (eds.): Review of Child Development Research, Vol. 1. New York, Russell Sage Foundation, 1964.
15. Mead M: A cultural anthropologist's approach to maternal deprivation. In Deprivation of Maternal Care. A Reassessment of its Effects. WHO Public Health Pap 14:1, 1962.
16. Whiting JWM, Whiting BB: Contributions of anthropology to the methods of studying child rearing. In Mussen PH (ed.): Handbook of Research Methods in Child Development. New York, Wiley, 1960.
17. Neubauer PB (ed.): Children in Collectives, Childrearing Aims and Practices in the Kibbutz. Springfield, Ill, Thomas, 1965.
18. Bowlby J, Ainsworth M, Boston M, et al.: The effects of mother-child separation: A follow-up study. Brit J Med Psychol 29:211, 1956.
19. Dennis W: Causes of retardation among institutional children: Iran. J Genet Psychol 96:47, 1960.
20. Lewis H: Deprived Children. (The Mersham Experiment). A Social and Clinical Study. London, Oxford Univ Press, 1954.
21. Prugh DG, Harlow RG: "Masked deprivation" in infants and young children.

In Deprivation of Maternal Care. A Reassessment of its Effects. WHO Public Health Pap 14:1, 1962.
22. Clarke AM, Clarke ABD (eds.): Mental Deficiency. The Changing Outlook. London, Methuen, 1958.
23. Susser M: Community Psychiatry. Epidemiologic and Social Themes. New York, Random House, 1968.
24. Dittman L (ed.): Early Child Care: The New Perspectives. New York, Atherton, 1968.
25. Caplan G: Clinical observations on the emotional life of children in the communal settlements of Israel. In Senn MJE (ed.): Problems of Infancy and Childhood. New York, Josiah Macy Foundation, 1954, pp 98–99.
26. Rabin AI: Growing Up in the Kibbutz. New York, Springer, 1965, pp 194, 195, 213.
27. Ruppin A: The Agricultural Colonization of the Zionist Organisation in Palestine. London, Martin Hopkinson, 1926.
28. Infield HF: Co-operative Living in Palestine. London, Kegan Paul, Trench, Trubner, 1946.
29. Eisenstadt SN: Israeli Society. London, Weidenfeld and Nicholson, 1967.
30. Spiro ME: Children of the Kibbutz. A Study of Child Training and Personality. New York, Schocken, 1965.
31. Darin-Drabkin H: The Other Society. London, Victor Gollancz, 1962.
32. Weingarten M: Life in a Kibbutz. Jerusalem, Zionist Organization Youth and Hechalutz Department, 1955.
33. Irvine E: Observations on the aims and methods of child rearing in communal settlements in Israel. Hum Rel 5:247, 1952.
34. Gewirtz HB, Gewirtz JL: Visiting and caretaking patterns for kibbutz infants: Age and sex trends. Am J Orthopsychiatry 38:427, 1968.
35. Pelled N: On the formation of object-relations and identifications of the kibbutz child. Isr Ann Psychiatry 2:144, 1964.
36. Bowlby J: Attachment and Loss, Vol. 1. Attachment. London, Hogarth, 1969, p 316.

10
Change and Discontinuity in Life Experience

Discontinuity in a community's life style may result from a sudden event or from long-term influences. The longer the period over which the change takes place the less noticeable is its effect on the individual, but it may have measurable effects on a cohort that has gone through the experience together. The discontinuity may be related to a single event or a cluster of factors. Both the time element and kind of cause are of relevance to our understanding of the impact of these changes on the health picture. We will discuss different kinds of change, i.e., cultural change itself, migration, sudden events, and common life crises.

CULTURAL CHANGE

Cultural change itself is a determinant of community health, since it involves a demand on the groups involved to adjust, adapt, or cope. With the increasing pace and spread of technologic development, industrial urbanization, migration, and different frameworks of living, all aspects of culture are involved and cultural change has become a feature of community living. Two illustrative case examples of the relevance of cultural change for health will be briefly reviewed here.

An anthropologic study of the social structure of the Tallensi of Northern Ghana was conducted in the 1930s by Meyer Fortes.[1,2] Some 30 years later, in 1963, he and his wife (a psychiatrist) revisited the Tallensi and spent 3 months with them, reporting on the change which he noted and the extent of psychosis which accompanied this change.[3]

Among the main features of change was the disparity between the continuance of a highly stable family system and the change in social life beyond the immediate family. In the 1930s the internal family system included major economic and educational functions and had been highly integrated with the extrafamilial system, i.e., the neighborhood, religion, and clan. Thirty years later not only had the family structure and value system persisted, but even the homesteads had undergone only minor change and had remained on the same sites occupied by the same families as before. In contrast, extrafamily activities had changed considerably. A high proportion of children were at school, avenues for earning a living had widened beyond the family subsistence farming, and there were clerks, teachers, and a number of men going into the cities of Ghana for work.

From his observations, Fortes makes several inferences which are pertinent to our present considerations of cultural change.

> Among the Tallensi, the remarkable stability of their family system in the face of quite significant social changes is, I think, to no small degree due to the very benevolent character of their form of patriarchy. This comes out most obviously in the upbringing of infants and young children. Men and women take equal delight, and show equal affection and indulgence, in looking after their young children. Corporal punishment is very rare. Obedience to parents is built into the domestic routine and the value system rather than enforced by coercion. Individuals, even quite young children, have a large measure of independence within the framework of duty to the family.
>
> To sum up, the more or less self-contained traditional society which I knew so well in the middle thirties is now wide open. The impression is inescapable, when I cast my mind back for comparison, that the Tallensi are at a critical point of transition in their social history. Their traditional social structure and way of life is on the brink of far-reaching transformation.
>
> In regard, more particularly, to their family system, formerly it was integrated with the wider society by bonds of kinship, marriage, neighborhood, and religious association; the same bonds in fact that bind its members together internally. What seems to be emerging now is a distinct cleavage and incompatibility between the still relatively stable, traditionally constituted, patrilineal family in its internal organization and value system, on the one hand, and the external social, economic, and ideological sphere in which individual members of a family can play a role divorced from traditional norms. . . . This seems to be a very recent development, going back some ten years at the most. It is significant that in the majority of my wife's cases psychotic breakdown was associated with experiences undergone in this extrafamilial sphere of social life, whether in the urbanised and alien south or even at home. This is where the stresses in modern conditions that precipitate mental illness among a tribal people like the Tallensi emanate from.[3]

It is often difficult to separate the effects on health of cultural changes from those of the social disorganization and disintegration that so often accompany such changes. In order to distinguish between these processes it is theoretically desirable to study a community which is undergoing gradual change without evidence of social disintegration, one in which there is a high degree of community solidarity and stability of community networks of relationships. Abramson[4] studied the health of adolescent girls in relation to cultural change in such a community, the Marshlands Indian community of Durban. This was a poor community, and while ethnically heterogeneous in its internal composition of differing Indian Hindu groups, it was homogeneous in contrast to the other major distinctive groups of the city, namely Africans, who were predominantly Zulu, and Europeans, who were mainly of British origin. Marshlands was thus a distinctively Indian slum neighborhood on the outer edges of the city. While poor, the community did not evidence the "culture of poverty" described by Lewis and discussed in Chapter 12. In fact, it was a community in which the outstanding features were family solidarity and a high degree of community participation in many associations, and although the role expectations and behavior of girls and boys were changing, roles of women and men were strongly influenced by traditional conceptions. Abramson carried out a study of adolescent girls, aged 16 to 17 years, who were living at home with their mothers in this neighborhood. The girls and their mothers were interviewed separately and they did not know of their respective responses. The interviews were structured questionnaires concerning health and traditionalism.

There was no relation between the traditionalism scores of the girls and their health indices.

> Evidence of ill health, with special reference to emotional disturbance, was found to be associated with a discrepancy, in either direction, between the traditionalism of the daughter and that of her mother. Where the mother was traditional compared with other mothers, there was more evidence of ill health among girls who were relatively modern than among those who were relatively traditional. Conversely, where the mother was relatively modern, there was more evidence of ill health among traditional girls, or among girls who were considerably *more* modern than their mothers. There was evidence that ill health was associated, also, with a disharmony between role prescriptions and the actual role enactment in the home.[4]

Abramson's comments on the implications of his findings are pertinent to community health care.

> In respect of community health education, the findings illustrate two important possibilities. First, that a program directed towards one age group rather than towards the community as a whole may endanger intergenerational adjustment, and may carry hazards to the solidarity of the family and the community. Secondly, that the less well-adjusted members of a community may be among those who are particularly likely to accept changes from their family norms, and may as a result become exposed to added stress. The importance of these considerations must vary with the actual program goals and their emotional connotation. In this community they are likely, for example, to be highly significant if the educational

objectives involve changes in the role of the adolescent girl, but of little relevance when the aim is a change in dental health practices.[4]

MIGRATION

Mental Disease and Migration

The possible health implications of migration were highlighted by the pioneer reports of Ødegaard[5,6] on the relatively high rate of admissions to mental hospitals of Norwegian-born immigrants in Minnesota, when compared with rates in Norway itself and with rates of native-born in Minnesota. He considered that one of the reasons for this difference was that migrants include a higher than expected proportion of prepsychotic persons, especially those who will become schizophrenics. Another factor was the process of migration itself, namely persons who migrated were more likely to break down, because of their hardships and emotional difficulties, compared with the native population and with those Norwegians who did not migrate. Continuing these studies on mental hospitalization and migration within Norway itself[7] he found differences between Oslo and the rest of the country. In Oslo, immigrants had higher rates of admissions to mental hospitals than did natives of Oslo, a finding similar to the previous reports on Norwegian immigrants in the United States. However, in rural areas and other towns of the country, those born in the area had higher rates than did immigrants, but these differences were smaller.

A considerable number of studies have been undertaken and, not unexpectedly have yielded differing results. The definition of migration and criteria for recognition of mental illness have varied considerably, and many of the earlier studies did not control for such factors as age and sex, or social class and economic status, which may be associated with both mobility and with mental illness. Thus if migrants to the cities of a country consist predominantly of particular age groups in which the rate of mental illness is highest, it might be expected that migrants would have a higher rate of hospitalization for mental disease than the native population. The general pattern in the United States, where the mass of the studies have been undertaken, was one in which foreign-born immigrants, or United-States-born migrants to the cities, have higher rates of admission to mental hospitals than do the native-born.[8–13] However, there are important exceptions to this pattern in which the reverse has been found,[14,15] and inconsistencies have been found between people of different race and origin, and possibly in times of migration.[16]

Murphy's analysis of Israel,[12] from relevant data and studies,[17,18] provides interesting contrastive relations between mental hospitalization and migration. Age-standardized first-admission rates to mental hospitals in the year 1958 indicate no differences, when all mental disorders were combined, between native-born Israelis and immigrants born in Europe and America. There were higher rates for schizophrenia among native-born Israelis than among the immigrants. On the other hand, Jewish immigrants from Asian countries and Africa had higher admission rates than did the native-born Jews and European-American immigrants for schizophrenia alone and for "all mental disorders" combined.

Post–World War II immigrants to Canada also reflect a different picture from that of the earlier findings in the United States. The immigrant group, which is mainly urban, resembling the Canadian urban population in its occupational distribution, had a lower incidence of mental hospitalization than did the native Canadians when compared by Murphy in 1958. This difference was much less marked when admissions for psychoses only were compared.

By studying the apparently conflicting results it appears that there is more involved than methodologic problems, although these are of considerable importance. The migration process involves important components, each of which may be relevant to our understanding of the apparent inconsistencies when rates of breakdown and mental hospitalization in native populations and different immigrant groups are compared.

Eisenstadt[19] considers the characteristics of such migratory movement as consisting in three aspects or stages.

> First, the motivation to migrate—the needs or dispositions which urge people to move from one place to another; second, the social structure of the actual migratory process, of the physical transition from the original society to a new one; third, the absorption of the immigrants within the social and cultural framework of the new society.

It is obvious that each of these aspects has relevance for mental health.

The motivation to migrate usually involves a turning away from the migrant's family, community, or wider society to another society, in expectation of improvement, be it economic improvement, chances for new friendships, more identification of feeling with the receiving society, or the hope of overcoming frustrations and limitations felt in his existing situation. Such emigrating groups will probably include a number of people whose maladjustment is a reflection of ill-health, especially mental health. The proportion of these cases among different migrating groups is likely to vary considerably according to the selective factors operating in relation to particular migrations.

The second aspect, namely the social structure of the migration process, might be expected to influence the rate of breakdown at least in the extent to which it provides support and cushioning during the usually stressful process of absorption and adaptation to new language, customary practices, and basic values. This requires consideration of the nature of the immigrant group as well as that of the absorbing or host society. The possible importance of group membership as a determinant of differences in rates of mental hospitalization has been reviewed by Murphy in several studies.[12,20,21] "In British Columbia, the only province that has a real Chinatown, the Chinese have the lowest hospitalization rate of all ethnic minorities. In Ontario, where the Chinese are scattered throughout the province in "penny" numbers and have no real focus, they have the highest rate of all ethnic minorities."[12]

He reported a similar finding in Britain, where the incidence of mental hospitalization of Polish refugees was inversely related to the size of the group.[20]

The third aspect, namely the absorption of immigrants into the social and cultural setting of the new society, will influence rate of breakdown to the extent that its challenges are beyond the coping capacity of the immigrant, bearing in mind the initial motivation for migration and the social structure of the migration process. Thus the social distance between the former kind of life and the new setting will determine the amount of social change demanded. This may be an important factor in breakdown as represented by mental hospitalization. The high rates associated with Norwegian migration into Oslo, in contrast to that of the rest of the country, and of African and Asian Jewish immigrants in Israel in contrast to European and North American immigrants, are suggestive examples of this.

To elucidate the role of migration as a determinant of mental illness, as distinct from hospitalization, a community-based epidemiologic study is needed. This would establish any differential mental health status of natives and migrants, whereas hospitalization rates measure something different, i.e., breakdown and one particular way of handling it. In their study of mental health in midtown Manhattan, Srole and his associates[22] were able to define two extreme types of immigrant. The one was from small towns, villages, and rural areas of Europe of low socioeconomic status, and the other was from large or medium-sized European cities of higher socioeconomic status. There were significant differences in mental health, standardized for age, between these two types of immigrant, the rural type having a higher rate of mental illness as measured by the criteria for the proportion considered to be impaired.

Evidence of an association between migration and emotional disturbance has been reported, in a small industrial town of some 5,000 people situated in a rural area in North Carolina,[23] in a study comparing first and second generation workers in a manufacturing plant. Other studies with similar evidence were conducted among university freshmen students at the Hebrew University, Jerusalem, in which native-born students were compared with foreign-born students of similar ethnic type,[24] and in an area of Jerusalem in which native-born and immigrant groups were compared.[25] In each of these studies the Cornell Medical Index (CMI) was used;[26] it has been found to be a useful indicator of emotional state.[27,28] In each of these studies the migrant group evidenced a higher rate of emotional disturbance as indicated by the frequency of higher scores on the CMI.

Lung Cancer and Rural-urban Migration

Migration from rural areas to metropolitan cities has been found to be associated with a higher-than-expected risk of lung cancer in the United States.[29,30] Of particular interest in the present context is the finding that only the migrants from rural to urban areas had a higher mortality rate from lung cancer, adjusted for age and smoking history, than did well-established residents of the place to which they migrated. The critical question is not so much whether migration is a causal factor of lung cancer but why farm migrants differ from others. A similar question is central to our understanding of the apparent inconsistencies found in mental hospitalization studies reviewed above. It is not so much whether migration per se is a cause of breakdown and mental hospitalization, but why the association between migration and mental hospitalization differs in different situations.

Coronary Artery Disease in Migrant Populations

Differences in the rates of various diseases among migrant populations and natives are to be expected when the migrant groups come from countries in which the disease patterns differ from those of the host country, or when the migrants represent a highly selected segment of the population from which they have migrated.

Thus, in the 1950s, when it was debated whether the increase in coronary heart disease in various countries was real or apparent, the observations on Japanese, and Yemenite Jewish, migrant populations were important. Gordon's[31] observation regarding the low mortality from coronary heart disease in Japan, the higher rate among Japanese in Hawaii, and the still higher rate in the Japanese of California pointed to change in way of life as a major cause of coronary heart disease mortality. This was also strongly suggested by the report of Toor et al.[32] that recent Yemenite Jewish immigrants to Israel had a very low mortality rate from arteriosclerotic degenerative heart disease, compared with the higher rate among those Yemenite Jews who had immigrated some 20 years earlier. Later reports have confirmed these earlier observations.[33]

Chronic Bronchitis in Immigrants

In contrast to the findings in mortality from coronary heart disease are those of chronic nonspecific lung disease reported by Reid and associates.[34] British-born immigrants to the United States had a mortality rate from nonspecific lung disease (chronic bronchitis, bronchiectasis, and emphysema) of less than one-fifth the rate in Britain itself, and comparable with that of United States natives. The findings of their postal questionnaire investigation confirmed this trend towards the rates of native-born Americans: British immigrants reported an unexpectedly low level for both "persistent cough and phlegm" and "chronic bronchitis," lower than native-born Americans. Selective factors in the British migrant population do not appear to have been responsible for this striking finding.

Migrant populations bring with them both genetic and life experience attributes from their country of origin. The picture of health and disease which they present may be characteristic of their native country, or they may represent a selected group differing from others in health as well as in other features. On the other hand, their health syndromes may be a direct result of the process of migration itself. In summary, the focus in community health studies investigating migrant populations involves consideration of the following factors which may be causal of the migrant populations' health status.

I. The process of migration itself
   A. Crisis and change involved in migrating
   B. Change in the environment
   C. Change in behavior as in changing dietary habits
II. The health of the group before leaving home
   A. Reflection of the health of the population from which it emigrated
   B. Selective factors differentiating it from others at "home."

CRISES

Sudden Community-wide Disaster

In addition to their immediate effects, community-wide disasters may also have an impact of a longer-term nature, the health implications of which are not always obvious.

One summer night in 1968, 3,000 houses in Bristol, England, were flooded by a heavy rain. Bennet[35] took the opportunity to carry out a long-term study of the later implications for health of the flooded community. He found a 50 percent increase in the number of deaths, from 58 in the 12 months before the flood to 87 in the 12 months after. This increase in mortality in the flooded homes was in marked contrast to the absence of change in the rest of Bristol; it was more marked in men than in women, especially in the age group 45 to 64 years.

The people who had been flooded showed a considerable rise in attendance at the general practitioner in the 12-month period after the flood compared with the same period before the flood (81 percent increase in males; 25 percent increase in females), while the nonflooded control group showed no such rise in attendance. The same trend was noted in hospital referrals and hospital admissions. The reasons for admission to hospital did not reflect any direct expected consequences of flooding, but covered a wide range of diagnoses.

Common Life Crises

Floods are not the lot of all people, but there are events of a stressful or even distressing kind which are more general experiences. Separation from loved ones and close friends is a universal experience, while other changes of a less distressing kind and not necessarily a part of everyone's life are nevertheless common events. The common sudden changes which are of epidemiologic interest as probable causes of illness include those concerned with love, work, and play; e.g., separation, deprivation or loss of significant and meaningful others by death, and migration. Examples of such common occurrences include dissolution of the family or any closely knit primary group; separation of individuals from one group and the process of entrance to new groups; and work and school changes.

In addition there is the role of sudden loss of ability to fulfill normal roles expected by self and by others, whether because of sudden illness such as an episode of myocardial infarction, or psychotic breakdown and its stressful challenge to adjustment.

Study of life history in epidemiologic investigation was, and still is, predominantly focused on investigation of exposure to a postulated specific agent of disease and of the situations in which this agent may have been introduced and transmitted in a population group. More limited has been its use in determining whether changes and events in life situations as such cause illness or breakdown. Obtaining information and systematically gathering the data for analysis in epidemiologic investigation of this kind is at its beginning. This subject is considered further here because of its potential importance in epidemiology and community medicine.

The work of Holmes in his earlier studies of tuberculous disease in relation to life crisis and stressful experiences is discussed in a later chapter. Following these studies Holmes, Rahe, and their associates have been developing a method of measuring the clustering of life events and changes and have been testing its usefulness in exploring the relations between life crises and illness.

Life crisis and sudden change in life situation can, theoretically, affect any one or all of the phases of development of a disease in the individual or community. Thus sudden disorganization in social functioning might lead to differences in exposure to infection, and the various phases of response, namely response to exposure, infection, and outcome of illness, might be differently affected by distressing or otherwise stressful experience. Expanding our epidemiologic model to various health conditions involves consideration of the following:

1. The presence of factors necessary to initiate the condition, but not necessarily sufficient in themselves to cause its expression in illness.
2. The factors which determine the expression or gradient of the condition, ranging from those which are protective to those which cause breakdown in illness or death.
3. The factors which determine later effects of the initial state or the outcome and complications of illness.

These phases may sometimes be caused by a single overwhelming factor such as a massive dose of radiation, poison, or infection in which the necessary initiating cause is also sufficient to determine expression and outcome in death. But most often this is not the case; communities are seldom completely wiped out by a single event or cause. There are differences in expression between individuals and between segments of a population group. Most necessary initiating causes such as the tubercle bacillus are not sufficient in themselves to cause disease. There is variation in expression and differential distribution of mortality, morbidity, and other responses.

The epidemiology of each phase may be distinct and the role of sudden change in life situation may play a different part in each of these epidemiologies. Distressing or stressful experiences may play a role in determining the differential mortality rates of tuberculosis, leprosy, or coronary heart disease. The role of these experiences in determining illness breakdown in persons at risk for these diseases may be similar despite the fact that the pathologies of the diseases and their risk factors are different. Thus without being sufficient cause for specific disease, they may be necessary or at least contributory to breakdown. It is precisely because of the possible wide spectrum of their effects that methods of study of such life events are important at this stage of development in epidemiology.

An Approach to Measurement of Change in Life Situation. If common life experiences such as those outlined above are to be investigated with respect to their effects on health, we need measuring instruments of the change itself. Holmes and Rahe[36] have used a "Schedule of Recent Experience" (SRE) in their investigations of life change and health. While the particular questions asked, and the relative importance attached to each, will probably not be universally applicable, their way of developing the questionnaire is of much potential use in community medicine.[37]

The authors refer to the life chart, devised by Adolf Meyer, as the root of this type of research, in which he arranged life events along with health and disease in a biographic way.[38] The use of such life charts in understanding the social processes, and especially the life chart associated with a patient's illness, can be extended to epidemiologic understanding of relations of life changes and crises to health and disease in a community.

The use of recent experiences only by these researchers, i.e., up to some 5 years before interview rather than the whole life history, is based on the tuberculosis studies of Holmes and his associates in which they found that life changes tended to cluster in the two years preceding the onset of tuberculosis.[39] This is in accord with the report by Hinkle and Wolff that "clusters of illness of all sorts often occurred in periods when the subject was experiencing significant difficulty in his attempts to adapt to the conflicting demands (as related to his own needs) of his total environment."[40] In their use of life crisis history in a study of multiple sclerosis in Israel, Antonovsky and Kats[41] found that recent crises were more related to onset of illness in 50 cases compared with their matched controls.

How many of the life changes occurring around the time of an illness are really a result, rather than a cause, of the illness episode? The question is not one to which a definitive answer should be expected. While life changes or life crises may precede illness, it should also be expected that illness will itself have effects on routine daily living and that these effects will last for varying periods of time after the illness. In the pilot testing of their Schedule of Recent Experiences (SRE) in its relation to changes in health, Rahe and Holmes[42,43] studied a group of 88 resident physicians of a hospital. The initial retrospective study involved answering questions of the SRE as well as listing by year of occurrence all "major health changes" they had experienced over the previous 10 years. Later the same physicians were contacted again and asked about the illnesses and other health changes they had experienced since the initial test. The generalizations that may be made from their findings in both the retrospective and prospective studies include the following:

1. There was a strong association between magnitude of the life crisis and change in health status; the greater the magnitude of the crisis score the greater the chances of illness or other health changes.

2. Not all persons reporting life crisis, including a number with a high crisis score, experienced illness within a period of two years following the crisis.
3. The relationship between life changes and health changes, or stated differently, between life crisis and disease, is not specific. Particular events are not associated with particular illness outcomes. It is more the combination of life changes, providing a total life crisis score, that determines change in state of health. Furthermore, the health changes include a wide variety of conditions. Acute and chronic disease, illnesses from infection, and parasitic diseases are very common. So-called "psychosomatic" conditions, psychiatric and allergic disorders, are no more frequent than conditions requiring surgery, musculoskeletal disorders, and accidents.

Among the more important implications for epidemiology arising from studies of the relations between life events and health or disease is that of giving separate consideration to the event or life change itself from its effects, namely psychologic or somatic. The concept of psychosocial as an entity may only serve to further cloud an already fuzzy area, providing "soft" data as distinct from the data gathered by observations of more definable entities for which criteria can be set. Table 10-1 is illustrative of this process.

TABLE 10-1. Association Between Life Crisis and Health

Change in life experience (life crisis) ⇄ Change in health status

UNDERSTANDING THE ASSOCIATION BY
INVESTIGATION OF THE INTERVENING VARIABLES

Social event or change → INTERVENING PROCESSES → Health change

Study of
psychologic and somatic
processes which translate
social change into
health change

REFERENCES

1. Fortes M: The Dynamics of Clanship Among the Tallensi. London, Oxford Un Press, 1945.
2. Fortes M: The Web of Kinship among the Tallensi. London, Oxford Univ Press, 1949.
3. Fortes M, Mayer DY: Psychosis and Social Change among the Tallensi of Northern Ghana. Cahiers d'Etudes Africaines 21, Vol. 6. Hague, Netherlands, Mouton, 1966, pp 9, 17.
4. Abramson JH: Observations on the health of adolescent girls in relation to cultural change. Psychosom Med 23:156, 1961.

5. Ødegaard Ø: Emigration and insanity. Acta Psychiatr Neurolog (Suppl) 4:1, 1932.
6. Ødegaard Ø: Emigration and mental health. Ment Hyg 20:546, 1936.
7. Astrup C, Ødegaard Ø: Internal migration and mental disease in Norway. Psychiatr Q (Suppl) 34:116, 1960.
8. Malzberg B: Social and Biological Aspects of Mental Disease. Utica, NY, State Hospitals Press, 1940.
9. Malzberg B: Mental disease among the native and foreign-born white populations of New York State, 1939–1941. Ment Hyg 39:545, 1955.
10. Malzberg B: Migration and mental disease among the white population of New York State, 1949–1951. Hum Biol 34:89, 1962.
11. Lee ES: Socioeconomic and migration differentials in mental disease, New York State, 1940–1951. Milbank Mem Fund Q 41:249, 1963.
12. Murphy HBM: Migration and the major mental disorders. A reappraisal. In Kantor MB (ed.): Mobility and Mental Health. Springfield Ill, Thomas, 1965, Chap. 1, p 25.
13. Struening EL, Rabkin JG, Peck HB: Migration and ethnic membership in relation to social problems. Am Behav Sci, 13:57, 1969.
14. Parker S, Kleiner RJ: Mental Illness in the Urban Negro Community. New York, The Free Press, 1966.
15. Kleiner RJ, Parker S: Social-psychological aspects of migration and mental disorder in a Negro population. Am Behav Sci 13:104, 1969.
16. Lazarus J, Locke BZ, Thomas DS: Migration differentials in mental disease. Milbank Mem Fund Q 41:25, 1963.
17. Halevi HS: Mental Illness in Israel; Admissions to Mental Hospitals and Institutions for In-patients during 1958. Mimeograph report. Jerusalem, Ministry of Health, 1960.
18. Sunier A: Mental Illness and Psychiatric Care in Israel. Mimeograph report. Amsterdam, 1956.
19. Eisenstadt SN: The Absorption of Immigrants. London, Routledge and Kegan Paul, 1954, p 1.
20. Murphy HBM: Flight and Resettlement. Paris, UNESCO, 1955.
21. Murphy HBM: Culture and mental disorder in Singapore. In Opler KM (ed.): Culture and Mental Health. New York, Macmillan 1959.
22. Srole L, Langner TS, Michael ST, et al.: Mental Health in the Metropolis: The Midtown Manhattan Study. New York, McGraw-Hill, 1962.
23. Cassel J, Tyroler HA: Epidemiological studies of culture change. I. Health status and recency of industrialization. Arch Environ Health 3:25, 1961.
24. Kark E, Zaslany A, Ward B: The health of undergraduate students on entry to the Hebrew University in Jerusalem. Isr Med J 22:147, 1963.
25. Abramson JH: Emotional disorder, status inconsistency, and migration. A health questionnaire survey in Jerusalem. Milbank Mem Fund Q 44:23, 1966.
26. Brodman K, Erdmann AJ Jr, Wolff MG: The Cornell Medical Index Health Questionnaire (Manual). New York, Cornell Univ Medical College, 1956.
27. Abramson JH: The Cornell Medical Index as an epidemiological tool. Am J Public Health 56:287, 1966.
28. Abramson JH, Terespolsky L, Brook JG, et al.: The Cornell Medical Index as a health measure in epidemiological studies. A test of validity of a health questionnaire. Brit J Prev Soc Med 19:103, 1965.
29. Haenszel W, Loveland DB, Sirken MG: Lung-cancer mortality as related to residence and smoking histories. I. White males. J Nat Cancer Inst 28: 947, 1962.

30. Haenszel W, Taeuber KE: Lung-cancer mortality as related to residence and smoking histories. II. White females. J Nat Cancer Inst 32:803, 1964.
31. Gordon T: Mortality experience among the Japanese in the United States, Hawaii, and Japan. Public Health Rep 72:543, 1957.
32. Toor M, Katchalsky A, Agmon J, et al.: Serum-lipids and atherosclerosis among Yemenite immigrants in Israel. Lancet 272:1270, 1957.
33. Stenhouse NS, McCall MG: Differential mortality from cardiovascular disease in migrants from England and Wales, Scotland and Italy, and native-born Australians. J Chronic Dis 24:423, 1970.
34. Reid DD, Cornfield J, Markush RE, et al.: Studies of disease among migrants and native populations in Great Britain, Norway, and the United States. III. Prevalence of cardiorespiratory symptoms among migrants and native-born in the United States. In Haenszel W (ed.): Epidemiological Approaches to the Study of Cancer and Other Chronic Diseases. National Cancer Institute Monogr 19. Washington, DC, US Dept of Health, Education, and Welfare, Public Health Service, 1966.
35. Bennet G: Bristol Floods 1968. Controlled survey of effects on health of local community disaster. Brit Med J 3:454, 1970.
36. Holmes TH, Rahe RH: Booklet for Schedule of Recent Experience (SRE). Seattle, Wash, Univ of Washington School of Medicine, Dept of Psychiatry, 1967.
37. Holmes TH, Rahe RH: The social readjustment rating scale. J Psychosom Res 2:213, 1967.
38. The Collected Papers of Adolf Meyer, Vol. 4. Mental Hygiene. Baltimore, Johns Hopkins Press, 1952.
39. Holmes TH: Multidiscipline studies of tuberculosis. In Sparer PJ (ed.): Personality, Stress and Tuberculosis. New York, International Univ Press, 1956.
40. Hinkle LE, Wolff HG: Health and the social environment. Experimental investigations. In Leighton AH, Clausen JA, Wilson RN (eds.): Explorations in Social Psychiatry. New York, Basic Books, 1957, Chap. IV, p 126.
41. Antonovsky A, Kats R: The life crisis as a tool in epidemiological research. J Health Soc Behav 8:15, 1967.
42. Rahe RH, Holmes TH: Life crisis and disease onset. II. Qualitative and quantitative definition of the life crisis and its association with health change. Mimeograph report. Seattle, Wash, Univ of Washington School of Medicine, Dept of Psychiatry, 1966.
43. Rahe RH, Holmes TH: Life crisis and disease onset. III. A prospective study of life crisis and health changes. Mimeograph report. Seattle, Wash, Univ of Washington School of Medicine, Dept of Psychiatry, 1966.

11
Social Disorganization and Anomie

In other chapters of this book increased rates of tuberculosis, streptococcal infection and disease, schizophrenia, and other disorders have been considered in relation to various social factors such as poverty, migration, minority status, family, and social disorganization. The independent effects of these social variables and the ways in which they influence health are not easily determined. Mortality rates from cerebral vascular disease in the black population of North Carolina have been found to vary with levels of social disorganization in the counties of this state.[1] The indices of social disorganization used were the following:

1. Family instability, as measured by the percentage of primary families with only one parent present.
2. The percentage of all children under 18 years of age not living with both parents.
3. Separation or divorce, as measured by the percentage of ever-married women now divorced or separated.
4. Illegitimate births, as a percentage of all births.
5. Men on "prison road camps," as a rate per 10,000 population of all men sentenced to prison road camps.

Ranking the counties of the state according to the degree of social breakdown, as measured by these indices, a relation was found between social disorganization and the stroke mortality rates in black men and women, at all ages from 35 through 74 years. The biggest differences were found in the younger age groups, aged 35 to 44 years. In their investigation, Neser et al. were able to demonstrate that the association was not likely to be a result of poverty, which was shown not to be associated with stroke mortality in this segment of the population living in the various counties of North Carolina. They suggest that their findings "tend to support the notion that social disorganization may enhance susceptibility to disease, especially in subordinated members of society," . . .[1] but they stress the indirect or ecologic nature of their study and therefore the need for further investigation using more direct case-control studies.

Evidence of this kind is accumulating and the possible influence of culture, particularly with respect to its value-system, will be reviewed here. The specific aspect that will be considered is the role of anomie as an intervening variable or causal link between social or family disorganization and disease rates in a community.

The relevance of culture to a community's health may be observed when the value-system by which people regulate their behavior is disturbed. While social control of behavior involves an operative legal system, even more important is the acceptance, by members of the community, of formal and informal rules. Reciprocal role behavior between members of a group depends upon the individuals who are involved in various social situations behaving in ways that are mutually expected and acceptable to each participant. Acceptance of social control is thus not a mere passive yielding to force but rather the result of a process of socialization or internalization of the value patterns of the community.[2] Where this process of social control fails we can speak of anomie or social disintegration. The concept of the regulation of individual behavior by society as a factor that determines suicide was developed by Durkheim. His analysis of the variation in suicide rates in different countries of Europe, in different socially-defined groups within various countries, and at different times during the 19th century led him to look beyond individual predispositions towards the "social concomitants of suicide." Among these he isolated two interrelated social factors. One was the degree of integration of the social groups of which the individual forms a part. Two forms of suicide, "egoistic" and "altruistic," were related to this factor, the former varying inversely with the degree of integration of the society and the latter occurring "when social integration is too strong. . . ." The second social factor Durkheim considered was the extent to which society regulates its individuals. He described anomic suicide in contrast to "egoistic" and "altruistic" suicide, "in its dependence, not on the way in which individuals are attached to society, but on how it regulates them."[3]

Acute economic crises, financial disasters, and catastrophes, as well as more fortunate crises with rapid increase in wealth, were associated with increase in suicide. On the basis of these observations, of which he presents a number of examples, Durkheim conceived a generalization, full of meaning for epidemiology over 70 years later.

> If therefore industrial or financial crises increase suicides, this is not because they cause poverty, since crises of prosperity have the same result; it is because they are crises, that is, disturbances of the collective order. Every disturbance of equilibrium, even though it achieves greater

> comfort and a heightening of general vitality, is an impulse to voluntary death. Whenever serious readjustments take place in the social order, whether or not due to a sudden growth or to an unexpected catastrophe, men are more inclined to selfdestruction.[3]

In addition to acute crises, for which Durkheim postulated a state of anomie as a cause of suicide, he also considered the chronic state of anomie that prevailed during a time of expanding trade and industry. At such a time there was little regulation of behavior by society and little readiness to accept any constraints, especially among employers. Suicide rates among industrial and commercial occupations were very much higher than in agriculture, "where the old regulative forces still make their appearance felt most and where the fever of business has least penetrated."[3]

Postulating external constraint as the explanation of his findings in a study of suicide in Chicago, 1959–1963, Maris argues that lack of external constraint is a single influence to which Durkheim's anomie and egoism refer. "Integration is the structure aspect and regulation the normative aspect of external constraint."[4]

The epidemiology of various forms of deviant behavior, of which suicide is but one, needs more understanding of social process if it is to extend beyond description of individual characteristics and the distribution of cases. This has much relevance to the present discussion on causal relationships between social values, behavior, and health. Merton's extension of the concept of anomie is illustrative of the kind of contribution which sociologic theory can make to epidemiology, and through it to family and community medicine, especially community mental health care.[5] In his analysis of social structure and anomie Merton focuses on two important elements of culture. Culture defines both the legitimate goals or aspirations of members of the society and the acceptable ways or practices of striving toward these goals. A well-balanced emphasis on both the goals and institutionalized means of attaining them is characteristic of stable societies and he postulates that the type of adaptation of individual members is related to the stability of the society.

In societies in which there is imbalance between the degree of emphasis on goals and ways of attaining them, the behavior of individual members will be affected accordingly. Thus, where the focus is on goals, with less stress on acceptable behavior in gaining these ends, individuals will pursue less valued means.

> In this context, the sole significant question becomes, which of the available procedures is most efficient in netting the culturally approved value? The technically most effective procedure, whether culturally legitimate or not, typically becomes preferred to institutionally prescribed conduct. As this process of attenuation continues, the society becomes unstable and then develops what Durkheim called "anomie" (or normlessness).[5]

Breakdown in normative control is at the core of social disorganization or social disintegration and its relation to health is not readily studied in isolation. In his description of the sick society, Halliday[6] stressed the importance of discipline in the functionally integrated or socially healthy group. He related chronic diseases and other personal health indices, physical and psychologic, to the functioning of the group as a whole. His analysis of a mining community of Britain in the period between the two world wars illustrates this approach.

He viewed high sickness rates, falling output per worker, and increasing absenteeism as social pathology; i.e., "as various 'medical' expressions of the loss of the sense of social purpose by the group."[6] Associated with these were other industrial and economic indices of disequilibrium, such as growing unemployment, epidemics of strikes, and the drift from industry. Halliday's observations on changes in personal behavior included indicators of antisocial behavior, increasing juvenile delinquency, broken homes, increasing suicide and loss of self-respect.

He thought that the increase in psychologic ill-health of the miners themselves was probably reflected in the sickness rates of their wives as well, but he had no measure of this. Burns, in her study of infant and maternal mortality in a coal-mining county of England in 1930, provided evidence of this.[7] After an examination of the British Registrar General's special report on occupational mortality in 1931, she wrote, "it may be seen that during the reproductive period, despite the special industrial hazards of the male, *it is more dangerous to be a miner's wife than to be a miner*. Both puerperal and nonpuerperal death-rates in these women are high."

Halliday's concept of the socially healthy was that of the functionally integrated group, i.e., a group that is productive and satisfying. When a group loses the characteristics of being "functionally integrated" it becomes disintegrated, i.e., it loses its coherence, it suffers dispersal, and it ceases to be able to fulfill its social functions. He regarded this as socially unhealthy. Members of such a disintegrated group or "sick community" reflect its social ill-health by being emotionally disintegrated (psychologically unhealthy).

The concept of social disintegration was used by Leighton and his co-workers in their epidemiologic studies of psychiatric disorder and sociocultural environment.[8] Like Halliday, they have used concepts of equilibrium and disequilibrium, and integration and disintegration, but in a more objective context. Central to their concept of integration-disintegration is the idea that it is the sharing of sentiments that "makes it possible for groups of people to live together in some agreement about what is right and good and what is expected."[9] Beliefs and values are included in the term "sentiments" which provides a clue to the understanding of the relation between culture and personality.

Choosing the small community as the unit of study, the Leightons and their co-workers investigated the relation between community disintegration and the prevalence of psychiatric disorders. In their comparative studies between communities in Stirling County, North America, and between different Yoruba villages in Nigeria, they found that in these very different cultural settings there was an association between social disintegration and the prevalence of psychiatric disorder.[9,10]

They have given considerable attention to finding and defining indicators of sociocultural disintegration of a community. Three sorting indicators were found sufficient in the Stirling County study. They were extensive poverty, cultural confusion, and widespread secularization. Durkheim's concept of anomie has bearing on the latter two indicators of disintegration and are interpreted in this way by the Leightons and their associates.

They consider that communities that are markedly disintegrated will have a high frequency of broken homes, few and weak associations, few and weak leaders, few patterns of recreation, a high frequency of hostility, a high frequency of crime and delinquency, and weak and fragmented networks of communications.

With suitable adaptation to the style of living of Yoruba villagers, poverty, cultural confusion, and secularization, along with other indicators, were found useful in discriminating between integrated, intermediate, and disintegrated communities.[9]

REFERENCES

1. Neser WB, Tyroler HA, Cassel JC: Social disorganization and stroke mortality in the Black population of North Carolina. Am J Epidemiol 93: 166, 1971.
2. Parsons T: The Social System. New York, Free Press, 1951.
3. Durkheim E: Suicide: A Study in Sociology. Translated by JA Spaulding, G. Simpson. London, Routledge and Kegan Paul, 1952, pp 246, 257, 258.
4. Maris RW: Social Forces in Urban Suicide. Homewood, Ill, Dorsey Press, 1969, p 179.
5. Merton RK: Social structure and anomie. Revisions and extensions. In Anshen RN (ed.): The Family: Its Function and Destiny. New York, Harper and Brothers, 1949. Also published in Merton's Social Theory and Social Structure, rev. ed. Glencoe, Ill, Free Press, 1957, p 231.
6. Halliday JL: Psychosocial Medicine: A Study of the Sick Society. London, Heinemann Medical Books, 1949, p 185.
7. Burns CM: Infant and Maternal Mortality. Newcastle upon Tyne, Kings College, University of Durham, Dept of Physiology, 1942, p 6.
8. Leighton AH: My Name is Legion: Foundations for a Theory of Man in Relation to Culture. The Stirling County Study, Vol. 1. New York, Basic Books, 1959.
9. Leighton AH, Lambo TA, Hughes CC, et al.: Psychiatric Disorder Among the Yoruba. New York, Cornell Univ Press, 1963, p 34.

10. Leighton DC, Harding JS, Macklin DB, et al.: The Character of Danger: Psychiatric Symptoms in Selected Communities. The Stirling County Study of Psychiatric Disorder and Sociocultural Environment, Vol. 3. New York, Basic Books, 1963.

12
Poverty, Culture and Health

Throughout history poverty has been associated with disease and pestilence, malnutrition and retarded growth, delinquency, and other social pathologies. It still is. As expected, the poor are usually classified in the lower classes of any social class system, being concentrated in the lowest class, class V, and to a lesser extent in class IV. Epidemiologically there is more to it than simple terminology. In many studies social class V stands out as different. In the studies by Hollingshead and Redlich of psychiatric illness and social class in New Haven the rate of schizophrenic psychoses increased with decline in social class. However the difference between the lowest social class, class V, and classes I and II was very much greater than that between social classes III and IV and the upper classes. The ratios were as follows (they have been calculated from the figures for age- and sex-adjusted rates of class status and rate of different psychoses per 100,000 population).[1]

Social class V: Social class I and II—8.1:1
Social class IV: Social class I and II—2.7:1
Social class III: Social class I and II—1.5:1

Ratios of the differences were similar in less commonly diagnosed psychoses, namely psychoses due to alcoholism and drug addiction where the respective ratios were 7.5, 2.1, and 1.9:1. The respective ratios for organic psychoses were 28.2, 5.1, and 2.7:1, and for senile psychoses 8.3, 2.9, and 1.5:1. The class differences in rates for affective psychoses were much less marked than that of the others but even in this group the lowest social class was outstanding.

In an extensive review of studies of the relation between social class and psychosis, Fried reported that the lowest social class groups showed the highest rates of psychosis.[2] This inverse relation between psychosis and lowest social class group does not necessarily represent the picture of a consistent linear increase in psychosis with decline in social class. While many of the studies did demonstrate a linear trend in the inverse relation, the findings were not as clear nor as consistent as for that of the lowest social class group and psychosis.

Figure 6-16, presenting social class differences in mortality from different causes in England and Wales, also points to distinctive features of the lowest social class in the 1949–1953 data. There is a very steep increase from social class III and IV to social class V in the mortality rate owing to such diseases as respiratory tuberculosis and pneumonia. Equally interesting is a U-type trend between class and mortality from diseases such as diabetes and vascular lesions of the nervous system. Thus the highest mortality rate of diabetes was in social class I but the next highest was social class V, not the intermediate classes. Ten years later, in the period 1959–1963, the steep increase in death rates of social class V was not only marked in respect of diseases such as respiratory tuberculosis and pneumonia. It was also evident for death from malignant neoplasms of the stomach, diabetes, nephritis and nephrosis, and vascular lesions of the central nervous system.

In the now classic study of John Boyd Orr on diet in relation to income in the United Kingdom, the curve showing decline in quality of diet with level of income drops sharply as it moves into the lowest income group of the population. This sudden change in the curve is readily noted for almost all constituents of the diet that were analyzed, i.e, protein, fat, calories, vitamins A and C, calcium, phosphorus, and iron (Fig. 12-1).[3]

The distinctiveness of social class V from other classes suggests a qualitative difference which may be characteristic of the class as a whole or of a particular segment of the people who are grouped together in this lowest social class. Lerner suggests that in the United States the poverty population be distinguished from the middle and working classes in order to study the relation between health level and socioeconomic status. While acknowledging the difficulties in defining the poverty population as a group, he states

> It has its own distinctive life style. This population is generally outside the mainstream of American life. Its levels of unemployment are typically high and income and educational attainment are low. Its family structure tends to differ from those of the other strata, being marked by a relatively weak paternal role, often involving prolonged absences.[4]

This approach may be especially helpful when focusing on health status and health care of poverty populations and the ways in which they differ from the other classes.

The broad groupings of social class have relevance for health in so far as they reflect class differences in characteristics of the populations

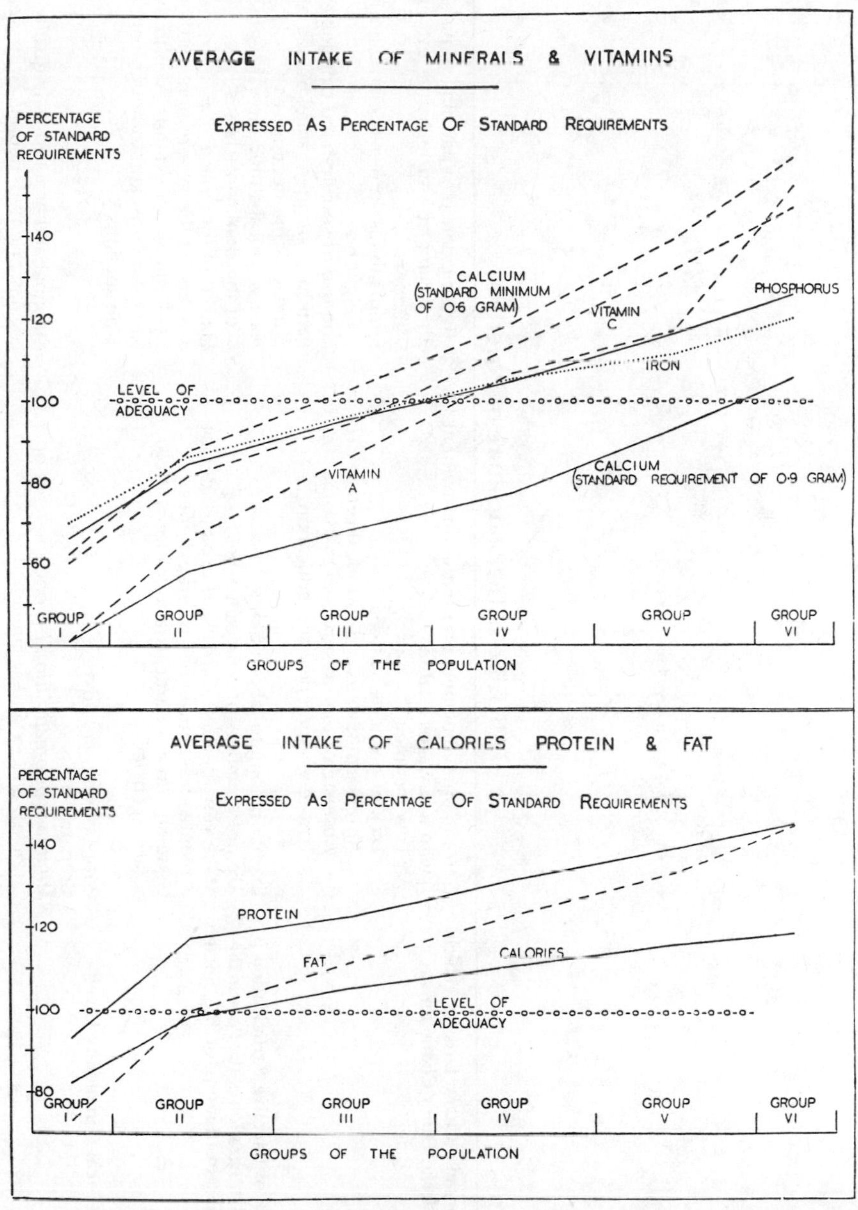

FIG. 12-1. Relationship between quality of diet and level of income, United Kingdom, 1937. Group 1 is the poorest group (From Orr.[3])

TABLE 12-1. The Subculture of Poverty

Economic Characteristics Which Underlie Other Characteristics:	Chronic unemployment and underemployment with low wages lead to Low income Lack of property ownership Absence of savings and chronic shortage of cash Absence of food reserves in the home Low level of literacy and education	High incidence of pawning of personal goods Borrowing at usurious interest from local moneylenders Spontaneous informal credit devices organized by neighbors The use of second-hand clothing and furniture Pattern of frequent small buying of food many times a day as the need arises
Lack of Effective Participation and Integration of the Poor in the Major Institutions of the Society	Do not belong to labor unions Are not members of political parties Make very little use of banks, hospitals, department stores, museums, or art galleries Generally do not participate in National Welfare Agencies	Have a critical attitude toward some basic institutions of the dominant classes Hatred of the police Mistrust of the government and those in high places Cynicism which extends even to the church Not class conscious although very sensitive to status distinctions
The Local Community Level	Poor housing, crowding Gregariousness *Minimum of organization beyond the level of nuclear and extended family* but in spite of this there may be: sense of community and esprit de corps in urban slums	Marginal and anachronistic quality Locally oriented people, with very little sense of history

The Family Level	Free unions or consensual marriages High incidence of abandonment of wives and children Trend towards female or mother-centered families with greater knowledge of maternal relatives A strong predisposition to authoritarianism Lack of privacy Absence of childhood as a specially prolonged and protected stage in life cycle Early initiation into sex Verbal emphasis on family solidarity, but rarely achieved	
Major Characteristics of the Individual	Strong feeling of marginality of helplessness of dependence and of inferiority	With high incidence of maternal deprivation, confusion of sexual identification, lack of impulse control, a strong present-time orientation Sense of resignation and fatalism High tolerance for phychologic pathology

(Adapted from Lewis.[5])

concerned. These characteristics may be summarized by the following indicators: (1) money available for use for such health essentials as food, water, and housing; (2) effective use of resources; and (3) health behavior.

The special features in the health of the lowest social class indicate the need for closer scrutiny of the factors responsible. The economic and educational components are obviously central to any measure of differences between classes, since they directly affect diet, housing, and so on. These factors may vary quantitatively through a community in a continuous distribution. However, the distinctiveness of the lowest social class suggests that the differences between it and other classes are also qualitative and these differences might be in both the genetic and life experience areas.

Oscar Lewis first suggested that the way of life of many groups of poor people, but not all, could be conceived as a subcultural entity and he studied the culture of poverty as other anthropologists investigate various social and culture groups. His concept of the culture of poverty[5] as distinct from poverty alone may be very meaningful for community medicine in the extent to which it reflects community characteristics that have a direct expression in the health of the community; it also presents a group of people having a value-system, behavior, and social structure in marked contrast to the middle-class orientations of the average health service system.

Lewis distinguishes between poverty and the culture of poverty. Poor people who are class conscious, active members of trade-unions, or who adopt a world outlook may be desperately poor, but are no longer part of the culture of poverty. He presents several examples of very poor communities which did not evidence major features of the culture of poverty.

> The Jews of Eastern Europe were very poor, but they did not have many traits of the culture of poverty because of their tradition of literacy, the great value placed upon learning, the organization of the community around the rabbi, the proliferation of local voluntary associations, and their religion which taught that they were the chosen people.[5]

The features of the culture of poverty are summarized in Table 12-1 which is an abstract of Lewis' description, using his terminology.

REFERENCES

1. Hollingshead AB, Redlich FC: Social Class and Mental Illness: A Community Study. New York, Wiley, 1958, Table 15.
2. Fried M: Social differences in mental health. In Kosa J, Antonovsky A, Zola IK (eds.): Poverty and Health. Cambridge, Mass, Harvard Univ Press, 1969.
3. Orr JB: Food, Health and Income, 2nd ed. London, MacMillan, 1937

4. Lerner M: The level of physical health of the poverty population. A conceptual reappraisal of structural factors. Med Care 6:355, 1968.
5. Lewis O: The culture of poverty. In La Vida (Introduction). A Puerto Rican Family in the Culture of Poverty—San Juan and New York. London, Secker and Warburg, 1967, p 45.

13

The Impact of Poverty and Malnutrition on Physique and Behavior Development

Historical change and geographic variation in the nutritional state of people are among the striking features of community health. Syndromes of malnutrition common at one period disappear in a succeeding one. Such has been the history of scurvy and of rickets in Europe.[1] The converse historical trend, in which nutritional disease syndromes become widespread where formerly they were uncommon, has also been described. Beri-beri became highly prevalent in 19th century Asia with the introduction of the steam-milling process and the resultant widespread use of polished rice. Pellagra spread to areas where maize had been introduced as the staple cereal: southern Europe, Africa, and the southern states of the United States.[2] At the present time kwashiorkor continues its spread through the child populations of extensive parts of the world as infant- and early-child-feeding practices change in a way leading to protein-calorie malnutrition.

Equally interesting is the geographic variation in the predominant syndromes of malnutrition. In each poor region of the world, a particular syndrome of malnutrition tends to predominate and while it may share certain features with those of other regions, the different combinations of clinical signs differentiate them from one another. Thus pellagra, which is a predominant nutritional disease among poor maize-eating Africans, presents the well-known skin, mucous membrane, and mental changes but also has some features in common with beri-beri, more especially peripheral neuritis. And yet it is readily distinguished from the clinical syndrome of beri-beri, which in turn is common among poor rice-eating peoples. Both diseases are the product of multiple deficiencies and imbalances in nutrition, but the different combinations of these deficiencies and imbalances result in a particular type of syndrome being predominant.

Change or variation in these combinations may therefore be expected to modify the clinical picture.

The primary factor determining nutritional status of a population is its diet. Historical change and geographic variation in the prevalence of nutritional disease or, conversely, of healthy growth and nutrition, may therefore be expected to be associated with change and variation in dietary practices.

Epidemiologic investigation of nutritional status, or of a particular syndrome thought to be essentially nutritional, involves several distinctive elements, each requiring well-defined criteria and standardized methods. These include the following:

Nutritional status: clinical, anthropometric, and laboratory investigations
Diet: food eaten, associated with investigation of availability and cultural, economic, and agricultural factors
Modifying factors: the phases of growth and development, age, exercise and work, sleep, reproduction and lactation, various diseases

ACUTE NUTRITIONAL FAILURE: CASE ILLUSTRATION: KWASHIORKOR

Since the name "kwashiorkor" was first introduced into the literature by Williams in her description of the disease,[3,4] the condition has been widely reported. It is likely that it has not only become more widely recognized but is more widespread as well. It is at present recognized as one of the outstanding clinical syndromes of protein-calorie malnutrition in young children. Common features include failure in growth, various dermatoses, edema, pathologic liver changes, and gastrointestinal disorders. Mental changes are a prominent feature, especially apathy, listlessness, and withdrawal, which resemble the results of maternal deprivation in institutionalized infants.[5,6]

In their survey of kwashiorkor in Africa, Brock and Autret obtained evidence from various workers indicating marked differences in the occurrence of the condition in different African communities. The differences appeared to be a result of the types of foods onto which infants were customarily weaned. Breast-feeding was characteristic of all communities and the kinds of other foods introduced determined the later occurrence of kwashiorkor. In communities such as the Masai of Kenya, the Watusi of Ruanda-Urundi, and the people of western Congo who weaned their children onto animal foods, milk, meat, or fish, there was no kwashiorkor. This was in contrast to their neighbors such as the Kikuyu of Kenya and Baganda of Uganda who weaned their children onto agricultural crops. Even among these communities there were differences. The Bahutu of the plateau areas of Ruanda-Urundi, who had plentiful supplies of beans and weaned their children onto bean dishes, had some kwashiorkor but less than might have been the case if no animal or plant protein foods had been used.

There is a variation in the clinical picture of kwashiorkor in different localities. The variation is no doubt related to differences in the degree of deficiency of various food elements in what is essentially a multiple deficiency syndrome. Thus, in some communities of Indonesia, India, and Jordan, xerophthalmia has been described as a common sign.[7,8] In African cases glossitis, angular stomatitis, cheilosis, and angular blepharitis have been marked features.[9,10] The degree and kind of anemia that may be associated with kwashiorkor will be affected by the nutritional deficiencies as well as by other disorders, especially infections and infestations such as malaria and hookworm. A mild nutritional anemia is common in kwashiorkor, with megaloblastic changes in bone marrow. Vitamin B_{12} levels are usually normal but folic acid is low, with most cases responding to small doses of folic acid.[11]

Imbalance and actual interference in absorption and availability of different food factors is suggested in Arroyave's review of the interrelations between protein and vitamin A. He suggests that in severe protein deficiency, vitamin A in the diet does not reach the liver and the vitamin A in the liver is not available for use. Thus a functional deficiency of vitamin A may occur in kwashiorkor, independent of its dietary intake. Furthermore, he points to the fact that in many developing countries such as El Salvador, children who have low protein and low vitamin A in their diet have a slow growth rate but often do not manifest kwashiorkor syndrome or xerophthalmia. Arroyave suggests that "If the rate of growth were accelerated by the supplementation with proteins alone, the clinical manifestations of vitamin A deficiency may suddenly become more serious."[12]

THE LONG-TERM EFFECTS OF CHILDHOOD MALNUTRITION AND KWASHIORKOR

Epidemiologically more is known of the distribution and causes of kwashiorkor than of its effects, especially its long-term effects. With advances in its treatment such as the use of high protein foods (e.g., skim milk, or powdered fish meal and beans in traditional dishes), the former very high mortality rate has been reduced considerably. Thus apart from the many children who have chronic malnutrition without developing an acute episode of kwashiorkor, there are now large numbers who live after such serious nutritional failure as kwashiorkor. Knowledge of the long-term effects of such malnutrition in infancy and early childhood is of considerable importance to a community's health, and in the case of a widespread disease like kwashiorkor such knowledge is vital to an appreciation of world health.

Long-term effects of malnutrition may result from several processes. First, the acute severe episode may cause permanent damage, and second, the causes of the malnutrition syndrome in early childhood may continue to operate after recovery from the acute illness. In communities in which the incidence of kwashiorkor is high it is reasonable to expect that widespread prevalence of malnutrition resulting from poor diet is not confined to early childhood. The crisis of change in diet from breast milk to poor-quality protein foods may precipitate the nutritional failure syndrome which is then called kwashiorkor, but malnutrition is more widespread than the mere incidence of the acute failure syndrome itself and extends throughout the community. In these circumstances it is difficult, if not impossible, to differentiate the effects of kwashiorkor as such from those of the malnutrition process as a whole. The results of control studies are likely to be inconclusive, because the control group is actually composed of people who are malnourished but did not happen to manifest acute failure. For these reasons the discussion which follows will not be confined to the effects of the kwashiorkor episode per se but will deal with the possible long-term effects of malnutrition of the kind in which kwashiorkor is sometimes precipitated. Retardation of growth and of mental development will be considered.

Growth and Nutrition

The association between physical growth in children and their nutritional status is so close that measurements of growth are recommended as objective indices in assessing nutrition of a group.[13] McCarrison's observations on diet and nutrition among different peoples in India and his tests of the effects of these diets on laboratory animals provided striking evidence of the potential effects of diet on growth and disease. Feeding laboratory rats foods resembling as closely as possible the diets of the different national groups, McCarrison demonstrated that the noticeable differences in physique of the various peoples were replicated in the growth and physique of the experimental animals.[14–16] Direct evidence of the effects of malnutrition itself on human growth is difficult to obtain because children who are malnourished are usually at a disadvantage in other respects as well. However, much evidence has accumulated through experimental supplementation of the diets of children, especially schoolchildren. Such experiments have consistently resulted in increased rates of growth.

A particularly important experiment was that reported by Corry Mann in 1926 of a 4-year controlled feeding trial in which children who were already receiving what was considered to be a good diet were given different supplements of equivalent caloric value. Those who received an extra one pint (0.56 liter) of milk daily made the greatest gains in height and weight.[17] These results have since been confirmed in many studies with obvious implications for redefinition of various diets for growth.

Following the pioneer work of Quetelet in Belgium,[18] anthropometric studies became increasingly used in nutritional and health assessments of children and adults. Both longitudinal (in which consecutive measurements are made on the same children) and cross-sectional studies have been extensively used. An early finding was a correlation between growth of children and the social class and economic conditions of their homes,[19] in which children of the nonlaboring classes, professional and other, were taller and heavier at almost all ages than those of the laboring classes. The correlation was consistent for English and American children and among different ethnic groups in the United States. A pioneer attempt to estimate the relation between food, health, and income on a national scale was reported by John Boyd Orr in 1936.[20] The association between diet and income was apparent, the differences being particularly striking with respect to animal foods, fresh milk, meat, fish, eggs, fruit, and vegetables.

More recently there has been an extension of studies relating diet, nutrition, and growth in a number of developing countries. Among many of these, deficiency in protein-rich foods is one of the outstanding features of diets in which there are multiple deficiencies. It is in these countries, too, that kwashiorkor has been commonly described. Evidence from these studies has been consistent; malnutrition has reflected itself in several aspects of growth retardation, namely retardation in the rate of growth in infancy and childhood, delay in age of maturation, and smaller final stature.

Writing of the growth of Mayan Indian children of preschool age in rural villages of Guatemala, Béhar concludes that

> the growth pattern of these village children coincides with that of children in most underdeveloped areas. Gain in height and weight is satisfactory for the first 3 to 6 months. The rates then drop and throughout the preschool years do not again approach the standard set by well-nourished children of an industrialized country where economic and social conditions are more favorable.[21]

This conclusion is reached after comparing the Guatemalan findings with those of studies in many other communities in different countries; Béhar refers, for example, to southern India, Thailand, New Guinea, Uganda, Mexico, and Chinese children in Malaya. At later ages in childhood, the spurt in growth before puberty, and the age of puberty itself were found to be delayed in poorer children compared with better-off ones.[22,23] In the Guatemalan studies, the difference in median age of menarche in girls of low and high socioeconomic status was greater than 1.5 years, the former being approximately 14.5 years and the latter just under 13 years of age. Guzman complements Béhar's remarks by the following statement.

> Children from low socioeconomic groups, in all racial groups studied, had lower growth levels than children of high socioeconomic status; and those children in turn differed little in all measurements from accepted standards for children of industrialized countries. Retarded bone development, late initiation of the prepubertal growth spurt, later menarche, and a lesser magnitude of maximum growth during puberty all indicated an altered function associated with growth retardation.[22]

It is undoubtedly these processes which combine to produce adults of relatively small stature in the developing countries of the world.

The epidemiologic features of this distribution of a nearly universal pattern of growth in developing countries vary from place to place and yet have much in common.

Breast-feeding is nearly universal and continues to varying ages, often well beyond one year and not infrequently to two years and over.

During the first 3 to 6 months of life breast milk provides the nutritional requirements for relatively satisfactory growth. It is also during this period that infants are less exposed to infection, more especially the infections associated with diarrheal episodes, and they retain their congenital passive immunity to various diseases.

There is considerable variation in the length of time that babies are solely breast-fed but after this period, between 3 to 6 months of age, breast milk alone will not usually provide sufficient nutrition for adequate growth. It is at this age that the growth curve of babies in these communities begins to fall below desirable standards. The standards used are often those developed from studies in the better-off industrialized countries or sometimes from studies of children from selected homes of well-educated and economically better-off families in the developing country itself.[24]

The period of weaning to other foods is critical and continues until 3 to 4 years of age. It is critical for several reasons. First the type of foods to which the child is weaned is important with respect to the amount and quality of animal or plant proteins that they contain. The evidence directly relating this factor to differential growth at this time is definitive. Second, this is a period of an increase in exposure to infection as well as a decrease in passive immunity acquired from the mother.

The relative absence of acute nutritional failure syndrome in children of school-age has been noted by many workers, and yet nonspecific signs of malnutrition are prevalent. It seems possible that the relatively slow rate of growth during this period creates less demand for food than in infancy and early childhood when growth rates are greater. Many years ago, Himsworth referred to this. "It is a commonplace that the state of nutrition influences growth; it is less readily recognized that growth can lead to malnutrition." He illustrated this by an experiment.

> Three groups of rats were given the same fat free carbohydrate diet in equicaloric amounts which supplied 500 mg of casein daily to each animal. A daily supplement of 50 mg of cystine was given to the rats of the second and third groups and those in the latter also received 5 mg of choline daily. Both groups receiving cystine grew more rapidly than the control group although all consumed the same amount of food. The livers of the control group contained slightly more fat than normal; those of the group receiving choline and cystine had a normal fat content throughout; those of the group given cystine alone developed gross fatty infiltration, while they were growing, and towards the end of this period an early diffuse hepatic fibrosis developed. But after growth had stopped, even though the supplement of cystine was continued, the fat content of the liver returned to normal and the early fibrosis resolved, for at subsequent autopsies, none was found. Apparently the acceleration of growth, consequent upon supplying adequate amounts of cystine, had outrun the supply of lipotropic factors in the diet and fatty infiltration had resulted to such a degree as to lead to hepatic injury.[25]

Nutrition, Physique of Women, and Reproductive Efficiency

The effects of malnutrition on growth and hence on stature and physique of adults may have its most serious repercussions on reproductive functioning. The Aberdeen studies of Baird, Thompson, and associates have become a landmark in our understanding of some of the associations between social and economic factors and outcome of pregnancy.[26–31] Women married to men of higher social class are taller than those married to men of lower social class, and have several other advantages such as better education and general health. Taller women were found to have lower rates of caesarian section at delivery, lower rates of low-birth-weight babies, and lower perinatal mortality. The excess of perinatal mortality among infants born of short women was caused by a number of disorders and not only by difficult labor.[28] Thus it is not only short women with abnormalities caused by earlier rickets, including pelvic abnormality, who account for this difference. The Aberdeen findings have in general been confirmed by those of the British nationwide perinatal mortality survey of 1958.[32]

While the differences in growth between girls of different social class and hence of their final stature are considerable even in a relatively well-off country such as the United Kingdom, the impact of long-term malnutrition on growth and adult physique in poorer and less developed communities

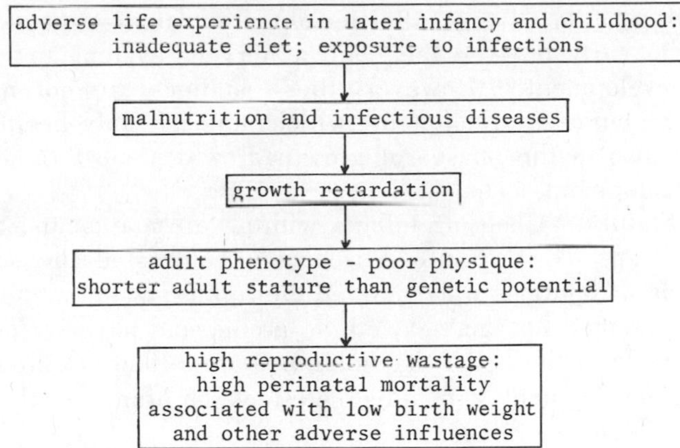

FIG. 13-1. The possible impact of early adverse life experience on later physique and reproductive efficiency.

must be expected to be very much greater. In general the birth weight of babies in Europe and North America is higher than that of Asian and African communities.[33] The extent to which this is a reflection of genetic differences between ethnic groups or of differences in life experience has not been studied in controlled comparative epidemiologic investigations. A hypothetical causal chain of associations, each stage of which needs testing in different communities, is shown in Figure 13-1.

Malnutrition and Mental Development

Mental development may be partly determined by nutritional status and an increasing amount of attention is being directed toward investigation of this possibility. It is difficult to differentiate the effects of malnutrition from those associated with causes of malnutrition itself such as poverty, poor education, and general neglect. Behavior changes are a clinical feature of kwashiorkor to which reference has already been made. These changes include varying degrees of apathy, the extreme case being minimal movement and an almost complete nonresponsiveness to environment.

An "accurate test of progress during treatment . . . is the return of interest in the outside world, the child becoming bright-eyed and following ward activities alertly."[6] While this apparent causal relationship between the child's mental state and his acute nutritional failure is readily appreciated, it is more difficult to relate subsequent mental development and behavior to either the acute episode of nutritional failure or continuing chronic malnutrition. There is now much evidence, from experimental animal studies, of the adverse influence of malnutrition—especially protein deficiency in early life—on the central nervous system and hence on behavior development.[34] However, these findings are not necessarily applicable to human development, which may not only be different in quality but also in the phases of growth at which most rapid changes in brain development occur.

Follow-up Studies. Choosing infants with severe marasmus, Stoch and Smythe of Cape Town, South Africa,[35–37] contrasted the subsequent development of 20 infants who survived their illness with the development of a group matched for age, sex, ethnic group, and poverty. They chose to study infants in the belief that malnutrition is likely to interfere with intellectual development by its adverse effects on brain growth in infancy and early childhood.

The differences between the two groups after 11 years of follow-up are summarized in Table 13-1 (the last measurements reported being for 1967).

TABLE 13-1

Height, weight, and head circumference (measured yearly)	The marasmic group had been consistently shorter, lighter, and smaller in head circumference
Developmental and intelligence tests (various tests) used at different ages at approximately two yearly intervals)	The marasmic group had markedly lower scores at all age levels
Educational progress	Most of the marasmic group lagged in grade appropriate for age
Cognition	Marasmic group had poorer grasp of concept of time
Motivation and personality tests	The marasmic group was inferior in each test

The marked inferiority of the "marasmic" group which was also evidenced by electroencephalogram findings, is notable, and it is tempting to relate the findings to the serious undernutrition in infancy. However, as the investigators themselves note "although both groups were drawn from the lowest socioeconomic level, the disparity of their living conditions was marked. Alcoholism, illegitimacy, and broken homes were the rule in the undernourished group, whereas the control group lived under more stable home conditions."[37] Thus, as is so often the case in severe nutritional failure of infancy and early childhood, dietary deprivation is one element of an overall syndrome of deprivation and this study does not succeed in delineating the influence of malnutrition as such from that of the general social deprivation.

A second study of similar kind is reported by Mönckeberg[38] of Chile. Fourteen children treated for severe marasmus in early infancy (age range on admission 1 to 5 months) were followed up for 3 to 6 years. After prolonged treatment the children were given regular free milk, 20 liters per month, with similar amounts for other infants and preschool children in the family. This effort to maintain a good standard of nutrition was successful to the extent that the general clinical appearance, and tests for total protein, albumen, hemoglobin, and hematocrit, were normal. Despite this, Gesell development tests remained below normal in most children, the retardation being especially marked in language development. The intelligence quotient (using Binet tests) was well below normal expectation in all 14 children. It was significantly lower than the average for Chilean preschool children of low socioeconomic status.

Cravioto[39,40] and his associates have reported on a comparative study of schoolchildren aged 6 to 11 years in a Guatemalan village. Measuring the height of all these schoolchildren, they compared the intersensory perception of the tallest and shortest quartiles. At each age the upper height quartile group was superior in various combinations of intersensory integration investigated, namely concordance or equivalence of perception of particular shaped geometric forms by "visual" and "haptic" perception (manipulation by finger and hands or manual exploration), and each of these with "kinesthetic" perception (passive movement of the arm through a cirucit which followed the shape being tested). The test used was that developed by Birch and Lefford.[41]

In this way an association was established between the stature of these rural children and their neurointegrative development. Using height alone as an indicator of malnutrition has been questioned. Being aware of this problem, and yet needing a simple and objective measurable index, the investigators present evidence suggesting that the relevance of height measurements in children varies under different circumstances. Thus in a group of upper-social-class urban schoolchildren there were also considerable differences in height but there were no differences in intersensory development; the errors made in recognition of identical forms were the same for the tallest and shortest quartile groups. Height may, therefore, be a good index of nutritional status in malnourished poorer communities, but not in upper-social-class or in better-off communities among whom other determinants, e.g., genetic factors, might be the most relevant. In this regard, too, it is of interest that Cravioto and associates did not find parental height significantly related to the height of the rural village children. This was in contrast to their finding of a strong association between paternal height and that of the children among upper-social-class urban groups.

Whether the inadequacy in intersensory integrative performance in the rural children was a result of malnutrition, or whether both poor integra-

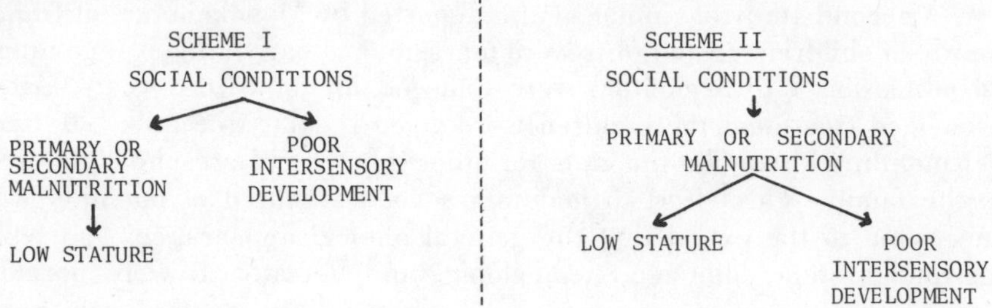

FIG. 13-2. Hypothetical relationships between social conditions, primary and secondary malnutrition, low stature, and poor intersensory development. (From Cravioto and associates.[39])

tion and growth differences are associated with more general subcultural differences, is a question requiring detailed consideration. These two alternatives can be analyzed most readily if they are considered diagramatically as two consequential schemata (Fig. 13-2).

While the evidence of various studies, including those cited above, suggests an association between malnutrition and poor physique on the one hand and retardation in mental growth on the other, it does not establish a causal relationship between them. In all epidemiologic studies there is need for considerable caution in inferring a causal relationship between two or more variables on the basis of an association in their occurrence. This is even more necessary in this case where the life situation may determine malnutrition, infection, and disease, and may also be relevant to mental growth. An association between social class and mental functioning is well known in more developed societies. The prevalence of mild mental retardation in adults and children[42–49] is very much higher in lower social classes. The converse of this is also true; not only is mild mental retardation less common in upper social classes but the prevalence of more highly intelligent people has been found to be greater in these classes.[42] In contrast to this social class effect on the distribution of less severe mental deficiency, severe cases tend to be distributed throughout all social classes without any significant class differences.[48] Furthermore, a very high proportion of these groups of severe mental retardation have evidence of brain damage. There is also evidence associating mother's education and the social class of her family of orientation (i.e., the home of her own upbringing) with her children's mental ability. This association has been found to be independent of other social variables.[39,40,47]

While experimental animal studies may produce more definitive evidence of malnutrition as a cause of central nervous system damage and retardation in growth of mental functioning, in human communities malnutrition is very closely associated with other poor social conditions which may themselves have a deleterious effect on mental growth. Malnutrition is a most important result of poverty and ignorance, but so are other conditions which may be potentially harmful to mental development. These other conditions may include infection and disease, lack of social interaction and language stimulation, large families with close spacing of successive children, inadequate personal health and medical care, and often a lack of prenatal care. This is reviewed further in Chapter 30, concerning a program for the promotion of growth and development.

Furthermore, there is the possibility that class differences exist in the genotype, and not only in differential phenotypic expression. This may be especially true in more developed countries.

Even in the absence of more definitive studies the case for action is very clear, but this does not gainsay the need for continuing investigation into the kind of relationship that exists between nutrition and different elements of growth, including the central nervous system and mental ability.

REFERENCES

1. Drummond JC, Wilbraham A: The Englishman's Food: A History of Five Centuries of English Diet. London, Jonathan Cape, 1939.
2. Terris M (ed.): Goldberger on Pellagra. Baton Rouge, Louisiana State Univ Press, 1964.
3. Williams CD: A nutritional disease of childhood associated with a maize diet. Arch Dis Child 8:434, 1933.
4. Williams CD: Kwashiorkor. Nutritional disease of children associated with a maize diet. Lancet 2:1151, 1935.
5. Brock JF, Autret M: Kwashiorkor in Africa. WHO Monogr Ser 8:1, 1952.
6. Jelliffe DB: Infant nutrition in the subtropics and tropics. WHO Monogr Ser 29:1, 100, 1955.
7. Patwardhan VN: Hypovitaminosis A and epidemiology of xerophthalmia. Am J Clin Nutr 22:1106, 1969.
8. McLaren DS, Shirajian E, Tchalian M, et al.: Xerophthalmia in Jordan. Am J Clin Nutr 17:117, 1965.
9. Kark SL: Adult and infant pellagra in South African Bantu. S Afr J Med Sci 8:106, 1943.
10. Gillman J, Gillman T: Perspectives in Human Malnutrition. New York, Grune & Stratton, 1951.
11. Woodruff C: Nutritional anemias in early childhood. Am J Clin Nutr 22: 504, 1969.
12. Arroyave G: Interrelations between protein and vitamin A and metabolism. Am J Clin Nutr 22:1119, 1969.
13. WHO Expert Committee on Medical Assessment of Nutritional Status. WHO Tech Rep Ser 258:1, 1963.
14. McCarrison R: Studies in Deficiency Disease. London, Henry Frowde and Hodder and Stoughton, 1921.
15. McCarrison R: Problems of nutrition in India. Nutr Abstr Rev 2:1, 1932.

16. McCarrison R: Nutrition and National Health. Cantor Lectures. London, Society of Arts, 1936. Republished as Nutrition and Health, 3rd ed. London, Faber and Faber, 1959.
17. Mann HCC: Diet for Boys During School Age. Special Report Series No. 105. Medical Research Council. London, Her Majesty's Stationery Office, 1926.
18. Quetelet A: Letters sur la Théorie des Probabilités Appliquée aux Sciences Morales et Politiques. Brussels, Hayez, 1946.
19. Roberts LJ: Nutrition Work with Children, rev. ed. Chicago, Univ of Chicago Press, 1935. Review of the early work of HP Bowditch, 1872–1891, and other early workers in USA; also a study by C Roberts, the physical development and proportions of the human body. St. Georges Hospital Reports 8:1, 1877.
20. Orr JB: Food, Health and Income, 2nd ed. London, MacMillan, 1937.
21. Béhar M: Prevalence of malnutrition among preschool children of developing countries. In Scrimshaw NS, Gordon JE (eds.): Malnutrition, Learning, and Behavior. Cambridge, Mass, MIT Press, 1968, p 37.
22. Guzman MA: Impaired physical growth and maturation in malnourished populations. In Scrimshaw NS, Gordon JE (eds.): Malnutrition, Learning, and Behavior. Cambridge, Mass, MIT Press, 1968, p 51.
23. Kark E: The menarche in African and Indian girls. In Kark SL, Steuart GW (eds.): A Practice of Social Medicine. Edinburgh, E & S Livingstone, 1962.
24. Collis WRF: Multifactorial causation of malnutrition. In Scrimshaw NS, Gordon JE (eds.): Malnutrition, Learning, and Behavior. Cambridge, Mass, MIT Press, 1968.
25. Himsworth HP: The Liver and Its Diseases. Oxford, Blackwell Scientific, 1947, p 67.
26. Baird D: The influence of social and economic factors on stillbirths and neonatal deaths. J Obstet Gynaec Brit Emp 52:339, 1945.
27. Baird D: Variations in reproductive pattern according to social class. Lancet 2:41, 1946.
28. Baird D: Social class and foetal mortality. Lancet 2:531, 1947.
29. Thompson AM: Maternal stature and reproductive efficiency. Eugenics Rev 51:157, 1959.
30. Thompson AM, Billewicz WZ: Nutritional status, maternal physique, and reproductive efficiency. Proc Nutr Soc 22:55, 1963.
31. Thompson AM: Historical perspectives of nutrition, reproduction. and growth. In Scrimshaw NS, Gordon JE (eds.): Malnutrition, Learning, and Behavior. Cambridge, Mass, MIT Press, 1968.
32. Baird G, Thompson AM: General factors underlying perinatal mortality rates. In Butler NR, Alberman ED (eds.): Perinatal Problems: The Second Report of the British Perinatal Mortality Survey. Edinburgh, E & S Livingstone, 1969.
33. Hytten FE, Leitch I: The Physiology of Human Pregnancy. Oxford, Blackwell Scientific, 1964.
34. Scrimshaw NS, Gordon JE (eds.): Malnutrition, Learning, and Behavior. Cambridge, Mass, MIT Press, 1968, Part 4.
35. Stoch MB, Smythe PM: Does undernutrition during infancy inhibit brain growth and subsequent intellectual development? Arch Dis Child 38: 546, 1963.
36. Stoch MB, Smythe PM: The effect of undernutrition during infancy on subsequent brain growth and intellectual development. S Afr Med J 41:1027, 1967.

37. Stoch MB, Smythe PM: Undernutrition during infancy, and subsequent brain growth and intellectual development. In Scrimshaw NS, Gordon JE (eds.): Malnutrition, Learning, and Behavior. Cambridge, Mass, MIT Press, 1968, p 279.
38. Mönckeberg F: Effect of early marasmic malnutrition on subsequent physical and psychological development. In Scrimshaw NS, Gordon JE (eds.): Malnutrition, Learning, and Behavior. Cambridge, Mass, MIT Press, 1968, Part 4.
39. Cravioto J, De Licardie ER, Birch HG: Nutrition, growth, and neurointegrative development. An experimental and ecologic study. Pediatrics (Suppl 2, Part II) 38:319, 1966.
40. Cravioto J, De Licardie ER: Intersensory development of school-age children. In Scrimshaw NS, Gordon JE (eds.): Malnutrition, Learning, and Behavior. Cambridge, Mass, MIT Press, 1968, Part 4.
41. Birch HG, Lefford A: Two strategies for studying perception in "brain-damaged" children. In Birch HG (ed.): Brain Damage in Children: The Biological and Social Aspects. Baltimore, Williams and Wilkins, 1964.
42. Burt C: A Study in Vocational Guidance. London, Her Majesty's Stationery Office, 1926.
43. Burt C: The Backward Child. London, Univ of London Press, 1937.
44. Clarke AM, Clarke ADB (eds.): Mental Deficiency: The Changing Outlook. London, Methuen, 1958.
45. Stein Z, Susser MW: The social distribution of mental retardation. Am J Ment Defic 67:811, 1963.
46. Susser MW: Community Psychiatry. New York, Random House, 1968.
47. Richardson SA: The influence of socioenvironmental and nutritional factors on mental ability. In Scrimshaw NS, Gordon JE (eds.): Malnutrition, Learning, and Behavior. Cambridge, Mass, MIT Press, 1968.
48. Penrose LS: A clinical and genetic study of 1,280 cases of mental defect. Special Report Series Medical Research Council No. 229. London, Her Majesty's Stationery Office, 1938.
49. Penrose LS: The Biology of Mental Defect, 3rd ed. London, Sidgwick and Jackson, 1963.

SECTION 3

Infection, Disease, and Community Health

INFECTION, DISEASE, AND COMMUNITY HEALTH—AN ILLUSTRATION OF CHANGING CONCEPTS OF CAUSE AND EFFECT

"Throughout nature, infection without disease is the rule rather than the exception."[1]

In our consideration of community determinants of health and disease little reference has been made to changing concepts of cause and effect. There is a basic dichotomy in ideas that various peoples have regarding the causes of disease, causes which arise from within the self and those that come from without. These beliefs in the endogenous and exogenous origins of disease parallel one another throughout history, sometimes one, at other times the other, dominating thought. Invasion by pathogenic agents includes beliefs in witchcraft, demon possession, microorganisms, and inhalation of irritants and poisons. In contrast to this are the endogenous causes of disease, brought on oneself through sin against the gods or one's fellow-men, and the concepts of disturbance in humoral balance, homeostasis, and regulatory processes.

The postulate that will be discussed here involves the following kinds of questions: Under what conditions does infection result in disease? What factors influence the severity and kind of expression of infections such as those by tubercle bacilli, plasmodium, or streptococcus hemolyticus.

The impact of infection on a community's health will be influenced by, and will influence, the syndrome of community health consisting in somatic and psychologic characteristics and the pattern of disease and disability. These elements of community health have been more fully discussed in Chapters 3 to 5.

The development of epidemiologic thought on the subject of infection, disease, and community health is considered here as an illustration of changing concepts of cause and effect (Fig. 14-1).

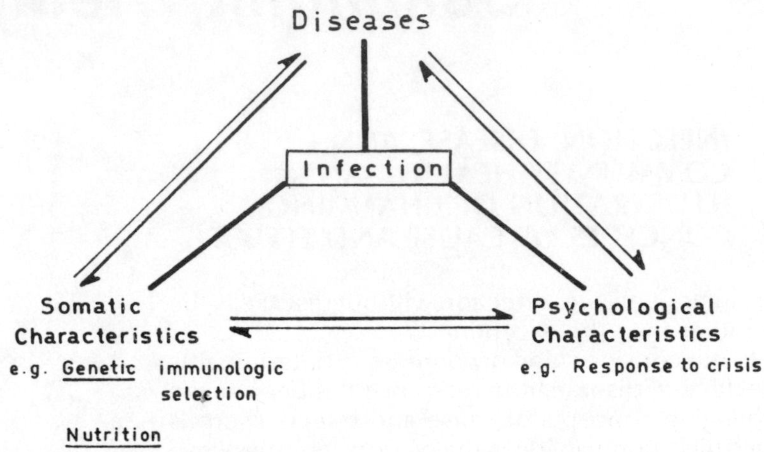

FIG. 14-1. A perspective of infection in relation to the epidemiologic determinants of its outcome in a community.

14

Specific Agents as Causes of Disease

The concept of diseases as distinct biologic entities, each caused by a specific agent, gained momentum during the 19th and 20th centuries in the discoveries of microbiology, nutrition, and biochemistry. The theory of a natural living agent as the cause of contagion was apparently first propounded in the 16th century by Fracastorius, a physician of Verona. In his book *De Contagione*,[2,3] published in 1546, he argued that disease is not caused by a "mysterious shadow or miasma, nor by obstructed humors" and postulated that contagion was caused by "a kind of seed or seminaria." These living substances were so small as to be invisible and were transmitted from one person to the next by actual bodily contact, through fomites, and through the air. They established themselves in the body of the victim by multiplying themselves, causing the same disease in him as they had caused in the person from whom they came.

At this time the concept of contagion became generally accepted in Italy and in fact throughout much of Europe. Its profound influence is evidenced in the laws made by a number of cities in Italy and elsewhere, especially in attempts to control tuberculosis. These laws included compulsory notification of cases with instructions to the local authorities as to what should be done with patients, their clothing, and the rooms in which they slept; as to the disposition of the patients and their personal belongings; as well as to the houses in which they lived. In the course of time the contagion theory of tuberculosis fell into disrepute and the law was no longer in force. It was even sometimes rescinded, as in the case of Florence in 1754. A more detailed account of this legislation, as well as the change of theory from contagion to heredity, is given in *The White Plague*.[4]

Later workers who contributed further observations on agents spreading disease were Kircher in the 17th century and Plenzis in the 18th century. The former referred to the natural transmission of disease by insects, suggesting that flies which fed on diseased and dying persons then deposited their material on food, thereby transferring the disease to others. Plenzis postulated that the germ does not only reproduce in the body but in suitable circumstances it would reproduce and live outside the body. However, these observations were not embodied in basic medical thinking until much later in the 19th century.

The focus of epidemiology on epidemic disease and "fevers" in the 19th century was no doubt due to the high prevalence rates and severity of these diseases at that time in Europe. The concept of the existence of specific causal agents for these diseases and, more especially, of living organisms as the specific agents, was founded on converging developments in biologic and medical knowledge. Definition and delineation of various "fevers" as distinct biologic entities was a necessary process in the growth of such concepts. Landmarks in this kind of development were Sydenham's differentiation of scarlet fever from measles in the late 17th century and well over a century later, in the early 19th century, Bretonneau's recognition of diphtheria as distinct from scarlet fever. Both made claims which later became important in epidemiology. Sydenham noted a secular trend in the expression of epidemics (i.e., the same diseases in different years will differ "as chalk from cheese"), running different courses and needing different treatment, but he did not consider separate specific causes of each disease. Bretonneau, on the other hand, claimed that different disease entities have different causes, each being the result of an organism, a specific transmissible agent.

Two very different types of study are among the outstanding milestones in the orientation of epidemiology toward living organisms as specific agents of disease. One, by Henle, was essentially an armchair discussion of a thesis based on a meditative review of existing knowledge drawn from different, but relevant, fields of study. The other, by Snow, was a report of observations on cholera in London, with interpretation of the findings and subsequent testing of the inferences by further observation. Owing to their importance, the reflections of Henle and the observations of Snow are summarized here.

JACOB HENLE: *ON MIASMATA AND CONTAGIA*

Not very long before the discoveries of Pasteur and Koch ushered in the age of bacteriology and established the germ theory of disease, the climate of medical opinion was to consider "miasmata" and "contagious matter" as distinctly different and separate causes of disease. In his essay, *On Miasmata and Contagia*, published in 1840, Henle[5] wrote of the academicians of his day, quoting them as saying that "the miasma is a noxious matter, originating externally and mixed with the air, which enters the body, and produces disease even in infinite quantity, in the manner of poisons. The contagious agent on the other hand is a material which is formed by a disease and which occasions the same disease in others." His rebuttal of this concept is summarized below. It is a major landmark in the history of medical thought and much of his reasoning was later embodied by Koch in the development of the germ theory of disease.

1. The contagious agent as cause of disease
   a. An organism with the ability to multiply
   b. When excreted by a sick person and communicated to healthy individuals, it produces the same disease in them
   c. The causal agent, and not the disease, reproduces itself
2. Entrance of the organism into individuals
   a. Disease begins with entrance of the organism
   b. Organisms enter the body through accessible mucous membranes or injured skin
3. Incubation period
   a. Following entrance of the organism, time is needed for it to multiply or develop sufficiently to produce clinical signs
4. Vehicles of contagion
   a. Organic material such as pus, mucus, blood, and excreta, which contain the infectious agent but are not otherwise infectious
5. Carriers
   a. Henle did not develop the modern concept of a carrier but recognized that there were individuals who externally carried the contagious agent without being affected by it
6. The unity of contagion and miasma
   a. Refutation of the dual concept of miasmatic diseases and contagious diseases
   b. Replaced dual concept by that of a specific living organism with the ability to multiply.

JOHN SNOW: *ON THE MODE OF COMMUNICATION OF CHOLERA*

The great pandemics of cholera which spread through Europe in the 19th century were an added challenge and stimulus to those seeking to understand epidemic diseases and fevers. It was during the second of these pandemics that John Snow carried out his studies of several local epidemics in London.[6] He first published his observations in 1849. His investigations became a model of epidemiologic method, involving descriptive observations regarding the distribution of the disease in different groups, on the basis of which he hypothesized as to its cause. His inferences concerning method of spread of the disease were tested by analytic study and, finally, by his use of an opportunity to conduct a natural experiment in which he was able to investigate the differential incidence of new cases and mortality rates in houses supplied by different water supplies.

It will be noted that his framework of thinking was almost completely agent-oriented. People are studied with respect to the way they become infected and how they might spread the disease rather than as hosts to infecting organisms. When the environment is considered it is as the vehicle of transmission of the organism, such as in the contamination of water.

As far as possible the summary of Snow's theories has been arranged in more or less the same order as that of Henle's work.

1. The specific agent as cause of disease
   a. Material which has the property of multiplying in people
   b. It passes from the sick to the healthy
   c. Probably has the structure of a cell
2. Entrance of the organism ("morbid material") into individuals
   a. The disease begins when the morbid material is swallowed into the alimentary canal, which is the first part affected.
3. Incubation period
   a. Period of reproduction of the organism (morbid material)
4. The spread of the disease
   a. Disease is spread by people
   b. Situations which favor the spread of the disease
      1. Pollution of foods by hands of those in contact with patient, without washing of hands before handling food
      2. When once introduced, cholera spreads where there is crowding of families in single rooms, where they live, sleep, eat, and wash together
   c. Water-borne epidemics: This is dealt with in more detail as it illustrates the importance of the natural experiment in epidemiology

At that time London's supply of water was by wells with pumps and by pipe reticulation of Thames river water. Snow's investigations included an epidemic which he associated with contamination of a pump well (the Broad Street pump), and several epidemics with a differential distribution in various districts. His examination of the records of the 1832 epidemic and his personal investigations of epidemics in 1849, 1853, and finally 1854 led him to conclude that widespread occurrence of cholera could only be due to the water supplies. This is illustrated in Figure 14-2, prepared from the detailed data presented by Snow, in which variation and change in water supplies were related to each epidemic.

Snow's observations on the means of transmission of cholera and his postulation of the specific causal agent were made many years before the discovery of the cholera vibrio. It was only some 30 years later, in 1883, that Koch discovered the cholera vibrio and then 10 years after that he established the fact that apparently well persons could excrete this pathogenic agent. The importance of this discovery for epidemiology

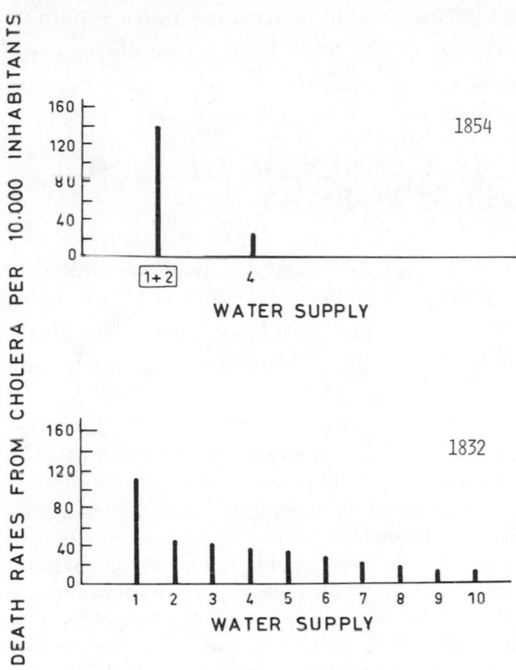

FIG. 14-2. Snow's investigations of cholera in London, illustrating the death rate from cholera according to water supplies of districts. The water supply companies are shown by numbers. 1832: The numbers 1 to 10 represent groupings of the various districts of London according to their main sources of water supply, arranged in descending order of the death rate from cholera. In general, the lesser the pollution of water at its source the lower the death rate. Thus districts supplied with water drawn from points high up the river Thames, and hence less polluted, had lower mortality rates. This was so in each of the succeeding epidemics—1849, 1853, 1854. The figure directs attention to a comparison between two groups of districts, according to their sources of water supply in 1854, without showing each of the other groups of districts. 1854: Number 4 water company removed their water works in 1852 from its original site on the river to one where they obtained a supply of water unpolluted by the sewage of London. Snow emphasized the importance of this change and its impact on the death rate from cholera even in those districts where this company's water supplies were distributed to some homes and those of Companies 1 and 2 to other homes in the same streets. The 1854 epidemic afforded him the opportunity to test his conviction regarding the role of water supplies in the transmission of cholera. The General Board of Health obtained data on the population of these districts with lists of houses receiving their water from Companies 1 and 2 combined, leaving houses receiving water from Company 4 separate. The deaths recorded were compared with sources of water supply and it is on the basis of this natural experiment that he prepared the statistics from which the figure has been extracted. (Adapted from Snow.[6])

was that it recognized and underlined an additional source of infection, namely the carrier state. Furthermore, and possibly of even greater importance, was the fact that infection and disease were not synonymous; one could be well *and* infected. However, this aspect was less appreciated at a time when truly remarkable contributions were being made as a result of the new knowledge of the age of bacteriology that was ushered in by Pasteur and Koch.

SPECIFIC CAUSES OF DISEASE: THE GERM THEORY

The germ theory, in which particular diseases are linked to specific causal organisms, has continued to have a profound impact on medicine and its concepts of disease causation. In his discussion of the etiology of tuberculosis, Koch[7] laid down the criteria that had to be met to prove that a disease was caused by specific organisms.

> On the basis of my numerous observations I believe it to be proven that in all tuberculous lesions in humans as well as in animals, the bacteria identified by me as tubercle bacilli, are present and distinct from all other bacteria. From this coincidence of tuberculous lesions and bacilli, however, it cannot yet be concluded that both these phenomena are causally related, although no small measure of support for this assumption can be derived from the fact that the bacilli are mainly found in tuberculous processes which are active and disappear when the disease is arrested.
>
> In order to prove that tuberculosis is a parasitic illness brought about by the invasion of these bacilli and determined by their growth and multiplication, the bacilli have to be isolated from the body, reproduced in pure cultures until they become completely free from any product accompanying illness originating from the animal body, and, finally, by the inoculation of the isolated bacilli into animals, produce the same disease picture of tuberculosis which normally is obtained by inoculation of naturally-produced tuberculous material.

Satisfying these criteria has ensured exacting methods in bacteriologic investigations of causal association between an organism and a particular disease. His postulates have recently been summarized as follows: "(1) The organism must be found in all cases of the disease in question. (2) It must be isolated from it and grown in pure culture. (3) When the pure culture is inoculated into susceptible animals or man, it must reproduce the disease."[8]

The demand for a high degree of specificity of effect of an organism before accepting it as the cause of a particular disease has had a profound effect on causal theory in general and on epidemiology in particular. It has been extended to the investigation of other diseases. In this way, nutritional disorders have been related to deficiency or excess of single specific food factors, carcinomata to carcinogens, allergies to allergens, and various diseases to other specific noxious substances in the environment, e.g., dusts, pesticides, smog, and radiation.

In addition to finding the specific agent in cases of the disease, there is the task of determining the incidence over time of new cases of the particular disease in those exposed to the agent. Koch's third postulate as outlined above makes some provision for this, but it was originally on an experimental laboratory basis, using relatively simple controlled study methods. The association between disease incidence and the distribution of an infecting organism (or other agent of disease in a human population group) is a first-level consideration in epidemiology. The difference in response of different segments of the exposed population has been a main reason for shift from the concept of a single agent as *the* cause of a disease to an appreciation of multiple causation.

THE XYZ THEORY, OR AGENT, HOST, AND ENVIRONMENT

As is well known, the germ theory was not readily accepted even at a time when bacteriology was making a series of important discoveries. Among its critics were Von Pettenkoffer and Florence Nightingale. One aspect of the broad front of disagreement between Von Pettenkoffer and Koch has been recorded by Rosenau.[9] In the 1892 to 1893 epidemic of cholera in Hamburg, Koch isolated the "comma bacillus" (cholera vibrio) from the water supplies and thereby reached an understanding of the role of water supplies in the causation of cholera. Von Pettenkoffer held that the organism could not be regarded as the only cause of the disease. Thus, he argued, it might be harmful to people in India or Hamburg but not necessarily to people elsewhere. The people and the place in which they lived determined whether they would be diseased. In his argument he developed his XYZ theory, likening the process to fermentation. Fermentation needs yeast (X), the carbohydrate in which the yeast will function (Y), and a suitable temperature for the fermentation to take place (Z). He supported his views with equivocal results when he and his assistant drank pure cultures of cholera, thereby challenging Koch's third postulate

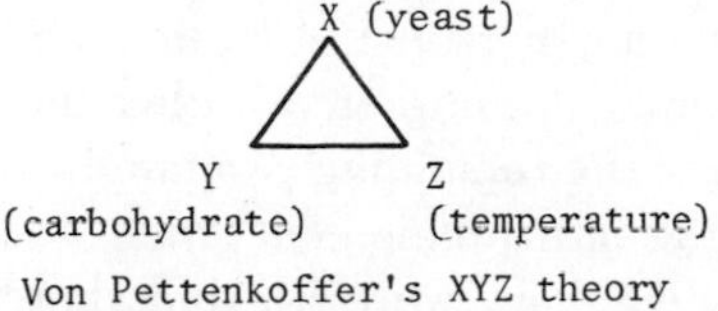

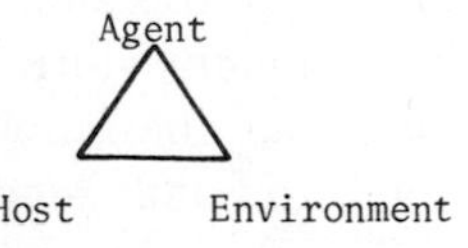

FIG. 14-3. Diagram illustrating the analogy between Von Pettenkoffer's XYZ theory and the later epidemiologic triangle.

as outlined above. Similar differing results were reported by others who repeated his personal experiment. As with so many of the great arguments between scientific opponents, the disagreement itself became a stimulus for further study, and with the passage of time and further study each of the opposing views were found to contain part of the truth or scientific reality. The analogy of the XYZ theory and the later, more commonly used, epidemiologic model is represented in Figure 14-3.

The model of interaction between agent, host, and environment ensures consideration of both the people and their environment in epidemiologic studies. Nevertheless in its focus on a single specific agent of each disease, and its sometimes restricted conceptualization of "people" as hosts to agents, this epidemiologic model has limitations.

The challenge put forward by Von Pettenkoffer was submerged in the welter of discovery of various organisms and the consequent advances in the control of infection. However, for a long time it has been known that the results of infection vary considerably; in fact, one of the earliest to describe this variation was Fracastorius in his reference to the changing picture of syphilis in Italy.

WIDENING CONCEPTS IN EPIDEMIOLOGY OF INFECTION, HEALTH, AND DISEASE

Dubos is among the most recent workers who has emphasized the importance of distinguishing between infection and disease: "various microbial agents including the classical pathogens can exist and persist in the tissues without manifesting their presence by pathologic disorders."[10] This, he states, "has long been known but grossly neglected." He refers to Koch's discovery of cholera vibrio carriers in 1893 as the first practical demonstration of the important role which such healthy people can have in the transmission of human disease. That an "epidemic" of the carrier state can take place in families with no case of illness during or before the epidemic period is well illustrated by a study of five families living in a city slum.[11] Stool specimens of the 26 individuals in these five families were repeatedly examined over a period of 16 months—in May, July, and September of 1967, and then monthly from January to August 1968. In July 1967, cholera vibrios were isolated in nine persons: a mother and two children in one family, a mother and child in another, a father and child in a third family, and one child in each of the remaining two families. Despite the presence of infection, none of the individuals concerned was ill at the time or had been ill before, no neighbors were ill, and there had been no known case of cholera in the neighborhood during the previous two years.

TABLE 14-1. Epidemiology of Group A Beta-Hemolytic Streptococcal Infection and Illness in a Population

PHASE I INITIATION AND TRANSMISSION	PHASE II RESPONSE TO EXPOSURE		PHASE III RESPONSE TO INFECTION		PHASE IV LATER EFFECTS
Exposure to streptococcal infection (The introduction and transmission of the organisms in a population group.)	Not infected		Returns to state of non-infected		Well—not infected or asymptomatic carrier
		Well	A 'well' carrier		Recurrence of infection or illness
	Infected		Immunity	Outcome	Rheumatic fever and rheumatic heart disease
		Illness			Glomerulonephritis
	Kinds of illness e.g.: respiratory, scarlet fever, skin, puerperal sepsis		Biologic gradient of infection and illness—varying degrees of severity		

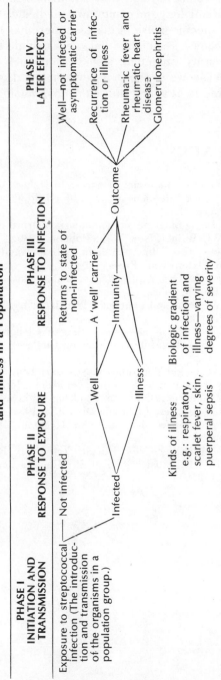

Phases: Each of these "phases" of a streptococcal infection in families or other groups has its epidemiology requiring investigation and different "levels" of action.

The full implications of such well-established facts have still to be incorporated in epidemiology and community medicine. Without detracting from the theory of specific cause of disease, there has been a broadening of the concept of causal association between a single specific agent and a distinct disease entity. Infection, disease from such infection, and the outcome of the disease are related but nevertheless distinct entities. This is illustrated in Table 14-1, which shows the epidemiology of streptococcal infection and illness.

REFERENCES

1. Dubos R: Evolution of microbial diseases. In Dubos RJ, Hirsch JG (eds.): Bacterial and Mycotic Infections of Man, 4th ed. Philadelphia and Montreal, Lippencott, 1965, p 32.
2. Fracastorii H: De contagione et contagiosis morbis et corum curatione. Translated by WC Wright. New York, Putnam, 1930.
3. Osler W: "Fracastorius." In An Alabama Student and Other Biographical Essays. London, Oxford Univ Press, 1908.
4. Dubos R, Dubos J: The White Plague: Tuberculosis, Man and Society. Boston, Little, Brown, 1952.
5. Henle J: On miasmata and contagia. Translated by GG Rosen. Bull Inst Hist Med 6:907, 1938.
6. Snow J: On the Mode of Communication of Cholera, 2nd ed. London, John Churchill, 1854. Reprinted in Snow on Cholera. New York, Commonwealth Fund, 1936.
7. Koch R: Die Aetiologie der tuberculose. Berl Klin Wochenschr 19:221, 1882. Quotation translated by D Pridan, Jerusalem, Israel.
8. Yerushalmy J, Palmer CE: On the methodology of investigations of etiologic factors in chronic diseases. J Chronic Dis 10:27, 1959.
9. Rosenau MJ: Preventive Medicine and Hygiene, 6th ed. New York, Appleton-Century, 1935.
10. Dubos R: Man Adapting. New Haven, Yale Univ Press, 1965, p 177.
11. Sen R, Sen DK, Chakrabarty AN, et al.: Cholera carriers in a Calcutta slum. Lancet 2:1012, 1968.

15 Community Infection and Disease

INFECTION AND TRANSMISSION OF THE INFECTING AGENT

The incidence or prevalence rates of infection are dependent on the exposure of a susceptible population group to specific infecting organisms. A continuing source of the agent is needed if the infection is to remain in the community. Its reservoir may be human or animal, and the channels of exit from the reservoir may be the respiratory or alimentary tracts, exposed surfaces, the skin and mucous membranes, or through milk. Flesh is an additional source of infection from animals.

Where the source of infection is human and the power of infecting is of short duration, an epidemic episode might be followed by no further infection. This has been recorded in many small or relatively isolated communities in which the reservoir of the infecting agent disappears and no new infection is initiated until contact is established with a source from outside the community. On the other hand, in those infections where the power of infection is of long duration and the chance of infection is enhanced by intimate and continued contact, as in infection with mycobacterium tuberculosis and Hansen, a small group such as a family or kin group can continue as the source of infection for considerable periods of time.

Transmission of the Agent

The main means of transmission include the following.

Contact—direct, indirect (droplet infection)
Airborne—droplet nuclei and dust
Vehicles—water, food, fomites
Arthropod vectors—infected vectors, vectors as mechanical carriers

The main channels of entrance of an agent to a new host are respiratory and oral, in addition to entrance through exposed mucous membrane and skin.

The social structure and functioning of a population group influences transmission of the agent. The frequency of contact between people of different segments of the community is obviously influenced by the network of relationships, especially those involving face-to-face contact. There are rural communities in which the homesteads, with extended family units living as joint families, are built as discrete units rather than in more compact villages. Neighboring homesteads may be some distance apart and their members are often not in one another's immediate network of relationships or primary groups. Instead, the homesteads of both conjugal and affinal kin may be the locus for day-to-day relationships between people and hence more useful for the study of exposure to infection. When infection enters a household its own members are exposed; there may be little or no spread to the wider community, and what spread occurs can often be traced through related kin groups.

COMMUNITY SUSCEPTIBILITY

"In any disease spread by direct contact it is probable that once a critical ratio between the immune and the susceptible members of the population is reached, infection tends to die out of its own accord."[1] This was well demonstrated in the community response to active immunization against diphtheria. Widespread continuing immunization programs not only reduced the cases of disease but also the carrier rate. The critical ratio between "immunes" and "susceptibles" is in effect that point at which "the chain of infection is broken." This point not only varies according to the infectivity of the organism but also with various characteristics of the community and its environment.

P. L. Panum: Observations During the Epidemic of Measles on the Faroe Islands in the Year 1846

The history of the community with respect to the specific agent of infection is a major determinant of its response. Panum's report on the measles epidemic among the Faroe islanders in 1846 has become a classic contribution to our knowledge of the response of a "virgin" population to an infection.[2,3]

Very soon after qualifying as a doctor of medicine at the age of 25 years, Panum was sent by the Danish government to the Faroe Islands in the North Sea. His function was to investigate the epidemic and provide medical help to the people. Closely following Hippocratic teaching, his investigation was oriented to the physical environment and mode of life of the people.

> When a physician is called to work in a place where climatic and dietary conditions are different from those to which he has been accustomed, his first problem is to study the hygienic factors which affect the state of health of the inhabitants. It is, in fact, these hygienic conditions which contribute towards the development and frequency of some diseases and the exclusion or rarity of others, and which more or less modify the symptoms of every disease; it is, indeed, these conditions that constitute the basis of the geography of disease, the special study of which subject will soon, perhaps, elevate it to the status of an independent science.

The health of the Faroe islanders *compared favorably* with that of the people of Denmark, in that "in Denmark more children under 10 years of age die than on the Faroes, and that . . . a far greater number reach the age of 70 years on the islands than in Denmark." In contrast to this he found that between 10 and 50 years of age "the mortality is higher on the Faroes than in Denmark" due to "the disproportionately greater number of people" who "meet violent death on the Faroes by drowning in the dangerous fjords, and by plunging down from the cliffs, than in level Denmark, surrounded by a calm sea."[2]

In seeking the reasons for the differences in health he examined his detailed description of the climate and geography of the islands and of the food, clothing, housing, activities, and occupations of the people. Regarding these conditions as more "injurious" than "beneficial" he was not able to relate the favorable health findings to these important "hygienic factors."

> After having thus reviewed the causes which at first glance would seem to be able to exert some effect on the favorable rates of mortality on the Faroes, without so far having found any factor to which, on closer scrutiny, might be ascribed any essential importance in this respect, we are led to accept the assumption that the entire or partial exemption of the Faroe islands from a number of diseases, especially those which are infectious, which decimate the populations of other countries, is the most important of all causes of the favorable rates on these Islands, and the high limit of life of the inhabitants.

Thus he notes that "scrofulosis and tuberculosis" are comparatively rare on the Faroes, malaria does not occur, and among the infectious diseases, "scarlatina has never, as far as I know, visited the Faroes, nor, probably, whooping cough," measles had not occurred since 1781, and smallpox since 1705. He concludes "the most essential cause of the favorable rates of mortality on the Faroes may be looked for in the freedom of these islands, because of their situation as well as their isolated condition as regards commerce, from many diseases which in other places—Denmark, for instance—very considerably increase the mortality."

The introduction of a new infection to such an isolated community is well illustrated in his study of the measles epidemic of 1846. "The first person on the Faroes who took the measles was a cabinetmaker. He left Copenhagen on the 20th of March and reached Thorshavn on the 28th; on the way he had felt quite well, but was attacked by measles early in April, on what day he did not know. Shortly before his departure he had visited some measles patients in Copenhagen."

There had been no case of measles in these island communities since 1781 and what followed the introduction of infection by this single case is an illustration of the impact of infection in a virgin population. Between April and September 1846 about 6,000 of the 7,782 inhabitants "were taken with measles." The following summarizes his main conclusions.

Susceptibility to Infection. While people of all ages were susceptible to infection he noted that recovery from measles insured people against a second attack.

> Of the many old people still living on the Faroes who had had the measles in 1781, not one, as far as I could find out by careful inquiry, was attacked the second time. I myself saw 98 such old people, who were exempt because they had had the disease in their youth. This was the more noteworthy in that a high age by no means lessened the susceptibility to measles, since, as far as I know, all the old people who had not gone through with the measles in earlier life were attacked when they were exposed to infection, while certain young persons, although constantly exposed, were exempt.

Transmission.

INCUBATION PERIOD. In his observations of outbreaks in 52 different towns of the islands he always found "that 13 or 14 days intervene between the reception of the contagion and the eruption of the rash."

CONTAGIOUS NATURE OF THE DISEASE.

> If, among 6,000 cases, of which I myself observed and treated about 1,000, not one was found in which it would be justifiable, on any grounds whatever, to suppose a miasmatic origin of the measles, because it was absolutely clear that the disease was transmitted from man to man and from village to village by contagion . . . it is certainly reasonable at least to entertain a considerable degree of doubt as to the miasmatic nature of the disease. . . .
>
> It is, in my opinion, not only theoretically justifiable to regard it on the whole as a contagious disease, but practically even necessary to do so. For if people think that the causes of the disease must be sought for as *generally dispersed in the atmosphere*, they can have no hope of protecting themselves against it.

QUARANTINE. "By cutting off communication with infected places, the residents of 15 listed places succeeded in keeping the measles entirely away" from their inhabitants.

Severity and Outcome. While people of all ages were susceptible to infection there were marked differences in the outcome of the disease as measured by mortality. By comparing the age-mortality rates for the period including the epidemic of measles with those usual on the Faroe Islands, he found

> that the measles, perhaps in connection with the epidemic of influenza which prevailed with it in the spring, was destructive to the young child

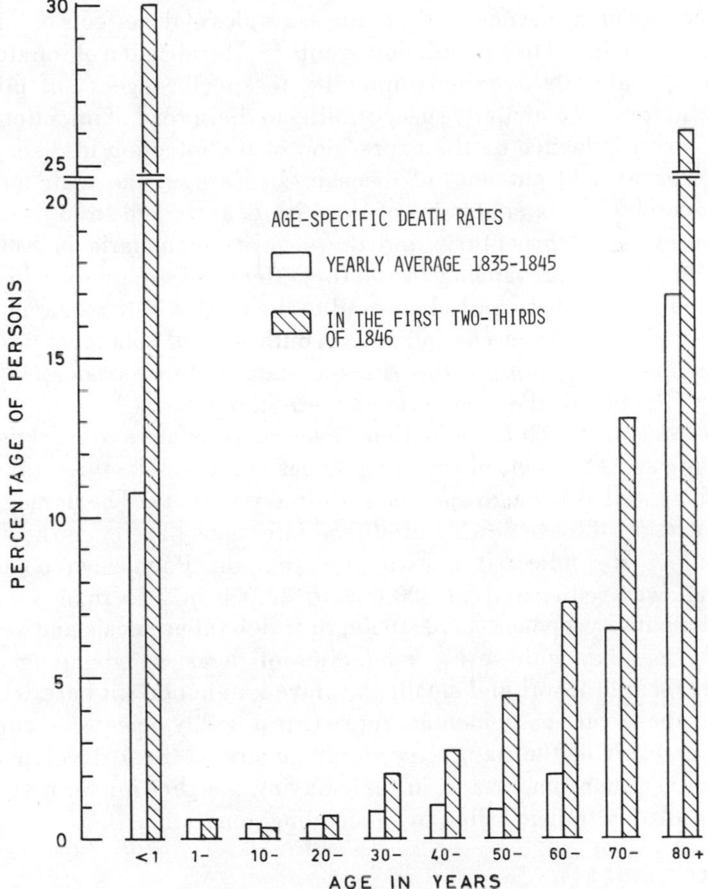

FIG. 15-1. Age-specific death rates for the first two-thirds of 1846, compared with the average of age-specific death rates between 1835 and 1845 (inclusive). (Adapted from Panum.[2])

under 1 year of age, but on the other hand, did not remarkably increase the mortality between the first and twentieth years of life, because the disease was less dangerous in this period; but that the mortality rose from the 30th year, until it became greatest for the age between 50 and 60 years, that is, five times as great as usual; besides which it then descended again after the 60th year—not because the disease was less dangerous for those still older, which was by no means the case—but because . . . those who had recovered from the disease in the last epidemic in 1781 were now immune.

Figure 15-1 is based on Panum's table comparing the rates of mortality of the respective age groups during the measles epidemic of 1846 with those usual on the Faroe Islands, i.e., the average annual mortality during the years 1835 to 1846.

There are many even more dramatic examples of the effects of infection when first introduced to a population group.[4,5] The absence of innate resistance or of naturally acquired immunity to specific agents of infection not only increases community susceptibility to the spread of infection itself, but has much influence on the expression of the infection in disease and on the severity and outcome of disease. In Europe, the high mortality rates from the cholera epidemics of the 19th century and from the plague epidemic of the 14th century, and the severity of malaria in European settlers in Africa, are analogous to the effects of smallpox when first introduced to the American Indians and to the effects of tubercle infection in Africa and on the American Indians. In outbreaks of poliomyelitis (1949)[5] in an Eskimo community of the Hudson Bay, and of measles (1952)[6] in southern Greenland, the same effects were illustrated.

The ways in which a population develops resistance to infection and to the more severe effects of resulting disease may well be through natural selection as well as through specific acquired immunity. The demographic effects of some of these newly introduced infections have been the subject of a number of studies. It is estimated that the Polynesian population of Hawaii was reduced from 300,000 to 37,000 in less than a century of contact with Europeans (1778–1860), in which tuberculosis and venereal diseases, together with severe epidemics of measles, whooping cough, influenza, scarlet fever, and smallpox, played an important part. The survivors of these various epidemics represent a highly select category, not only as a result of the natural immunity many of them developed but, possibly even more important, in their having a higher innate resistance. This is probably transmissible to succeeding generations.

REFERENCES

1. Wilson GS, Miles AA: Topley and Wilson's Principles of Bacteriology and Immunity, Vol. 2, 5th ed. London, Edward Arnold, 1964, p 1546.

2. Panum PL: Observations Made During the Epidemic of Measles on the Faroe Islands in the Year 1846. Translation by AS Hatcher. In Panum on Measles. New York, American Public Health Association, Delta Omega Society, 1940, pp 3, 34.
3. Dubos R: Man Adapting. New Haven, Yale Univ Press, 1965, Chap. 7.
4. Burnet FM: Natural History of Infectious Disease, 3rd ed. London, Cambridge Univ Press, 1962.
5. Peart AFW: An outbreak of poliomyelitis in Canadian Eskimos in wintertime. Can J Public Health 40:405, 1949.
6. Christensen PE, Schmidt H, Jensen O, et al.: An epidemic of measles in Southern Greenland, 1951. Measles in virgin soil. I. Acta Med Scand 144:313, 1952.

16

Some Genetic Considerations in the Epidemiology of Infection and Disease

TUBERCULOSIS

A question that arises for the epidemiologist in community medicine concerns the extent to which selection has played a role in human communities. Theoretical considerations suggest that a community which has a disease with a high mortality rate before reproductive age would, in the course of time, develop a genetic immunity by eliminating the highly susceptible elements. In those communities in which tuberculosis is common there is a very high infant mortality rate; this was certainly true of those countries which today have a relatively low rate of tuberculosis but which 100 or more years ago had a very high rate of tuberculosis. It is known that in a country such as the United Kingdom the majority of communities have been exposed to a history of tuberculosis for several hundred years; during the early phases of the Industrial Revolution, towards the latter part of the 18th and early 19th centuries, the tuberculosis rates in the newly urbanized communities reached epidemic proportions (Fig. 16-1).[1]

It might be expected that the modern descendants of the survivors of those days would have a higher natural resistance to infection with tuberculosis than did those generations who had a high mortality rate and than communities who have not gone through a similar selective process.

In conditions such as tuberculosis, in which genetic factors are thought to be of some importance, theoretically the genetic influence should be measurable by the variation in expression of the infection according to the genetic relationship of the people exposed. The closer the relationship, the closer the resemblance in their response to infection. Studies of twins

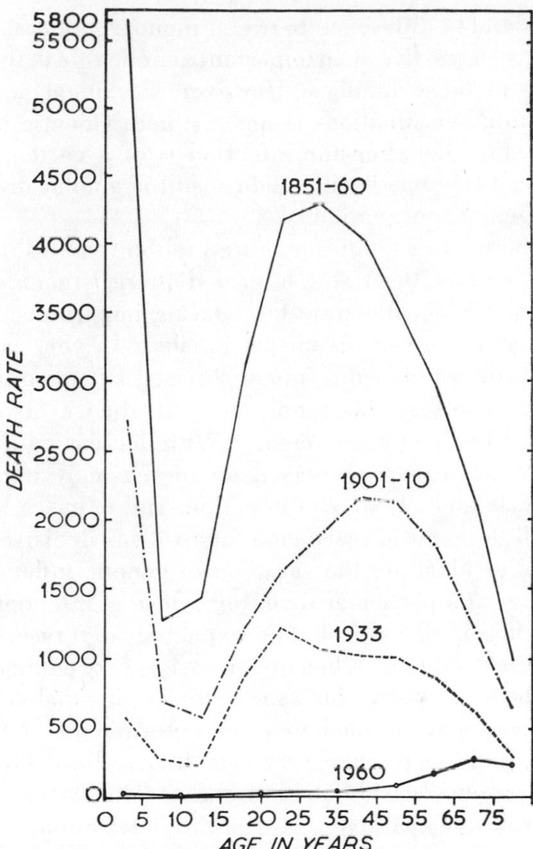

FIG. 16-1. Death rates per million from tuberculosis (all forms) at various ages, for England and Wales. (From Wilson and Miles.[1])

may have an important contribution to make in this regard. The genetic resemblance of monozygotic twins should result in a higher concordance rate of tuberculosis between them as compared with the concordance rates in dizygotic twins or other siblings. This is well illustrated in the New York twin studies.[2] The index cases for these family studies were one twin of a set, aged 15 years or over, with active pulmonary tuberculosis. In the families finally selected for investigation there were 78 monozygotic and 230 dizygotic twins. The tuberculosis morbidity rates in other members of the families of these index twin cases, corrected for age, were 87.3 percent of their monozygotic twins, 25.6 percent of their dizygotic twins, 25.5 percent in full siblings, 16.9 percent in parents, 11.9 percent in half siblings, and 7.1 percent in their spouses.

The considerable difference between monozygotic twin partners and others is strongly suggestive of an important genetic role in the development of tuberculosis in these families. However, uncritical generalization of this inference to other situations is not justified. Genetic influences may have an important role when the infection is of a certain type or dose. A massive dose of tubercle bacilli might result in similar disease in people with different genetic susceptibility.

Lurie's experimental studies in inbred rabbit families ranging through highly resistant strains, those with intermediate resistance, and those who were highly susceptible, illustrate the varying importance of the genetic factor according to dose of organisms inhaled. In very large doses, "it mattered very little whether the animal exposed belonged to the resistant family . . . or to a susceptible family. . . . All died in a relatively short time of a nodular caseous pneumonia."[3] With decreasing doses of bacilli, the natural genetic resistance played an increasingly important role in determining cause and outcome of infection, and in cases where the dose inhaled is small the natural resistance factor "was decisive."

These studies illustrate the variation of genetic influence depending on circumstances at a particular time, e.g., dose of infection. The genetic factor or influence in disease may be expected to vary according to the distribution of the condition. When the disease is very common, the genetic influence may be less obvious, but as it decreases in incidence and severity the genetic factor may be an important determinant of the expression of the disease, and again when very rare it may have little measurable effect. These various considerations influence the interpretation of the epidemiologic relevance of genetic factors in determining the distribution of an infectious disease like tuberculosis during a particular period in the history of a specific community.

Among the oldest medical beliefs is that of the association between physique and risk of developing tuberculosis. This belief could have easily arisen from the fact that the disease process itself leads to loss of weight and hence to thin or underweight tuberculous persons. The association between this type of body build and tuberculous disease could also be the product of a life situation conducive to both malnutrition and to exposure with the Mycobacterium tuberculosis.

The association between body build and tuberculous disease has been confirmed in the study of over 800,000 men enlisted in the US Navy between 1958 and 1967.[4] The median height of men who developed active tuberculosis was greater than that of all the recruits, and their mean weight on recruitment was less. Thus morbidity was increased in taller and lighter men. This is in contrast to infection rates, for which no difference was found according to height and weight. On the basis of their studies, Edwards and her co-workers have suggested that "physique and susceptibility to tuberculous disease are interrelated familial or stock traits."[4]

Another important mediator of the role of genetic influences in tuberculosis infection is that of the life situation and the state of health of the exposed community. Under certain circumstances, the life experience of a community may reinforce its genetic resistance to tuberculosis. With sudden change or deterioration in the life situation and nutritional state, the tuberculosis incidence may rise considerably. Rene and Jean Dubos describe the change in tuberculosis among the Jews of Europe "in the face of physiologic and social misery" suffered by them. Their resistance, thought to have been "acquired during centuries of urban life in the crowded ghettos of Central Europe proved of little help, . . ."[5] and among the Jews of Warsaw the tuberculosis death rate, which had been lower than among the non-Jewish population, increased greatly after the beginning of World War II. The increase was notable among the non-Jews as well, but that of the Jews was very much more marked, as evidenced by the figures, presented in Table 16-1, of the tuberculosis death rate per 100,000 population of Jews and non-Jews in Warsaw.

TABLE 16-1. The Tuberculosis Death Rate Per 100,000 Population in Warsaw

	JEWS	NON-JEWS
1938	71	186
1940	205	377
1942	601	425

Resemblance of genetic constitution and closeness of blood relationship is associated with a sharing of life experience. The possible meaning of this in determining the occurrence of tuberculosis in twins was explored by Simmonds in London.[6] Her studies extended to 202 pairs of twins in which at least one twin had tuberculosis. Both twins had the disease in 29.6 percent of the monozygotic and in 12.8 percent of the dizygotic twins. Monozygotic twins are thought to have closer contact with one another than do dizygotic twins and other siblings. Her study gave some support to this, especially in the case of monozygotic female twins of whom 68 percent were living together at time of diagnosis of the twin-index case, contrasted to 43 percent of female dizygotic twins. In order to assess the relative importance of contact between twins on the concordance of tuberculosis in twin studies, she distinguished between those living together at the time of diagnosis of the twin-index case and those who had been living apart for two or more years prior to the diagnosis of the index case. Table 16-2 is a tabulated summary of her findings.

The high concordance rate in monozygotic twins living together is striking and suggests the importance of physical contact between such twins in determining the concordance rate. The difference between the incidence of tuberculosis in monozygotic and dizygotic twins living apart

TABLE 16-2. Contact Between Twins as a Factor in the Concordance of Tuberculosis

AT TIME OF DIAGNOSIS OF TUBERCULOSIS IN THE INDEX CASE	MONOZYGOTIC CO-TWINS			DIZYGOTIC CO-TWINS		
	No.	No. with Tuberculosis	Percent	No.	No. with Tuberculosis	Percent
Co-twin living with index case	33	14	42.4	92	15	16.3
Co-twin living apart from index case for two or more years	22	4	18.4	58	6	10.3

(Adapted from Simmonds.[6])

from the index case was not significant, but this may be due to the very limited number of cases in this group.

Additional problems encountered in the interpretation of twin studies, to which Simmonds drew attention, include the need for careful definition of criteria in determining monozygotic versus dizygotic twins, and the inclusion of all twin pairs. Thus in studies of tuberculosis, unless particular attention is directed to each index case as to whether he is or has been a twin, there is likely to be a bias especially in the direction of concordance in monozygotic twin pairs, exaggerating the importance of inheritance.

GENETIC POLYMORPHISM AND INFECTION

Polymorphisms of health relevance include blood groups, such as the ABO and Rh blood group systems, various hemoglobinopathies, and an enzyme polymorphism known as glucose-6-phosphate dehydrogenase deficiency (G6PD deficiency).

Ford[7] has defined genetic polymorphism as "a type of variation in which individuals with sharply distinct qualities co-exist as normal members of a population. . . ." Hemoglobin polymorphism is common in many parts of the world where abnormal hemoglobins have a high frequency and together with normal hemoglobin Hb^A constitute various polymorphisms.[8] Among the genes which cause the formation of abnormal hemoglobin are Hb^S, the sickle-cell gene, common in a broad belt of Africa (from east to west through central Africa) (Fig. 16-2); the α- and β-thalassemia genes with high frequency in countries bordering the Mediterranean, western Asia, India, and Southeast Asia, as well as distinctive regions in west and central Africa (Fig. 16-3); and Hb^C, common only in certain regions of west Africa. The polymorphism may involve only two hemoglobins, Hb^A and Hb^S, but in areas where sickling trait is common Hb^C may also occur and the polymorphism may thus involve three alleles: Hb^A, Hb^S, and Hb^C.[9]

The epidemiologic relevance of these polymorphisms is related to the diseases with which the abnormal hemoglobins are known to be associated; namely sickle-cell anemia, thalassemia major (Cooley's anemia) or minor, and Hb^C anemia.[10] Their particular role in improving biologic fitness of the population under certain conditions may be of considerable relevance in areas of endemic Plasmodium falciparum malaria (Fig. 16-4).

While it is reasonable to believe that genetic selection is involved in the changing resistance of human population groups to infection, direct evidence of the genetic process is very limited. Examples have been given of the general selective processes at work through the survivors of epidemics which decimate populations when first exposed to the particular infection.

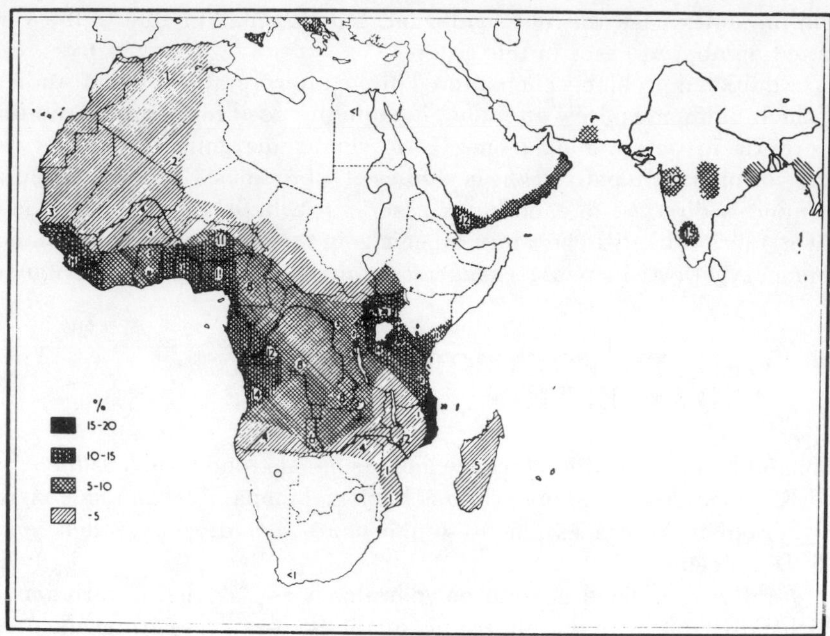

FIG. 16-2. Frequency of sickle-cell gene in Africa, Asia, and southern Europe. (From Allison.[9])

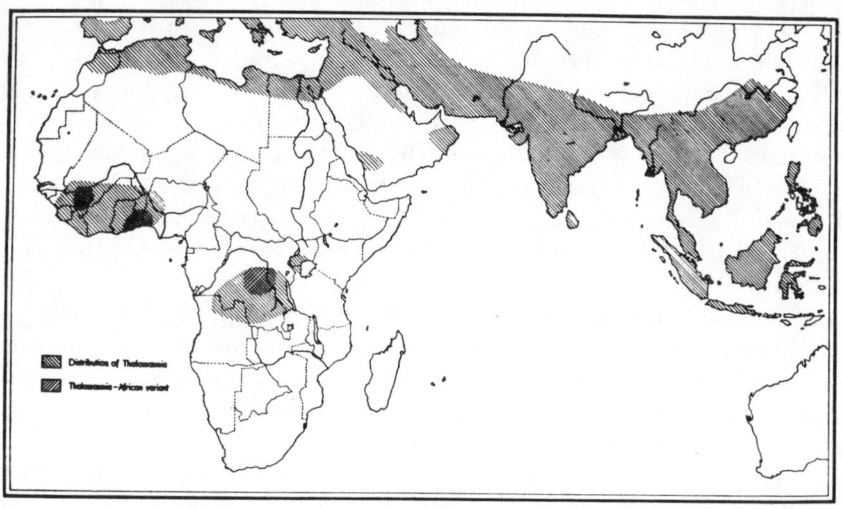

FIG. 16-3. Distribution of thalassemia in Africa, Asia, and southern Europe. (From Allison.[9])

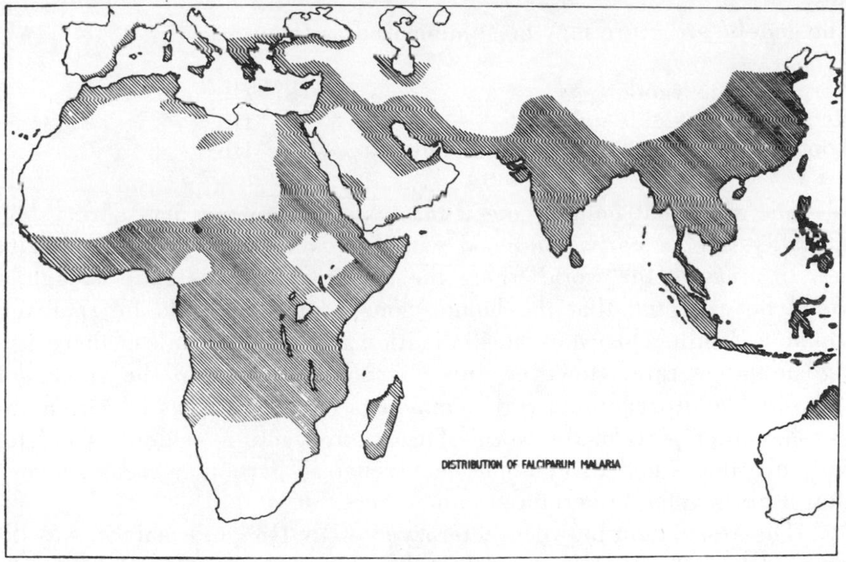

FIG. 16-4. The distribution of Plasmodium falciparum malaria in Africa, Asia, and southern Europe. (From Allison.[9])

The subsequent change that takes place in increasing resistance to these infections—protozoal, bacterial, and viral—is but indirect evidence of the probability that innate resistance plays an important role.

Further understanding of the relation between infection and genetic selection has been gained in the study of sickling and infection with the malarial parasite, Plasmodium falciparum. These investigations followed the suggestion by Haldane, in 1949,[11] that the heterozygote in certain hemoglobinopathies, such as thalassemia minor, may have certain advantages. They were made possible by the discovery by Pauling and associates in 1949 that there were different adult hemoglobins.[12] Sickle-cell hemoglobin could be distinguished from normal hemoglobin by differences in their electrophoretic mobility.

THE SICKLE-CELL TRAIT AND MALARIA

A hemoglobin abnormality is the basic genetic fact in persons with sickle-cell trait. Instead of normal hemoglobin—hemoglobin A (Hb^A)—a proportion of the hemoglobin is abnormal, thus producing hemoglobin S (Hb^S).

The genetic structure may be summarized as follows:

Normal homozygote	$Hb^A Hb^A$
Heterozygote: sickle-cell trait	$Hb^A Hb^S$
Abnormal homozygote: sickle-cell anemia	$Hb^S Hb^S$

The abnormal homozygote with sickle-cell anemia has a very high mortality rate in early childhood with relatively few survivors to adult life. In areas of the world where the frequency of this gene is high, it would be expected that the homozygous condition would be relatively common, leading to eventual elimination of the gene unless there is a high mutation rate. However, this has not been so and the sickle-cell trait (i.e., heterozygote) is very common in extensive parts of Africa and in some other parts of the world. The heterozygote is seldom associated with any illness and its common occurrence in particular areas suggests that it has a value in certain circumstances.

The association between heterozygote Hb^AHb^S and malaria was discovered by Allison in Uganda.[13–16] The heterozygote Hb^AHb^S has considerable advantages for survival in endemic Plasmodium falciparum regions of Africa when compared with the normal homozygote, Hb^AHb^A. Its distribution in Africa approximates that of Plasmodium falciparum.

A number of investigations in east and west Africa have been carried out and are supportive of Allison's findings. Table 16-3 is a summary of a review of the subject by Allison.[16] The prevalence of infection in children without the sickling trait is consistently higher than in those with sickle-cell trait and the difference between the two categories is generally even more marked when they are compared for heavy infection.

As might therefore be expected, there is a difference in mortality from malaria in the two categories of children.

A similar selective advantage of Hb^AHb^S was demonstrated in a comparative study of Nigerian children under 4 years of age with severe P. falciparum malaria, i.e., high fever (over 40C or 103F) with convulsions or coma, with parasite counts of 100,000 or more per cc. Only 4 percent of 100 cases were heterozygous (Hb^AHb^S) versus 96 percent homozygous (Hb^AHb^A), in contrast to 18 percent heterozygous of 200 control children who attended the clinic for other purposes.[17]

It is difficult to conduct a cohort or prospective study of the two categories, especially in those areas in which malaria is endemic, but comparisons of findings in children who have died of malaria have often been undertaken.

African children with sickle-cell trait are rarely found among those who die from malaria, as indicated in Table 16-4.

The possibility of differences in reproductive performance between Hb^AHb^S and Hb^AHb^A mothers in areas where there is a high prevalence

TABLE 16-3. The Prevalence of Malaria Parasite P. Falciparum in 10 Studies of African Children*

COUNTRY	ALL CASES OF INFECTION	HEAVY INFECTION
Uganda	2.18	3.86
Uganda	1.55	2.63
Kenya	1.49	1.96
Tanganyika	1.54	1.66
Ghana (south)	1.47	4.11
Ghana (south)	1.10	3.05
Ghana (north)	5.00	1.47
Ghana (north)	2.79	—
Nigeria	1.02	—
Nigeria	1.98	1.99
Weighted mean relative incidence	1.46	2.17

Relative prevalence of infection in children without sickle-cell trait compared with those having sickle-cell trait (heterozygous) taken as unity.
**The ages of the children in the different studies varied, from below 4 years to below 10 years.*
(Adapted from Allison.[16])

of malaria has been studied. A number of workers have not found such a difference but Firschein[18] reported significant differences between the two groups of mothers in British Honduras, Central America. Controlling for age, he found that heterozygous mothers had more total births and more live births than homozygous women. The fertility ratio between the two groups was 1.45 for total births. Firschein considered the probability of this difference being the result of excess abortions in Hb^A Hb^A mothers, which might have resulted from malaria.

TABLE 16-4. Sickle-cell Trait in Children who Died of Malaria Compared with the Expected Mortality According to the Frequency of that Trait in the Population

	PREVALENCE OF SICKLE-CELL TRAIT IN POPULATION (%)	NUMBER OF DEATHS OF MALARIA	NUMBER OF DEATHS OF CHILDREN WITH SICKLE-CELL TRAIT	
			Expected	Observed
Uganda	20	16	3.2	0
Congo	23	23	5.3	0
Congo	25	23	5.8	1
Ghana	8	13	1.0	0
Nigeria	24	29	7.0	0

(Adapted from Allison.[16])

THE POSSIBLE ADVANTAGE OF G6PD DEFICIENCY AND THALASSEMIA

The frequency of the deficiency of the enzyme glucose-6-phosphate dehydrogenase (G6PD) and that of sickle-cell trait (Hb^A Hb^S) are positively correlated in African populations.[19,20] The parallel distribution of G6PD deficiency with that of sickle-cell trait in malarial areas has led to the suggestion that individuals with the enzyme deficiency may, like those with the sickle-cell trait, have some advantage in Plasmodium falciparum malarial areas. The evidence is conflicting but suggestive.[17] Similarly, the distribution of thalassemia in other areas of the world in which P. falciparum malaria occurs has suggested that thalassemia, like the sickle-cell trait, has its frequency distribution in certain areas because of its protection against malaria.[20] This possibility remains an hypothesis needing direct epidemiologic study.

PRIMARY IMMUNOLOGIC DEFICIENCY

Rapid advances in knowledge of immunologic abnormalities suggest that study of the genetic aspects of immune response to infection will make an increasingly important contribution to epidemiologic understanding of the distribution of infection in the community. While specific genetically determined immunologic deficiency diseases are not in themselves common disorders, the overall subject of the immune response to infection is receiving attention.[21]

Primary hypogammaglobulinemia was first described as an entity in 1952[22] and since that time it has been increasingly recognized and reported. Since the earlier investigations the concepts of immunoglobulin deficiency and abnormality has widened. Not only have a number of abnormalities been described but it is now probable that the difference between normal and abnormal is not of a simple qualitative nature with a bimodal distribution in the community, but rather one in which there is a gradient in the distribution of the blood serum levels of the particular immunoglobulins concerned. Thus, for example, the lower the immunoglobulin G, the more likely is the individual to be susceptible to repeated bacterial infections.[23]

In an illustrative study the serum immunoglobulin of children who had clinical evidence or a history of an unusually high number of infections was investigated.[24,25] Six hundred such children were compared with a number of so-called "normal" children. Forty-four percent of the "infected" children had one or more immunoglobulin concentrations outside normal bounds for their age compared with only 7.7 percent of the "normal" group.

The infections were mainly respiratory and many of the children had allergic manifestations including asthma, allergic rhinitis, eczema, and milk allergy. Their impression was that infections were somewhat more severe in the children with multiple immunoglobulin deficiencies but there was no evidence of any differences in the kind or site of the disease in the different categories of immunoglobulin abnormality. Here it should be noted that while the majority of the abnormalities—199 (76 percent)—had immunoglobulin deficiencies, 54 (24 percent) of the abnormals had elevations of one or more of the immunoglobulins. It is clear that there is a need for community studies of the distribution of immunologic abnormalities and their relation to infection in the community.

REFERENCES

1. Wilson GS, Miles AA: Topley and Wilson's Principles of Bacteriology and Immunity, Vol. 2, 5th ed. London, Edward Arnold, 1964.
2. Kallman FJ, Reisner D: Twin studies on the significance of genetic factors in tuberculosis. Am Rev Tuberc 47:549, 1943.
3. Lurie M: Resistance to Tuberculosis: Experimental Studies in Native and Acquired Defensive Mechanisms. Cambridge, Mass, Commonwealth Fund, Harvard Univ Press, 1964, p 142.
4. Edwards LB, Livesay VT, Acquaviva FA, et al.: Height, weight, tuberculous infection, and tuberculous disease. Arch Environ Health, 22:106, 1971.
5. Dubos R, Dubos J: The White Plague: Tuberculosis, Man and Society. Boston, Little, Brown, 1952, p 195.
6. Simmonds B: Tuberculosis in Twins. London, Pitman Medical, 1963.
7. Ford EB: Genetic Polymorphism. London, Faber and Faber, 1965, p 11.
8. Huehns ER, Shooter EM: Human haemoglobins. J Med Genet 2:48, 1965.
9. Allison AC: Abnormal haemoglobin and erythrocyte enzyme deficiency traits. In Harrison GA (ed.): Genetic Variation in Human Populations. Oxford, Pergamon, 1961.
10. Levin WC: "Asymptomatic" sickel cell trait. Blood 13:904, 1958.
11. Haldane JBS: Disease and evolution. La Ricerca Scientifica (Suppl) 19:68, 1949.
12. Pauling L, Itano HA, Singer SJ, et al.: Sickle-cell anemia, a molecular disease. Science 110:543, 1949.
13. Allison AC: Protection afforded by sickle-cell trait against subtertian malarial infection. Brit Med J 1:290, 1954.
14. Allison AC: The distribution of the sickle-cell trait in East Africa and elsewhere, and its apparent relationship to the incidence of subtertian malaria. Trans R Soc Trop Med Hyg 48:312, 1954.
15. Allison AC: Aspects of polymorphism in man. Cold Spring Harbor Symp Quant Biol 20:239, 1955.
16. Allison AC: Polymorphism and natural selection in human populations. Cold Spring Harbor Symp Quant Biol 29:137, 1964.
17. Gilles HM, Fletcher KA, Hendrickse RG, et al.: Glucose-6-phosphate dehy-

drogenase deficiency, sickling, and malaria in African children in South Western Nigeria. Lancet 1:138, 1967.
18. Firschein IL: Population dynamics of the sickle-cell trait in the Black Caribs of British Honduras, Central America. Am J Hum Genet 13:233, 1961.
19. Motulsky AG: Metabolic polymorphisms and the rate of the infectious diseases in human evolution. Hum Biol 32:28, 1960.
20. Motulsky AG: Current concepts of the genetics of the thalassemias. Cold Spring Harbor Symp Quant Biol 29:399, 1964.
21. WHO Scientific Group: Genetics of the Immune Response. WHO Tech Rep Ser 402:1, 1968.
22. Bruton OC: Agammaglobulinemia. Pediatrics 9:722, 1952.
23. Medical Research Council Working Party. Summary Report: Hypogammaglobulinemia in the United Kingdom. Lancet 1:163, 1969.
24. Buckley RH, Dees SC, O'Fallon WM: Serum immunoglobulins. I. Levels in normal children and in uncomplicated childhood allergy. Pediatrics 41: 600, 1968.
25. Buckley RH, Dees SC, O'Fallon WM: Serum immunoglobulins. II. Levels in children subject to recurrent infection. Pediatrics 42:50, 1968.

17
Nutrition, Infection, and Disease

Malnutrition and high rates of infectious disease often occur together in poor communities. The features which characterize such communities are well known to be important determinants of the spread of infection and of malnutrition. Poverty usually involves deficiencies in housing, sanitation, and water supplies as well as in food, and the ignorance that accompanies poverty includes ignorance of protection against infection and of healthy feeding practices. The human and environmental defects which together lead to infection and malnutrition are so inextricably interwoven in poverty that it is seldom possible to separate those which are responsible for malnutrition from those which are responsible for disease from infection. While an association between nutritional deficiency diseases and infectious diseases is therefore to be expected, it is difficult to establish a causal relation between nutrition and infection, more especially to establish the role of nutritional status in determining the acquisition of infection and the biologic gradient of infection.

War-time conditions have from time immemorial been associated with famine and epidemics of infectious disease. Tuberculosis is among the diseases in which we expect a rise. Because the nutritional changes commonly occur together with much social disorganization, it is difficult to associate the rise in the occurrence of tuberculosis with change in the nutritional state only. In a review of the problem, René and Jean Dubos discussed the changes in mortality from tuberculosis in Denmark through the years of World War I (1914 to 1918).[1] Denmark was not one of the countries itself at war in World War I. It was not occupied by any of the opposing armies and there was no obvious social disorganization during the war years. And yet, following a long period of steady decline in the tuberculosis death rate, there was a marked increase in this rate in 1915 until 1917. During 1915 to 1917 Denmark exported very large quantities of meat and dairy products to the United Kingdom, thereby reducing sharply the amount of meat consumed by the average Dane. In 1917 submarine warfare interrupted the flow of exports to the United Kingdom from Denmark. As a consequence there was a rise in the consumption of these foods in Denmark and, of interest to our present discussion, a decline in the tuberculosis mortality rate. Dubos considered this particular case, in which a population's nutritional balance changes during the period when war is going on around it but not within it, to be perhaps the nearest example we have of the commonly accepted association between nutrition and tuberculosis.

WEANLING DIARRHEA

The weaning process is associated with an acute diarrhea of infants and young children, in which there has been noted a striking synergism between nutrition and infection.[2–8] In a series of studies of rural communities in less developed countries, Gordon and his associates have investigated the relationship of these two factors in diarrheal disease.

Each of the following factors may play a role in the production of diarrhea in infants and young children.

1. Diarrhea is possibly a result of infection through insanitary practices in preparation of foods. In these circumstances the contrast between children who are only breast-fed and those who are ingesting other foods, would be very marked. The infecting agent, if indeed there is always an infecting agent, is not commonly found. Shigella, salmonella, and Escherichia coli are found in varying proportions of cases in different epidemics but usually constitute a minority of cases. Whether these specific pathogens when found are indeed the causal agent of the diarrhea is not established. No differences are found in the clinical picture of cases of diarrhea in which one of these microorganisms is found and those in which they are not. Furthermore, while there is a marked difference in the severity and general clinical picture of acute diarrheal disease in infants and young children of better-off communities and those of less developed or poorer communities, the infectious agents are much the same. These facts suggest that the main features of the clinical picture are not necessarily related to bacterial agents, but rather to viral infection and the characteristics of the children themselves.
2. For many years diarrhea was thought to result from parenteral infection as well as intestinal infection, and treatment was directed to the infection involved, such as otitis media. More recently, this diagnosis has been less common and the existence of such an entity has been questioned. This may represent a change in medical thinking, but on the other hand it may be a result of an actual change in the disease picture of infants. Such cases of parenteral diarrhea may well have been com-

mon in generations of children whose nutritional state was not as sound as that of the present-day infant in better-off communities. In addition, more infections of the respiratory tract in infants are readily controlled by the use of antibiotics which may well be preventing the type of purulent otitis media that was so common in pediatric units 20 to 30 years ago. The possibility that such parenteral disease is still associated with diarrhea in poor communities and in less developed countries is worthy of further epidemiologic investigation.

3. A mere change in the nature of the food might produce sufficient disturbance to precipitate the diarrhea, more especially if the foods introduced cannot be adequately digested by the infant. An example of this was found by the author in a rural African community in which neonatal diarrhea during the first week of life was a common cause of severe illness and death. Careful examination of possible causes revealed the fact that the baby was not put to the breast until the colostrum had been replaced by a free flow of milk or until the umbilical stump had separated. During this period, which was often as long as one week, the older tradition had been to feed the babies on a special preparation of cow's milk. With the considerable decline in cattle in this community, a special infant feed composed of a cereal, maize, was prepared in the form of a drink and it was this that was fed to the babies. As

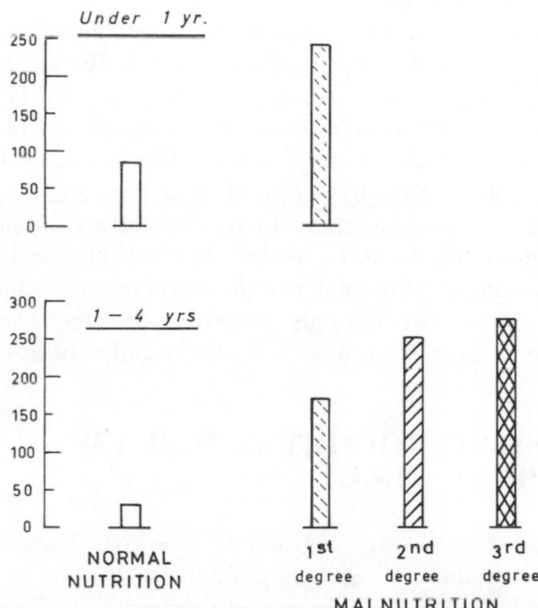

FIG. 17-1. Attack rates of acute diarrheal diseases in rural Guatemalan children, according to nutritional status. Cases per 100 children per year. (Adapted from Gordon et al.[4])

this practice was not deeply rooted in the culture of the community, an intensive educational program led to the disappearance of this unusual form of neonatal diarrhea.

4. Nutritional deficiency might be a common cause of the diarrhea. The rural studies of Gordon and his associates in Punjab, northern India, and of Gordon, Scrimshaw, and their associates in Guatemala, have focused on the nutritional aspect of acute diarrheal disease in these communities. Diarrhea in well-nourished children of better-off communities is usually a short, sharp illness with prompt full recovery. In the communities they studied it is usually not an isolated episode but one in which the acute diarrhea is less sharply defined; the child tends to remain ill and may have several more episodes of diarrhea. Following the initial diarrhea there is a period of prolonged illness, with irregular recurrences of loose stools and an increase in malnutrition. This may be interspersed with acute episodes of diarrhea. They found that the greater the degree of malnutrition, the higher the incidence of acute diarrheal disease (Fig. 17-1).[3]

In both the Punjab and Guatemala studies there was increased incidence of diarrheal disease during the process of weaning. This was first noted with the introduction of additional foods to breast milk and its highest incidence was at the time when the process of weaning was being completed, i.e., when the child was being taken off all breast milk onto a completely independent diet.

The concept of weanling diarrhea as an epidemiologic entity is an interesting example of the shift in focus from a single causal agent of disease to an interest in the interaction between several factors, with an increasing emphasis on the role of the host himself. In fact, as Gordon and his associates indicate, while weanling diarrhea must be considered as an epidemiologic entity, it results from a number of causes and is itself composed of several diseases which occur during the period of weaning from breast-feeding to other foods.[5] The association is between the processes of weaning and infection and their synergistic action in determining nutritional status. This not only influences the frequency of episodes of acute diarrheal disease but also its severity and expression.

A FUSO-SPIROCHETAL DISEASE: TROPICAL ULCER

Fuso-spirochetal diseases are a group of infective diseases in which a variety of microorganisms, including fusiform bacilli, are found with spirochetes that are normal inhabitants of the mouth. The diseases include periodontal disease, ulceration of the mouth (which in its severe necrotic state is known as noma), and ulceration of the external genitalia. Rosebury[9] states that "fuso-spirochetal disease seems always to be superimposed on tissue damage induced by other agencies, including scurvy, pellagra, inanition or other nutritional disturbances; agranulocytosis or radiation injury; viral infections, including measles and primary herpes simplex."

Tropical ulcer, an ulceration of the skin and subcutaneous tissues, also belongs to this group of diseases. It has often been described in epidemic form in developing countries as one of the fuso-spirochetal diseases in which a nutritional component is thought to be an important determinant. Whatever may initiate an epidemic, a number of observers have suggested nutritional deficiency as a determinant of its distribution in a community. This association was commented upon many years ago by a number of workers when contrasting the incidence or prevalence of tropical ulcer in different communities having different dietary habits.

Lowenthal[10] noted that there were many more cases among poorer Ruanda than among the Baganda of Uganda and he suggested that the initial vesicle of tropical ulcer was a product of tissue necrosis related to the subjects' general malnutrition. A higher prevalence was noted among the vegetarian Akikuyu than the meat- and blood-eating Masai of Kenya.[11] Similar differences were found between two different groups of the Atongole of Uganda, namely the fish-eating Opami and the non-fish-eating Ajuluku.[12] In Sudanese tribal groups with different eating habits, tropical ulcer was less common amongst cattle-raising people than others.[13,14]

In a previously unpublished study conducted by the author during the course of an epidemic of tropical ulcer in an African subtropical hyperendemic malaria area, a closer study of the relationship of nutrition and tropical ulcer was possible. Of interest were the schoolchildren of two contrasting communities living very near to one another but under markedly differing conditions. The first group, with a relatively high prevalence of tropical ulcer (17.1 percent), lived in flat bush country in contrast to the second group (2.9 percent), who lived on the slopes of a nearby mountain. The state of health and nutrition was also markedly different. The children living on the hill slope were obviously in a better nutritional condition than the others and had a markedly lower prevalence of malaria and bilharzia. The contrast in prevalence of tropical ulcer in these two

TABLE 17-1. Tropical Ulcer in Schoolboys of the "Flats Area" According to Nutritional Status

NONSPECIFIC CLINICAL NUTRITIONAL SIGNS	TROPICAL ULCER PRESENT	NO ULCER FOUND	TOTAL NO. OF CHILDREN
Follicular hyperkeratosis and/or angular stomatitis	25 (37.9%)	41	66
Neither of the above signs	14 (12.5%)	98	112
Total	39	139	178

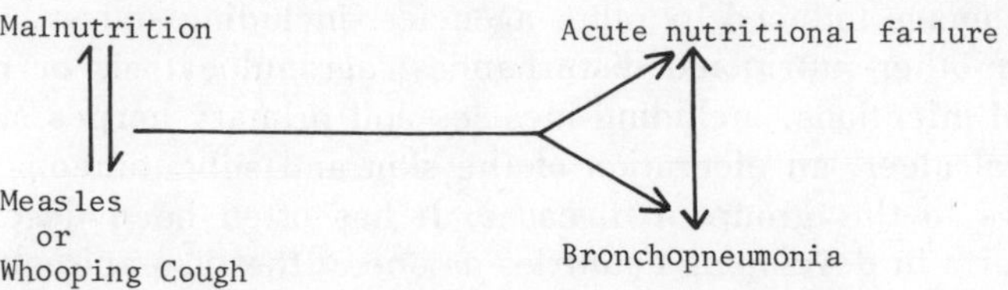

FIG. 17-2. The relation between malnutrition and disease.

communities of children is similar to those of the other earlier studies reported above. Further analysis of the findings in individual children of the high-prevalence area itself indicates a significant association between the prevalence of tropical ulcer and clinical signs of malnutrition. Table 17-1 shows that 37.9 percent of the boys with such signs had tropical ulcer, whereas only 12.5 percent of those not manifesting signs of malnutrition had tropical ulcer. This difference, although highly significant, does not indicate a cause and effect relationship of malnutrition and tropical ulcer, but provides direct evidence of an association between the two, confirmation of the impression formed in comparing different communities.

There are many other illustrations of a relation between malnutrition and infectious disease. In fact, so commonly do they occur together that it may be too-readily generalized that nutritional deficiency is a cause of disease from infection, e.g., measles and whooping cough. It may well be that measles and whooping cough are more severe diseases in malnourished communities than in those of better nutritional status; there is much supportive evidence of this.[15] The effects of these diseases on undernourished children might be to precipitate a serious acute nutritional failure syndrome, like kwashiorkor. This relation may be expressed in an oversimplified diagram (Fig. 17-2).

A more general causal relation between poverty, malnutrition, infection, and disease may be expressed as in Figure 17-3.

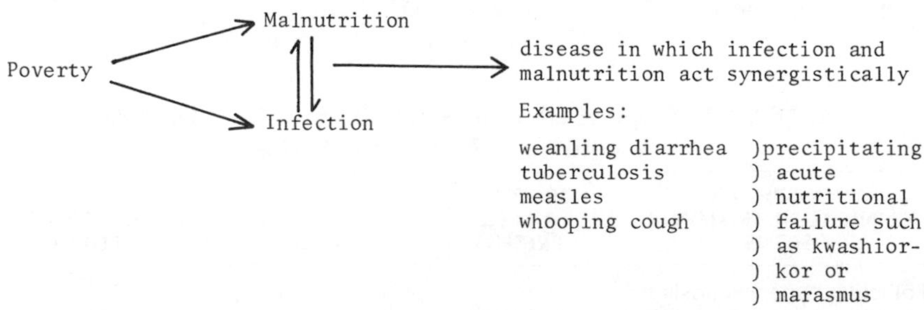

FIG. 17-3. The relation between poverty, malnutrition, infection, and disease.

While the associations shown in Figures 17-2 and 17-3 may indeed represent a causal network, the mechanism of association is not understood and progress towards such understanding has been slow and often confusing. Furthermore, reviews by experts in the respective fields of microbiology and nutrition indicate that what may be true for some diseases may not be so for others.[6,16,17]

REFERENCES

1. Dubos R, Dubos J: The White Plague: Tuberculosis, Man and Society. Boston, Little, Brown, 1952.
2. Gordon JE, Chitkara ID, Wyon JB: Weanling Diarrhea. Am J Med Sci 245: 345, 1963.
3. Gordon JE, Béhar M, Scrimshaw NS: Acute diarrhoeal disease in less developed countries. I. An epidemiological basis for control. Bull WHO 31:1, 1964.
4. Gordon JE, Guzman MA, Ascoli W, et al.: Acute diarrhoeal disease in less developed countries. II. Patterns of epidemiological behaviour in rural Guatemalan villages. Bull WHO 13:9, 1964.
5. Gordon JE, Béhar M, Scrimshaw NS: Acute diarrhoeal disease in less developed countries. III. Methods for prevention and control. Bull WHO 31:21, 1964.
6. Scrimshaw NS, Taylor CE, Gordon JE: Interactions of nutrition and infection. Am J Med Sci 237:367, 1959.
7. WHO: Nutrition and Infection. WHO Tech Rep Ser 314:1, 1965.
8. Hanson JDL, Wittman W, Moodie AD, et al.: Evaluating the synergism of infection and nutrition in the field. In Scrimshaw NS, Gordon JE (eds.): Malnutrition, Learning, and Behavior. Cambridge, Mass, MIT Press, 1968.
9. Rosebury T: Bacteria indigenous to man. In Dubos RJ, Hirsch JC (eds:) Bacterial and Mycotic Infections of Man, 4th ed. Philadelphia and Montreal, Lippincott, Chap. 1, p. 326, 1965.
10. Lowenthal LJA: Tropical ulcer as a deficiency disease. Lançet 2:889, 1932.
11. Orr JB, Gilks JL: Studies of Nutrition. The Physique and Health of Two African Tribes. Medical Research Council Special Report, No. 155. London, Her Majesty's Stationery Office, 1931.
12. de Courcey-Ireland MG, Hoskin WR, Lowenthal LJA: An Investigation into Health and Agriculture in the Teso District of Uganda, 1937. Agricultural Department of Uganda, Colonial Office.
13. Cruikshank A: Tropical diseases of the Southern Sudan. Their distribution and significance. East Afr Med J 13:172, 1936.
14. Corkill NL: Tropical ulcer. Observations on its treatment and cause. Trans R Soc Trop Med Hyg 32:159, 1938.
15. Scrimshaw NS, Salomon JB, Bruch HA, et al.: Studies of diarrhoeal disease in central america. VIII. Measles, diarrhoea, and nutritional deficiency in rural Guatemala. Am J Trop Med Hyg 15:625, 1966.
16. Dubos R, Schaedler RW: Nutrition and infection. J Pediatr 55:1, 1959.
17. Dubos R: Man Adapting. New Haven, Yale Univ Press, 1965, Chap. VI.

18

Family and Infection

There are a number of diseases well known to occur more often in some families than in others. The familial aggregation of tuberculosis and leprosy has long been recognized, as has the clustering of acute infectious diseases in family epidemics.

The introduction and spread of infections in families is dependent upon the nature of the microorganism, the dose to which the family members are exposed, and their susceptibility. Familial factors determining this are the size of the family, its age and sex composition, the genetic immunologic potential, previous experience, and state of health of the family members. Equally important is intra- and extrafamily functioning, such as family relationships and outside contacts of members in their various activities.

A measurement of spread of an infection or an infectious disease in families, known as "the secondary attack rate," was apparently first developed by Chapin of the United States in his studies of the effectiveness of removal to isolation hospitals of primary cases of scarlet fever and diphtheria in Providence, Rhode Island, 1896 to 1913.[1] The secondary familial attack rate is the percentage of other susceptible members of families who become infected or contract disease during a defined period of time from the date of onset of a primary case in the family. It is calculated as follows.

Secondary familial attack rate:

$$\frac{\text{No. of susceptible contacts in the family developing disease}}{\text{Total no. of susceptible contacts in the family}} \times 100 \text{ in a defined period of time}$$

or

Secondary familial infection rate:

$$\frac{\text{No. of susceptible contacts in the family who become infected}}{\text{Total no. of susceptible contacts}} \times 100 \text{ in a defined period of time}$$

Secondary infection and attack rates in groups of families would normally be age- and sex-specific and may extend to other variables depending upon the particular condition and the purpose of the investigation. The data required include:

1. The date of onset of the primary case.
2. Family contacts—number, age, sex, susceptibility.
3. The number of secondary infections or cases of disease occurring in the family during the observation period.
4. Definition of the observation period. The incubation period of a disease would obviously influence this and in diseases with prolonged incubation periods (e.g., leprosy) the observation would extend over many years.

The family member introducing the infection into the home, i.e., the "primary" case, will naturally vary according to the nature of the infection, the differences in immunity of family members to the condition, and their life situations at home and out of home. In their studies of home infection in a selected group of families in Cleveland, Ohio, Dingle and his associates[2–7] found that the father was responsible for introducing respiratory infection into the home less often than any other member. Taking 1.0 as the frequency with which the father was the primary case they found the following frequencies: mother, 1.22; preschool children, 2.01; schoolchildren aged 6 years and over, 2.06; and schoolchildren below 6 years, 3.01. Fathers also had the lowest secondary attack rate, namely 17 percent, followed by schoolchildren aged 6 years and over, 24.3 percent; mothers, 27.4 percent; schoolchildren under the age of 6 years, 37.5 percent; and preschool children (those not yet at any school), 49 percent. In this last group infants under 1 year of age had less respiratory illness than those aged 1 to 4 years.

In contrast to these Cleveland studies an investigation carried out in Paddington, London,[8] found that in addition to children attending school the youngest child or those not yet at school were the main introducers of infection into the family. The living and housing conditions of the children in this second study were different from those of families studied by Dingle. Most of the families in the Paddington study were living in crowded neighborhoods where young children were easily exposed to the risk of infection. This is in contrast to the Cleveland families, who belonged to higher socioeconomic strata living in separate homes.

Family size is an important determinant of secondary attack rate. As expected the larger the families the higher the incidence of infection in the home and in each individual.[3] This is probably the result of the existence of a greater number of individuals who can introduce infection and in certain circumstances a greater possibility of crowding which would at least increase the possibilities of transmission. The incidence of infection in a family will depend on the frequency of introduction of the infection into the family, as well as its transmission between members of the family. The earlier studies of common respiratory infections depended upon clinical manifestations, i.e., observable infection in symptoms or signs of illness. The limitations imposed by this are being overcome by more recent serologic immunity studies.[9]

Morris[10] has demonstrated the increased mortality rate from respiratory infection in England and Wales, from 1949 to 1950, in comparing the infant mortality from bronchitis and pneumonia in families of different size. The postneonatal mortality rate increased with increase in size of family in each social class and was especially marked in large families with young mothers.

Not only do factors such as age, sex, and size of family determine the acquisition of infection and the occurrence of infectious disease in families, but it would appear that other factors have an important role to play in determining differences in susceptibility of different families and of different individuals in families. Of interest in this regard is the considerable number of individuals who, even when intimately exposed to an infection such as hemolytic streptococcal infection in the home, do not acquire the infection. Differences in individual and family susceptibility to infection and disease have been demonstrated by the Cleveland family studies and by those of Harvey and Dunlap.[11-13]

Thus with respect to families as a whole, as well as to their individual members, mere exposure to a given series of infections cannot account for the diversity in family experience and types of streptococci. Individual and family susceptibility factors must play a large part in determining the acquisition of the organisms. There is no linear relation between infection rates and the illness rate.[11-13] In fact, many individuals with a high carrier rate show less tendency to acquire overt infection than do noncarriers, suggesting that the carrier state produces type-specific immunity which protects against later illness from infection by the specific type of streptococcus.

These studies pose challenging questions of an epidemiologic nature, indicating that different factors are involved in the epidemiology of acquisition of infection, the epidemiology of the carrier state, the epidemiology of streptococcal illness in those infected, and the severity of the illness and its outcome. This is illustrated in Table 14-1 of Chapter 14.

REFERENCES

1. Frost WH: The familial aggregation of infectious diseases. First published in Am J Public Health, and Nation's Health 28:7, 1938. Also included in Maxcy FK (ed.): Papers of Wade Hampton Frost, M.D. New York, Commonwealth Fund, 1941.
2. Dingle JH, Badger GF, Feller AE, et al.: A study of illness in a group of Cleveland families. I. Plan of study and certain general observations. Am J Hyg 58:16, 1953.
3. Dingle JH, Badger GF, Feller AE, et al.: A study of illness in a group of Cleveland families. II. Incidence of the common respiratory diseases. Am J Hyg 58:31, 1953.
4. Dingle JH, Badger GF, Feller AE, et al.: A study of illness in a group of Cleveland families. III. Introduction of respiratory infections into families. Am J Hyg 58:41, 1953.
5. Dingle JH, Badger GF, Feller AE, et al.: A study of illness in a group of Cleveland families. IV. The spread of respiratory infections within the home. Am J Hyg 58:174, 1953.
6. Dingle JH, Badger GF, Feller AE, et al.: A study of illness in a group of Cleveland families. V. Introductions and secondary attack rates as indices of exposure to common respiratory diseases in the community. Am J Hyg 58: 179, 1953.
7. Dingle JH, Badger GF, Jordan WS: Illness in the Home. Cleveland, Press of Western Reserve Univ, 1964.
8. Brimblecombe FSW, Cruikshank R, Masters PL, et al.: Family studies of respiratory infection. Brit Med J 1:119, 1958.
9. Monto AS: A community study of respiratory infections in the tropics. III. Introduction and transmission of infections within families. Am J Epidemiol 88:69, 1968.
10. Morris JN: Uses of Epidemiology, 1st ed. Edinburgh and London, E & S Livingstone, 1957.
11. Harvey HS, Dunlap MB: Risk to children exposed in home to respiratory bacteria. Am J Dis Child 103:777, 1962.
12. Dunlap MB, Harvey HS: Multiple types of streptococci in the home. Am J Dis Child 107:85, 1964.
13. Harvey HS, Dunlap MB: Carrier state in relation to streptococcal disease. Am J Dis Child 107:240, 1964.

19

Social and Personal Crisis in Infection and Disease

The history of many peoples extends through periods of relative social equilibrium and more or less orderly change, interspersed with episodes of social disorganization or even chaos and dispersal. Epidemics of infectious, nutritional, and mental diseases have been an outstanding feature of this disorganization. The decline of certain diseases over long periods of time is well illustrated in the history of tuberculosis in Europe and in descendants of Europeans in other continents—North America, Oceania, and parts of Africa. It is estimated that in the mid-19th century the mortality rate from tuberculosis in Europe and North America reached its peak and was higher than 500 per 100,000.[1] It then began to decline, and except for the two world wars when it increased in Europe, the decline was continuous.

In a number of countries, following World War II, the decline has continued and there has been a striking decrease in the mortality rate from tuberculosis. In the Jewish population of Israel there has been a similar marked decrease in both mortality and morbidity (Fig. 19-1).[2] This is despite the mass immigration of Jews from many countries, especially those coming from the misery and travail of Hitler's Europe, and those poor and uneducated immigrants who came from the Arab countries of the Middle East and North Africa. This decrease has not been consistent. While there has been a marked decrease in all age groups, the decline in older adults is less than among children and younger adults.

Positive tuberculin reactions at different ages in men and women do not necessarily bear a consistent relation to the incidence of new cases in these groups. In 1949 mass BCG vaccination was introduced in Israel and was preceded by tuberculin testing of the population to be immunized. During the first year of the BCG mass vaccination (November 1949 to November 1950) over 365,000 persons were tuberculin tested.

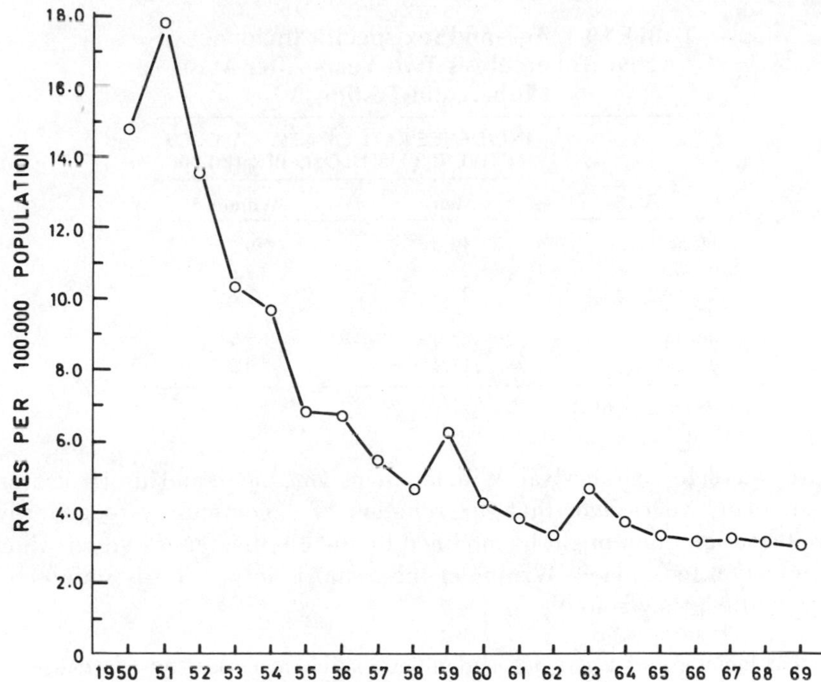

FIG. 19-1. Mortality from tuberculosis in the Jewish population of Israel. Rates per 100,000 population. (Adapted from Israel Central Bureau of Statistics.[2])

While the vast majority of men and women were tuberculin positive (over 90 percent of men and over 80 percent of women) there was a marked sex difference in the incidence of new cases of tuberculous disease. This was especially so among adults over the age of 35 (Table 19-1).[3]

It is clear that breakdown with active disease is a phenomenon beyond infection itself requiring epidemiologic investigation over and above that of infection. Similar consideration must be given to mortality from a disease like tuberculosis.

Change in the mortality rate from an infectious disease may be the result of any one of the following: (1) change in the infection rate; (2) change in the disease rate; and (3) change in the severity of the disease and in its outcome.

We have previously discussed the impact of a new infection on virgin communities, noting their high susceptibility to infection and to severe illness from the infection. However, there is variation in response between different communities which goes beyond the biologically acquired immunity determined by previous exposure or by innate immunity determined

TABLE 19-1. Age- and Sex-specific Incidence of Active Tuberculosis Two Years After Mass Tuberculin Testing

	INCIDENCE RATE OF NEW CASES OF ACTIVE TUBERCULOSIS PER 100,000	
AGE	Men	Women
60 and over	19.0	9.7
55–59	23.2	7.5
50–54	22.5	7.8
45–49	19.2	9.8
40–44	17.9	7.7
35–39	15.3	9.7

(From Gruschka.[3])

by previous selective survival. With much insight, Lister and his associates[4] noted, many years ago, that the reaction of a community to a newly-introduced infection might be modified by the circumstances under which the infection took place. Writing of tuberculosis in previously uninfected communities, they stated

> that members of isolated communities exhibit a marked susceptibility to tuberculosis when brought into contact with infection; and that, although the infection may be fairly well tolerated under natural or tribal conditions, this susceptibility is fraught with extreme danger when exposure to infection is accompanied by a sudden change in occupation, food, housing, and mode of life.[4]

It is in these circumstances that infection results in epidemics of the severe generalized form of tuberculosis described by Borrel[5] among African Senegalese tribesmen arriving in France in World War I, and the similar devastation of American Indian communities of the Canadian plains in the 19th century.[6]

Some 20 years ago observations on tuberculosis patients of Seattle, Washington, added further insight into the possible association between social disequilibrium, stressful life experiences, and breakdown with disease.[7] The ecologic studies of Holmes and his associates went well beyond mere confirmation of the well-known association of tuberculosis with poverty. In general, the wealthier neighborhoods of the city had the lowest incidence of the disease. However, the rates for nonwhites living in these neighborhoods, who composed only 1 percent of the population living in these areas, were higher than that of nonwhites in all other areas of the city. The central business area of the city consisted mainly of adults; nearly two-thirds of its population were 35 years of age and over, with unmarried men predominating. This area had a high incidence rate of the disease and also the highest proportion of advanced cases, amongst whom many had been living alone. The nonwhites, who constituted 14 percent of the population in the central area, also had a high incidence rate of tuberculosis, but despite the adverse circumstances the rate was lower than that of the nonwhites living in the wealthiest areas of the city. Compared with the high incidence of tuberculosis in nonwhites living in the wealthier areas and those of the central business area, there was a markedly lower rate of tuberculosis among those living in areas immediately beyond the city business area. A distinguishing feature of those areas was the settlement of the nonwhites in particular neighborhoods.

Holmes and his associates made a number of more direct observations, among which the following social factors operated in cases of tuberculosis.

1. Mobility: There was a very high residential and occupational mobility of patients.
2. Social isolation: Almost a quarter of the cases admitted to the tuberculosis hospital of the city had been living alone in one room for at least 2 years before their admission to hospital.
3. Increase of stressful experience: In many cases there was a gradually increasing incidence of stressful experiences culminating in serious life crises in the 2-year period preceding hospitalization. These included changes in residence and in jobs, loss of job and financial worries, social withdrawal, marital stress, drinking (alcoholism), and ill health.

Further understanding of the significance of these associations requires investigation of the mechanisms by which social disequilibrium is manifested in stressful life experiences, of their meaning in terms of the mental health of individuals, and how these psychologic factors cause infected persons to breakdown with illness. It is not so much a direct chain of causation that needs to be sought, but rather a field of interactions between social situations and psychophysiologic processes in which breakdown from infection may occur through change in the immunity-susceptibility regulating mechanisms.

We have seen that changes in life situations and life experiences are among the factors possibly determining susceptibility to infection. In the life of an individual or small group, like a family, these changes include the following:

1. Personal crises in family or friendship group, e.g., death, sudden injury, or illness of a family member or close friend; family disruption through divorce, separation, or sudden departure; or disruption of a close friendship.
2. Economic and occupational change, e.g., loss of a job, change in employment, acute financial worries.
3. Pressure to meet deadline, e.g., examinations and climax of preparation for the examination by students.

4. Residential mobility, e.g., movement of home from rural to urban area, from one country to another, from one neighborhood to another.

There is also a different type of disturbing or stressful experience that may have an important influence on the equilibrium established between an infecting agent and an individual or group. This involves a type of continuing or chronic stressful experience, such as the problems presented by status inconsistency and other inconsistencies—job versus ability; expectations of self versus self-estimate of ability to achieve; or continuing worries of a financial or personal kind. Parental deprivation, whether caused by death, separation, or divorce, may be associated with a higher-than-expected death rate from certain disorders. Among these is tuberculosis. Holmes[7] reported that 41 of 100 consecutive cases admitted to a tuberculosis sanatorium had been deprived of one or the other parent before the age of 18. This unexpectedly high figure may be the result of a number of factors. It may be related to the social class distribution of the patients, or it may be that the same disease was a cause of early death of one or the other of the patient's parents. It may also be that patients deprived of their parents in childhood are themselves living "alone" and hence more likely to need care in an institution. In fact, Holmes stated that no less than 20 of the 40 patients had themselves experienced a disrupted marriage. A much higher-than-expected proportion of tuberculotics who were admitted to the hospital had had a broken marriage by divorce or separation.

In studies of marital status and mortality, a wide variety of diseases have a much higher mortality rate in single and divorced persons than in those married. This is especially so among men. These diseases include several common infections, such as tuberculosis, pneumonia, and syphilis.[8] While they are of much interest in locating special risk groups, these associations between marital status and disease do not in themselves represent a cause-and-effect relationship.

Some clinical epidemiologic explorations have provided suggestive evidence of stressful family experiences determining the acquisition of infection itself, as well as of illness resulting from these infections. This was shown by Meyer and Haggerty[9] in a small-scale study of 100 persons in 16 lower-middle-class families over a 12-month period.

The investigators found a relation between acute stress and beta-hemolytic streptococcal illness as well as acquisition of a streptococcal infection without illness. In checking the time relationship of the stressful experience and infection, streptococcal illness and infection acquisition, as well as nonstreptococcal respiratory infections, followed acute stress in the majority of cases in which they were associated with stress. Of the total 56 cases of beta-hemolytic streptococcal illness, over one-third were associated with acute stress and, in these, stressful experiences preceded the illness in 17 of the 20 cases. While a lower proportion of beta-streptococcal infection acquisitions without illness (20 percent) and non-streptococcal respiratory infections (11 percent) were associated with stress, the stressful experience preceded the infection 4 times more frequently than it followed the infection.

"Chronic family stress" was rated on a scale of family functioning.[10] An association was found between long-term family disorganization or poor family functioning with the number of illnesses from streptococcal infection, the number of acquisitions of streptococcal infection, the anti-streptolysin-O response, and, to a lesser extent, prolonged carriers.

Families with evidence of acute crisis situations and of long-term stressful experience (social disorganization or poor functioning) may constitute high risk groups. Testing this hypothesis would be an interesting application of epidemiology to family and community medicine.

REFERENCES

1. Dubos R: Man Adapting. New Haven, Yale Univ Press, 1965.
2. Israel Central Bureau of Statistics: Publications on Causes of Death 1951, 1953, 1954, 1967 and Annual Statistical Abstracts of Israel. Jerusalem.
3. Gruschka T: Health Services in Israel: A Ten Year Survey 1948–1958. Jerusalem, Israel Ministry of Health, 1959.
4. Lister S: Tuberculosis Research Committee Report, Vol. 5, No. 30. Johannesburg, South African Insititute for Medical Research, 1932, p 20.
5. Borrel A: Pneumonie et tuberculose chez les troupes noires. Ann Inst Pasteur 34:105, 1920.
6. Ferguson RG: Studies in Tuberculosis. Toronto, Univ of Toronto, 1955.
7. Holmes TH: Multidiscipline studies in tuberculosis. In Sparer PJ (ed.): Personality, Stress and Tuberculosis. New York, International Univ Press, 1956.
8. Berkson J: Mortality and marital status. Am J Public Health 52:1318, 1962.
9. Meyer RJ, Haggerty RJ: Streptococcal infections in families. Pediatrics 29:539, 1962.
10. Bell NW, Vogel EF: Modern Introduction to the Family. Glencoe, Ill, Free Press, 1960.

SECTION 4

The Community Syndrome Concept

It is usual to speak of a clinical syndrome as consisting in a number of related signs and symptoms. The syndrome may be accounted for by a single underlying pathologic process. Thus many clinicians aim to explain their findings of various signs and symptoms by a diagnosis of one disease in the framework of a single pathology. However it should be recognized that clinical syndromes are often the product of several processes which, acting on one another, produce a final common expression.

Extending the use of the word "syndrome" to the description of health and disease in a community, we may speak of a community syndrome. The importance of this concept is both in its implications for epidemiologic thought and research, and in its potential meaning for the development of community medicine programs. A community health syndrome is an epidemiologic association between various health conditions. It can be defined as the concomitant occurrence of somatic or psychologic characteristics in the community, the distribution of these characteristics in relation to the disease picture, and the concurrent incidence or prevalence of certain diseases.

The expression of a particular disease is often determined by other diseases or health factors with which it occurs; e.g., there is a difference in the meaning of hypertension when it occurs in a community in which hyperlipidemia and coronary atherosclerosis are also common, from one in which these conditions are uncommon. In the former it is a high risk factor for acute myocardial infarction whereas in the latter it is not.

Another aspect of interest in the concept and definition of a community syndrome is the interaction or synergism between the component parts of the syndrome. One such example has been reviewed in Chapter 17, on the relation between malnutrition and infection in the production of weanling diarrhea, a syndrome which differs markedly from acute diarrhea in well-nourished infants.

A community syndrome may result from different causes, each having its effects on a particular element of the syndrome. On the other hand the causes, like the health syndrome itself, may constitute an interacting network of factors which together produce the syndrome. Categorical health programs are frequently directed at a single disease or a specific pathogenic agent of that disease. However, focus on a syndrome may often be more effective. Some of these approaches are discussed in Section 5, and more especially in Chapters 30 and 31.

Diagnosing a community syndrome requires careful definition of each of its components and should never be allowed to regress into easy generalizations about a community's health. The first step towards recognition of a syndrome is to list the facts about the community's health, using all available sources of information. In addition, specially planned surveys will be needed, including interviews and health examinations.

For practical purposes investigation of community syndromes can be built around common and important diseases in that community, especially those diseases which can be better treated or prevented if recognized in the context of the epidemiological syndrome of which they are a feature. Two contrasting syndromes are presented in the following chapters; one is the product of poverty in a rural peasant community undergoing rapid change, and the other is found in more affluent societies of the world.

20

A Community Syndrome of Malnutrition, Communicable Diseases, and Mental Ill-Health in a Rural Community

This is a case illustration from the author's own experience and investigations when initiating a community health center in a rural African community.

High up in the foothills of a mountain range which separates the countries of Lesotho and South Africa lives a community in which soil erosion was the outstanding environmental determinant of its poor health and perhaps the major obstacle in effective response to comprehensive community health care. It is a district of deep valleys with fast flowing rivers and rugged mountains stripped of their vegetation. In the valleys and lower slopes of the foothills of the mountain range are the poorly cultivated fields of the people—fields dominated by maize, the staple food. Cattle and goats graze on the scanty vegetation of the ridges and upper slopes of the mountains. In summer, the rainfall season, herdboys confine the grazing animals to these areas while the fields below are planted with crops to be reaped in the dry winter season. After reaping, the cattle graze on the stumps of maize and sorghum left by the reapers.

The countryside is at once beautiful, imposing, and tragic; beautiful in its grandeur and harshness, tragic in the devastation that has been wrought by soil erosion. Where once there may have been indigenous forest and lush veld, sheet erosion has exposed subsoil and rock, and gullies have torn their way through the grazing lands, past the lines of homes and deep into the fields below. The stimulus of the bracing climate at an altitude of 1,300 to 2,000 meters above sea level, the sunny days of winter with the cold winds that come from the snow-capped mountain range, and the summer rainfall and the mists that smooth the harshness of the steep mountain slopes present a physical challenge which others might have met differently. This community was overpowered by the challenge.

In considering the disharmony in the relations of the community and the soil, a brief review of a healthy soil cycle will be given. A healthy soil is one which maintains a vegetable and animal life to the maximum of the potentiality of its region. The soil, together with the vegetation and animal life, forms an integrated whole. Not only does vegetation depend for its growth upon the soil content, but the soil in its turn depends upon decaying vegetation and animal life for its nutritive powers. A rhythmic cycle is established between the soil and the life it sustains. This cycle has two essential phases involving growth of vegetation and animal life, and the excreta and products of decay of these forms of life. The process of decay and the return of the decaying products to the soil are essential for the process of growth. Without them there would be no humus formation, and without humus the living soil would be replaced by a sterile medium with loss of soil fertility. The link between growth and decay of living matter thus takes place in the soil, and where the processes balance one another, a healthy cycle is established.

While the place of humus in the maintenance of soil fertility has been well established, support has been given to a theory that goes further, claiming that food grown on soil rich in humus has qualities of health-promotion that are conveyed to those who eat such food.[1-4] A summary of the relationship which exists between the health of man, animal, plant, and soil fertility is presented in Figure 20-1. The key role of proper disposal

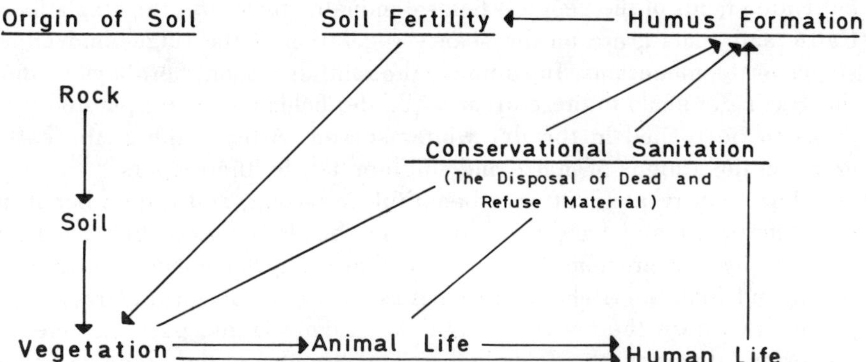

FIG. 20-1. A healthy soil cycle. Effects of vegetation: (1) binds the soil; (2) protects the soil from direct effects of wind, rain, and sun; and (3) promotes humus formation. Effects of humus formation: (1) soil fertility; (2) aeration; (3) water retention; and (4) immunity of plants to disease.

of refuse material in the formation of humus may be defined as conservational sanitation.

A cycle such as the one described allows for maximum food production in a particular area. A community which maintains an environment with such a healthy soil cycle is more than likely to be well nourished and have a high standard of health.

The main point in the soil cycle which was disturbed in this particular area was the natural vegetation.

The vegetation of extensive areas had been disturbed or completely removed by deforestation, overgrazing of pasture land, poor methods of cultivation of arable lands, bad drainage from houses, footpaths, roads, and railways. This resulted in exposure of the soil to the direct effects of sun, wind, and rain, and reduction of the quantity of organic matter in the soil.

The long dry winter season and the heavy rains of summer provided almost ideal conditions for rain and wind erosion of exposed soil. Depletion of soil humus, associated with these processes, meant reduced soil fertility and a loss of soil stability, which are the main elements of the process of soil erosion. The disturbance of the healthy soil cycle, thus begun, becomes a vicious spiral of increasing erosion and loss of fertility. Among the more obvious signs of the progressive deterioration of the soil were the following.

1. Forest land. There had been a considerable thinning out of forests in river catchment areas, and in many places complete deforestation had occurred.
2. Pasture land. The nature of the grasses was changing, with a patchy thinning out of grassland. In areas where these patches coalesced the vegetation was stripped by extensive sheet and gully erosion exposing subsoil and rock.
3. Ploughed, cultivated land. Most fields dried out very rapidly after rains, with caking of exposed soil and rapid run-off of water. On many fields there was deep gully formation and exposure of subsoil. Some of these were abandoned but most continued to be used and the crops were very stunted and diseased.

These signs of deterioration of the soil were reflected in several associated conditions; one was the failing food production which resulted in inadequate diet with consequent malnutrition. Another associated condition was the migration of men of working age to and from cities, with its impact on family relationships and the introduction of various diseases from the cities. (Fig. 20-2).

The measurable effects on food supplies, migration of men to work, and on the community's health are summarized in Tables 20-1–3.

1. Inadequate Food Production. (Based on measurements conducted

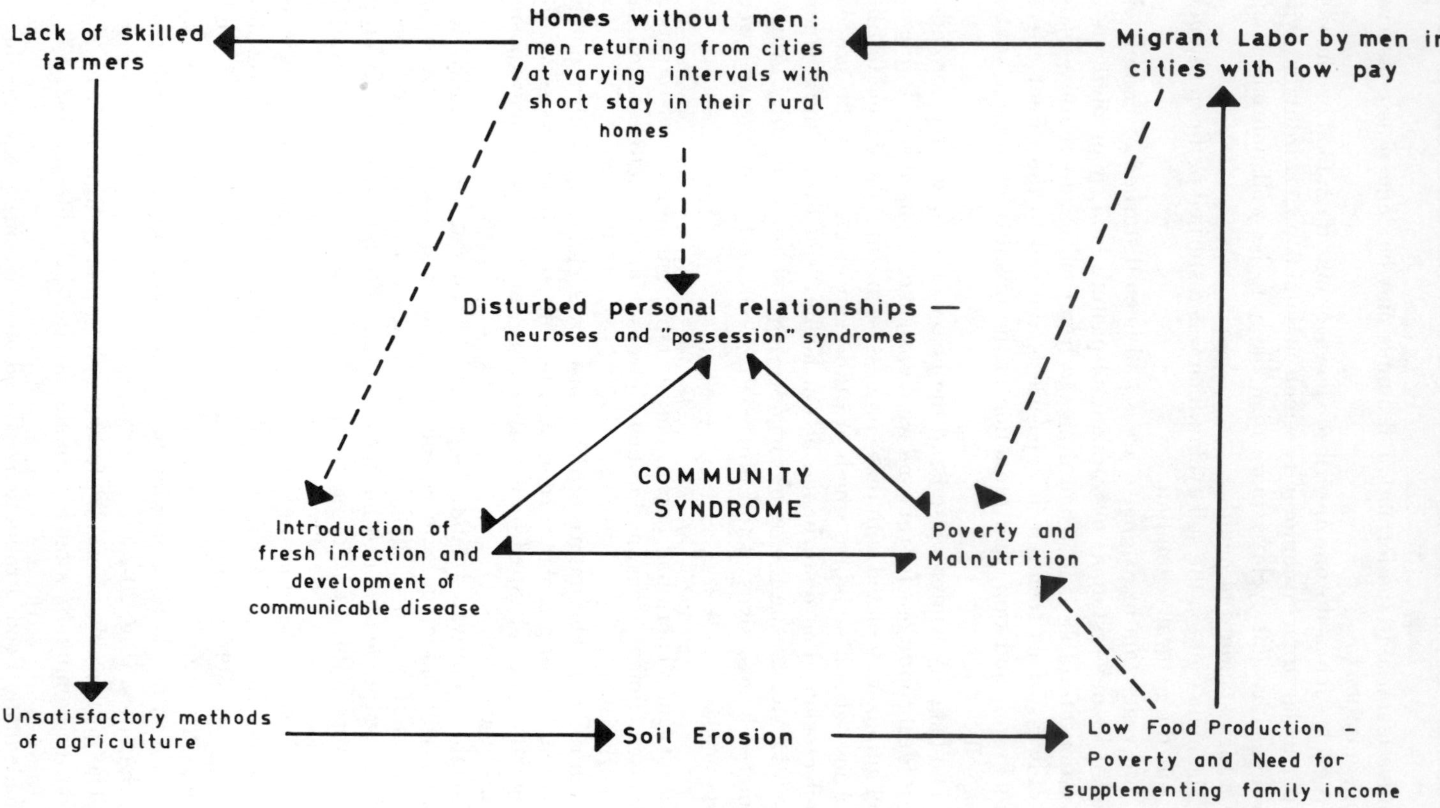

FIG. 20-2. The determinants of a community syndrome of malnutrition, communicable diseases, and mental ill-health in a rural area.

TABLE 20-1. Calorie Production

	AVERAGE PRODUCTION CALORIES AVAILABLE PER PERSON PER DAY*		LOWEST QUARTILE OF HOMES—AVERAGE OF "POOR" AND "GOOD" YEARS
	Poor Year	Good Year	
Staple cereal —maize	650	1,000	< 250 calories per person daily
Supplementary —sorghum	100	200	< 30 calories per person daily
—beans	20	30	0
Total	770	1,230	< 280

Calculated on basis of 365-day year following reaping of the mature crop.

TABLE 20-2. Milk Yield (3 Years Average)

	AVERAGE PRODUCTION AVAILABLE PER HOME PER DAY (AVERAGE 7 PERSONS PER HOME) (LITERS)	PERCENT OF HOMES IN WHICH THERE WAS NO MILK AVAILABLE	
		Worst Year	Best Year
Spring	0.15	92	87
Summer	2.20	59	48
Autumn	1.30	63	55
Winter	0.25	85	75

TABLE 20-3. Meat Available

	AVERAGE NUMBER PER HOME	PERCENTAGE OF HOMES HAVING NONE
Ownership of cattle	4.4	25
Ownership of goats	2.8	76
Ownership of pigs	0.8	50
Ownership of sheep	0.06	97
Ownership of poultry	9.3	4

by community health workers trained at the health center itself. The measurements used were gathered over 3 successive years.) This was a cattle-keeping, milk-eating community living in an area potentially suitable for cattle and milk production. The milk yield of cows-in-milk was very low, varying from an average of 1 liter per day in the winter and spring months to a maximum average of 2 to 3 liters in the best summer months of different years.

Cattle and goats were eaten on ceremonial occasions only, or when an animal died. Poultry was the most common meat eaten, although

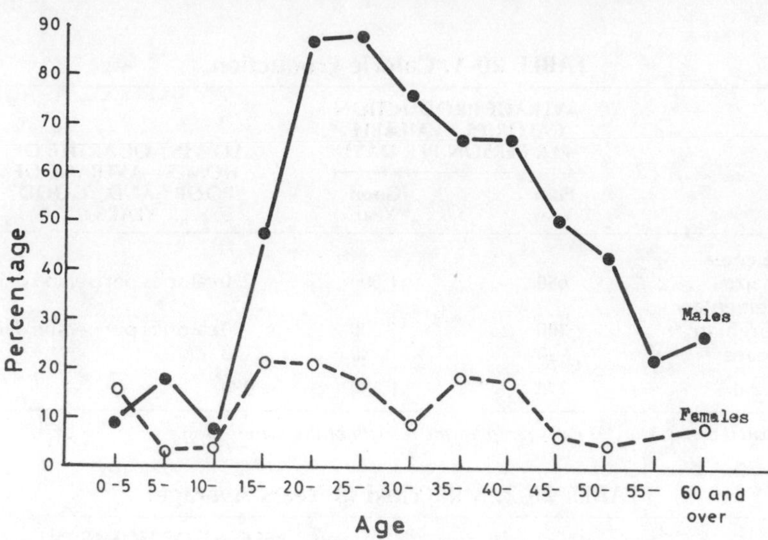

FIG. 20-3. The percentage of persons away from their rural home district for at least 1 month during the course of a year. (Adapted data from Kark.[5])

seldom eaten more than once a week even in the best-off homes. Eggs were rarely eaten.

2. Migration of men to work. There was a very high proportion of men away at work in various cities (Fig. 20-3). A special study of this was conducted by the health center in connection with its program of control of communicable diseases which were introduced by these men on their return home. In a more detailed study extending over 1 year, of 133 men who were away from their home district, it was found that no less than 42 (32 percent) were away from their homes for the whole year, and an additional 26 (20 percent) were away for over 9 months.
3. Malnutrition. Malnutrition was manifest in retardation in growth and in various nonspecific signs and symptoms. These were very common, with seasonal variation in prevalence. The main signs included follicular hyperkeratoses of the skin, and cheilosis and angular stomatitis, gingivitus and glossitis of the mucous membranes. The two common nutritional failure syndromes were kwashiorkor in later infancy and pellagra in older children and adults.
4. Communicable diseases. Of special interest were the communicable diseases brought in by men returning from work in the towns. These included venereal disease (especially syphilis), tuberculosis, typhoid fever, and dysentery.
5. Disturbances in personal relationships and behavior. The main disturbances of a serious nature were those between husbands and wives, and between women and their mothers-in-law. In this regard it must be noted that married women in this community lived in the family

home of their husbands. The main abnormal behavioral manifestations were various "possession" syndromes thought to be brought about by witchcraft, as well as neurasthenia.

The facts summarized in the above items are presented in Figure 20-2 as a community syndrome of malnutrition, communicable diseases, and mental ill-health in the setting of its network of causes of rural poverty, poor agricultural methods, soil erosion, migrant labor, and homes without men. Each aspect of the health syndrome was studied in more detail. Here we will present some of the somatometric data gathered in the course of a community medicine program conducted by this health center.

THE USE OF SOMATOMETRIC DATA IN COMMUNITY HEALTH APPRAISAL

The relevance of measures of height and weight in an appraisal of health status of a population is illustrated in a number of examples from this rural African community. These studies were undertaken as an integral part of the community medicine practice of the health center.[5] The following relevant aspects are presented: (1) the weight growth of well infants; (2) height and weight growth of schoolchildren; (3) weight change in pregnancy; and (4) height and weight of adults at different ages.

Weight Growth in Well Infants

Criteria in selecting well babies, judging by the mother's health, included the following.

1. Normal pregnancy and labor.
2. Nutritional status at least average. There were very few expectant mothers who did not manifest the signs of malnutrition that were common in the community.
3. Absence of disease such as syphilis (which was very common) and tuberculosis in the mother herself or other members of the home.

Criteria in selecting well babies, judging by the baby's health, included the following.

1. Normal birth, with no evidence of congenital deformity or congenital syphilis.
2. No severe illness during the first year of life. This excluded babies diagnosed to have had common diseases such as pneumonia, acute otitis media, whooping cough, primary tuberculous infection (tuberculin positive test), and acute nutritional failure.

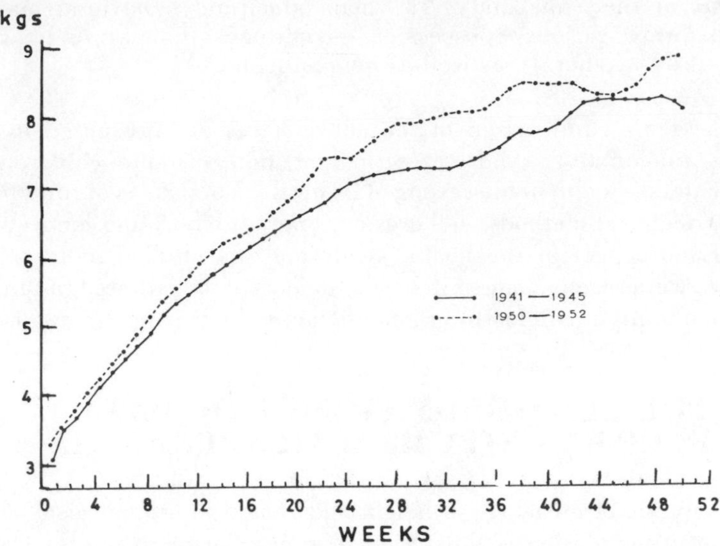

FIG. 20-4. Change in the weight curve of well babies associated with a health program in a rural African community. (From Slome.[7])

While the criteria were neither strictly defined nor rigidly applied, especially with respect to nutritional state, their application was very selective. Only 98 babies of several thousand attending the health center over a 5-year period were included in the first weight-growth curve of well babies in this particular rural community. Some 10 years later the same criteria were used and a new weight-growth curve of infants in the community was established. The change in the weight curve is shown in Figure 20-4. It is evident that well babies, as so defined, were superior in weight after 10 years of the health center program in the community, the details of which have been described elsewhere.[6,7] This superiority became more evident after the age of 5 months. The changing community picture, as represented by these two weight curves, may be interpreted with other variables as an indicator of improved infant health. In particular improved weight-growth was associated with a marked decline in the infant mortality rates in this community. The health center had to establish its own birth and death registration system to ensure the ongoing surveillance of health of the community and evaluation of its programs.

In considering the growth of the moderately well baby in this African rural community the increasing retardation in weight growth during the first year of life was noted. This was related to nutritional state and more generally to poverty, and was modified by a community health education program directed towards some of the specific defects in daily care of infants in the community, especially infant feeding and protection against infection.

The Height and Weight of Schoolchildren

Height and weight measurements of schoolchildren were included as an integral part of the periodic health examination of all children attending schools in the area. The results were compared with other communities and as expected, these children were shorter and weighed less than did those of better-off communities.[8] Their respective physiques relative to those of others are illustrated in Figure 20-5, where the changing stature of British children is compared with findings in this African community. As stated earlier, increase in the rate of growth of children has been noted in many countries where the standard of living has been improving over the 19th and 20th centuries. Britain is one of these countries, and three periods in which data are available for the height and weight of British children are compared with these children, namely 1820–1836,[9] 1909–1910,[10] and 1947,[11] the last period being approximately the same time as the rural African community was studied.

Karn used the ages 11 to 13 years for the purposes of her comparative study and for this reason Figure 20-5 shows these ages.

The average boy at school in this rural community appears taller and heavier when compared with British children studied in the period 1820–1836, of the same height and weight as British children of the period 1909–1910, and markedly shorter and lighter when compared with British boys of 1947. The relative growth curve among girls shows a similar trend, but the girls in this community generally compare more favorably with their British counterparts than do the boys.

With improvement in their standard of living, this African group might well have a similar secular trend toward more rapid growth and the attainment of greater stature. The comparison of their stature relative to others adds a dimension to health appraisal by which the "normal" child in the community may be perceived.

Weight Change in Pregnancy

Figure 20-6 shows the weight change in pregnancy of relatively "normal" or "well" women attending the prenatal sessions of the health center in this community.[12] The figure should be read with caution. The average duration of pregnancy at first attendance was approximately 22 weeks. The figure is based on the records of 116 women whose attendance and

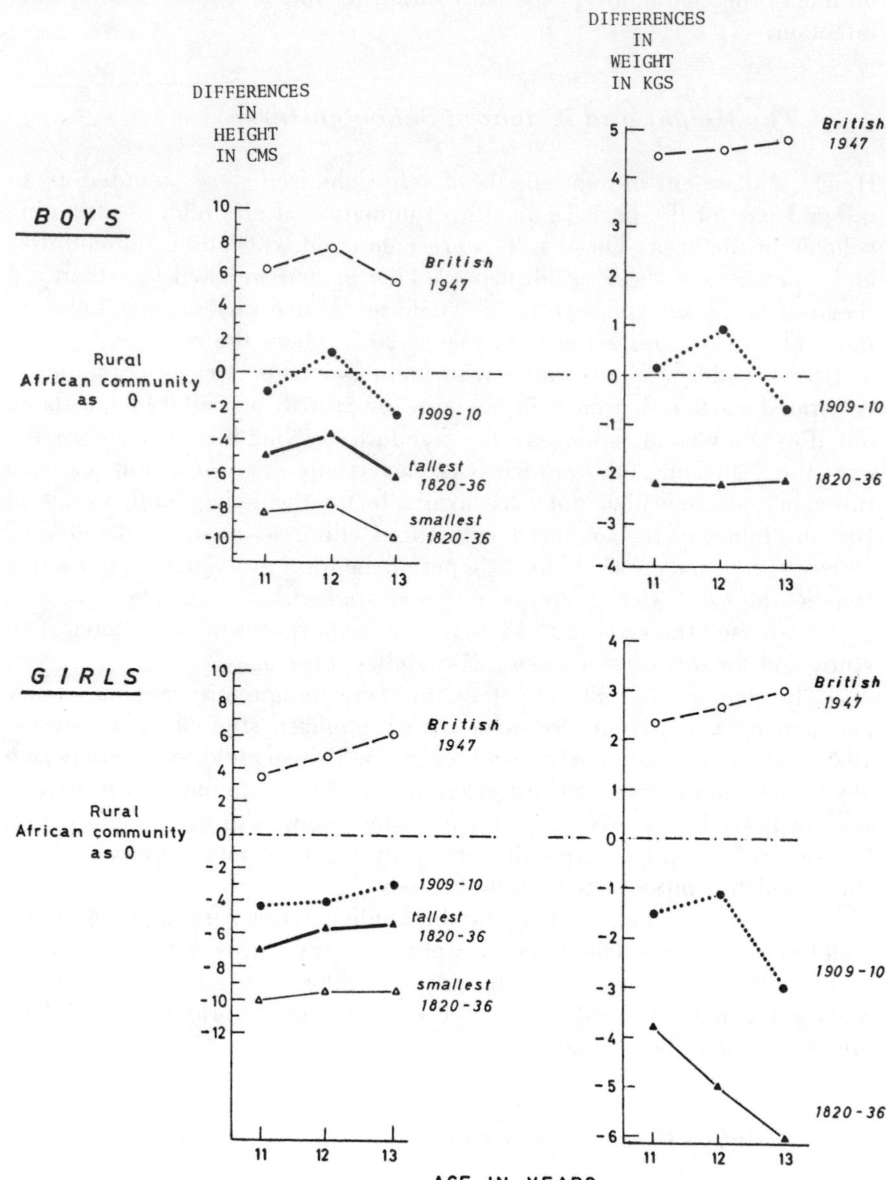

FIG. 20-5. The heights and weights of girls and boys in a rural African community (1945), compared with those of British children at different periods from 1820 to 1947. Using the African means as zero, the deviation of British children is shown in centimeters and kilograms. (Adapted from Kark and Kark;[8] Kark;[5] Karn;[9] Tuxford and Glegg;[10] and Daley.[11]

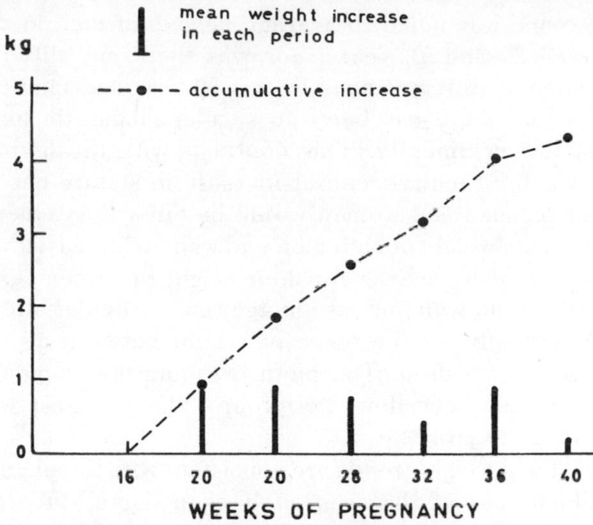

FIG. 20-6. The mean changes in weight of expectant mothers in a rural community. (Adapted from Kark.[12])

weight records allowed for measurement of change. Further analysis showed that during the first 4 months only 11 of the 31 women (35.5 percent) whose weights were known immediately before pregnancy gained over 1 pound (above 650 grams) in weight, whereas 13 women lost more than 1 pound. Even more striking was the finding during the last month of pregnancy, in which only 31 (52.5 percent) of the 59 women whose change in weight was known for this period gained more than 1 pound. In the intervening months (the fifth to the ninth, or the 16th to 36th weeks) a higher proportion of women gained weight, but there was a consistently high percentage whose weight did not change by more than 1 pound or who lost more than 1 pound. This varied between 23 and 45 percent of the women at different periods.

The limited change in weight during pregnancy is consistent with other findings of malnutrition in this community. While the individual women who accord with general findings may be regarded as in a state of normal pregnancy for their community, the community picture itself is an indicator of a low level of community health.

The Height and Weight of Adults

As might be expected, the men and women of this African community were relatively short and of low weight.[12] The height among men and women follows a normal distribution curve.

No difference was noted in average heights of men in different age groups between 20 and 70 years, nor was there any difference in the height of women at different ages in this 50-year age-span (Fig. 20-7A). This suggests that there has been no secular change in height of men or women of this community. This contrasts with the findings in communities in which a secular trend of increase in stature has been noted, in which younger men and women would be taller than older people. As expected, the mean weight of both men and women increased with increase in height, women being heavier for their height than men.

The weight trend with increase in age is of particular interest. Among men there is virtually no difference in weight between ages 20 and 59, after which there is a drop. The picture among the women was one of a steady decline in succeeding age groups, the youngest women being the heaviest (Fig. 20-7B).

The height and weight trends are consistent with the picture of malnutrition and high rate of diseases such as pellagra, tuberculosis, and

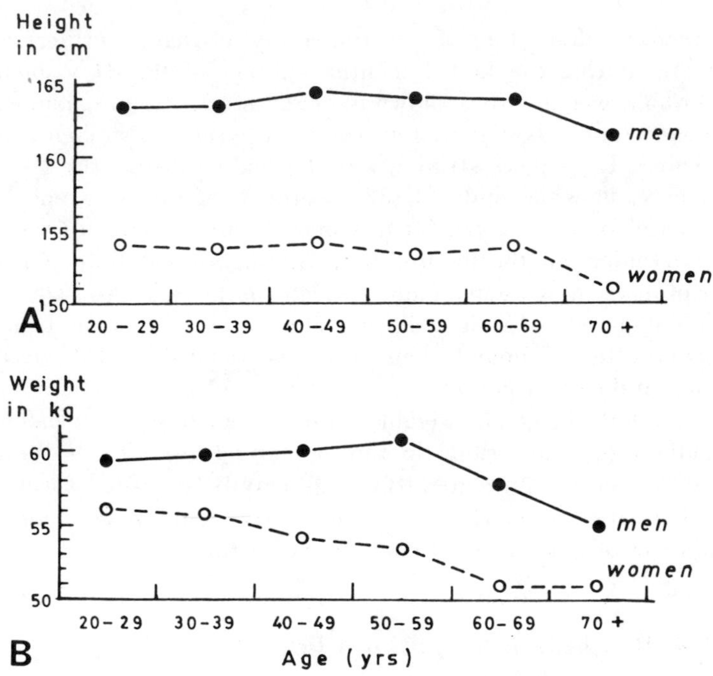

FIG. 20-7. The height and weight of men and women at different ages, in a rural African community. (Adapted from Kark.[12])

pneumonia. They are also compatible with the absence of clinical or overt occurrence of coronary heart disease, angina pectoris, or myocardial infarction; the rarity of diabetes mellitus; and a relatively uncommon occurrence of essential hypertension. Obesity too was uncommon, especially in middle-aged and older men and women.

SOME HEALTH-RELEVANT FEATURES OF POOR PEASANT COMMUNITIES

This rural community presents many of the characteristics of peasant societies among whom such diseases as coronary artery disease are rare. Some of the more important health-relevant features of these societies are summarized below and may be read alongside a similar summary of the health characteristics of those societies in which coronary artery disease is common. This is presented in the next chapter.

1. Mortality: High death rates from infectious diseases and nutritional failure
2. Disease
   a. Common diseases are diseases of malnutrition
      1. Generalized nonspecific signs of malnutrition as well as high occurrence of disease syndromes like pellagra, nutritional anemias, kwashiorkor.
      2. Nutritional liver disease, such as the extensive cirrhosis of liver described in malnutrition, in which there are high estrogen and lipoprotein lipase levels with consequent lower serum cholesterol.[13]
   b. Communicable diseases: high prevalence and incidence
      1. High rates of infection and infectious diseases of children, e.g., diarrhea, pneumonia.
      2. High rates of tuberculosis, and endemic 'tropical' diseases, e.g., malaria.
   c. Low occurrence of diabetes, atherosclerosis
3. Somatic characteristics
   Somatic characteristics of such a community could resemble very closely the detailed description given of height-weight changes of the peasant community outlined above. The features include relatively slow growth, late maturation, very little change in weight during the adult years (any change is quite often a decrease), low blood cholesterol with very little change with age, and low blood proteins.

REFERENCES

1. Picton LJ: Thoughts on Feeding. London, Faber and Faber, 1946.
2. Wrench GT: The Wheel of Health. London, Daniel, 1938.
3. Howard A: Farming and Gardening for Health or Disease. London, Faber and Faber, 1945.
4. Balfour EB: The Living Soil. London, Faber and Faber, 1943.
5. Kark SL: Nutrition and Adjustment in the Changing Society of Polela. Johannesburg, Doctoral Thesis, University of Witwatersrand, 1952.
6. Kark SL, Steuart GW (eds.): A Practice of Social Medicine. Edinburgh and London, E & S Livingstone, 1962.
7. Slome C: Community health in rural Polela. In Kark SL, Steuart GW (eds.): A Practice of Social Medicine. Edinburgh and London, E & S Livingstone, 1962.
8. Kark SL, Kark E: Growth of African urban and rural schoolchildren. In Kark SL, Steuart GW (eds.): A Practice of Social Medicine. Edinburgh and London, E & S Livingstone, 1962.
9. Karn MN: Summary of results of investigations into the height and weight of children of the British working classes during the last hundred years. Ann Eugenics 7:376, 1937.
10. Tuxford AW, Glegg RA: The average height and weight of English schoolchildren. Brit Med J 1:1423, 1911.
11. Daley A: Heights and weights of London school children. Med Officer 79: 292, 1948.
12. Kark SL: The height and weight of men and women in relation to age. In Kark SL, Steuart GW (eds.): A Practice of Social Medicine. Edinburgh and London, E & S Livingstone, 1962.
13. Spain DM: Problems in the study of coronary atherosclerosis in population groups. Ann NY Acad Sci 84:816, 1960.

21

Coronary Heart Disease and the State of Health of the Community

Coronary heart disease is the commonest single cause of death in some communities while in others it has not yet been reported as a cause of illness or death.

What are the differences in the states of health of such communities? It is apparent that they differ in many more respects than that of their coronary arteries. Atherosclerosis of the coronary arteries is part of a more general pathologic process affecting the arteries of the body. The extent and severity of the disease in the coronary arteries is not necessarily correlated with that in other arteries such as the aorta or cerebral arteries.[1] Until comparatively recent years atherosclerosis was regarded as a disease of aging, affecting middle-aged and older persons. One of the reasons for this was no doubt the age at which its effects were commonly manifested, whether in the pain of angina pectoris, in an acute episode of myocardial infarction, in sudden death, or in the chronic effects of several previous infarcts. While earlier workers had observed coronary atherosclerosis in younger men[2,3] little notice was taken of this fact. The report of a marked degree of coronary occlusion in the United States soldiers killed in the Korean War drew attention to its being already a well-established disease in very young American men. Over 12 percent of the men killed in action had occlusion of more than 50 percent of the lumen and in 5 percent of the men the occlusion was 90 percent.[4,5]

The other pathological process involved in coronary artery disease is thrombosis, which is responsible for a proportion of cases of coronary occlusion with myocardial infarction. The relation between thrombosis and atherosclerosis has been a much studied subject by pathologists.

Men who die following acute episodes of coronary artery disease may or may not have evidence of a recent thrombosis. Epstein[6] referring to several investigations,[7,8] noted that evidence of recent thrombosis was the exception in men who died of acute heart attacks.

Morris[9] has presented evidence of an historical kind, suggesting that the rise in incidence of myocardial infarction is related to an increase in occluding fresh, unorganized thrombus in the coronary arteries rather than a change in the amount or degree of coronary atherosclerosis. Examining the records of the department of pathology of London Hospital from 1907 to 1949, Morris found documented evidence of atheroma of the coronary arteries in the early as well as the later years. If there was any difference the condition was more marked in the earlier case records. The main change had been a marked increase in evidence of acute myocardial necrosis and recent thrombus. This points to luminal occlusive thrombosis as a cause of acute myocardial infarction over and above that caused by atheroma.

Studies in other places have not confirmed Morris' evidence. Spain[10] found "In all age categories the males from 1951 to 1955 showed a considerably greater degree of coronary atherosclerosis than those from 1931 to 1935." His analysis included autopsy reports of cases who had died from infectious disease in the earlier period and from accidents in the later period, i.e., they were relatively free of chronic disease.

It is clear that coronary occlusion usually occurs in coronary arteries affected by atherosclerosis. While thrombosis may be considered a most important complication of atherosclerosis, the factors determining its formation are not only the damaged wall of the artery but also that of blood flow and platelet aggregation. Viscosity of the blood, platelet stickiness, fibrin, and fibrinolysis have an important function in platelet aggregation and in stabilization of the aggregation into a thrombus by fibrin or its resolution by fibrinolytic action.

Any factors associated with the process of atherosclerosis and thrombosis are therefore central to our understanding of the epidemiology of coronary artery disease. Here we are especially concerned with other aspects of the health of the community. In the following discussion we will consider the various factors that may be involved in mutual interaction and which together may result in myocardial infarction. It is important to stress that an association between two or more factors does not in itself necessarily signify a cause-and-effect relationship between these particular variables.

What are the diseases and the somatic and psychologic characteristics that have been found to be associated with coronary artery disease?

Mortality: The pattern of mortality is one in which there is a relatively low death rate from infectious diseases and nutritional failure, and relatively long life with an increasing rate of death from atherosclerotic diseases, especially coronary artery disease.

Diseases: High rates of atherosclerosis and thrombosis, manifested as well in conditions other than coronary artery disease, i.e., cerebral vascular disease and peripheral vascular disease. Diabetes mellitus and hypertensive disease are also common, increasing with age.

Somatic characteristics: Rapid growth through childhood, early maturation, increase in weight during the adult years, high serum cholesterol increasing with age, high serum triglycerides and lipoprotein, high blood pressure increasing with age. High saturated fatty acid content of subcutaneous tissues.

Psychologic characteristics: Suggestive evidence of an association between personality and behavior with coronary heart disease.

Each of these aspects will be further considered in more detail.

SOMATIC CHARACTERISTICS

Epidemiologic data from different communities and population studies in various parts of the world indicate an association of one or more of the following somatic characteristics with coronary artery disease: serum cholesterol, blood pressure, and weight. The three striking features in the association of these variables with coronary heart disease are (1) their high levels, (2) their increase through young adulthood to middle age, and (3) in combination, the association with coronary heart disease is strengthened, especially the occurrence together of high levels of blood cholesterol and high blood pressure.[11,12]

Cholesterol Levels and Coronary Heart Disease

An outstanding feature in the epidemiology of coronary disease is the association between high levels of serum cholesterol and coronary artery disease. This has been demonstrated by indirect studies of differences between population groups as well as by direct studies of differences between individuals in defined communities.

A number of prospective studies have shown that elevated serum cholesterol levels in apparently healthy men are directly associated with subsequent incidence of clinical coronary heart disease. Figure 21-1, based on several such studies, is illustrative of this.[13–15]

The literature on differences between population groups has been summarized in a comparative analysis of 74 studies in a wide variety of countries.[16] The high correlation between serum cholesterol level and the occurrence of coronary artery disease is clearly shown in this analysis. The contrasting extremes are the findings in eastern Finland of a very high cholesterol level and high coronary heart disease level and, at the other end, Japan, in which there are very low cholesterol levels and low incidence of coronary heart disease.

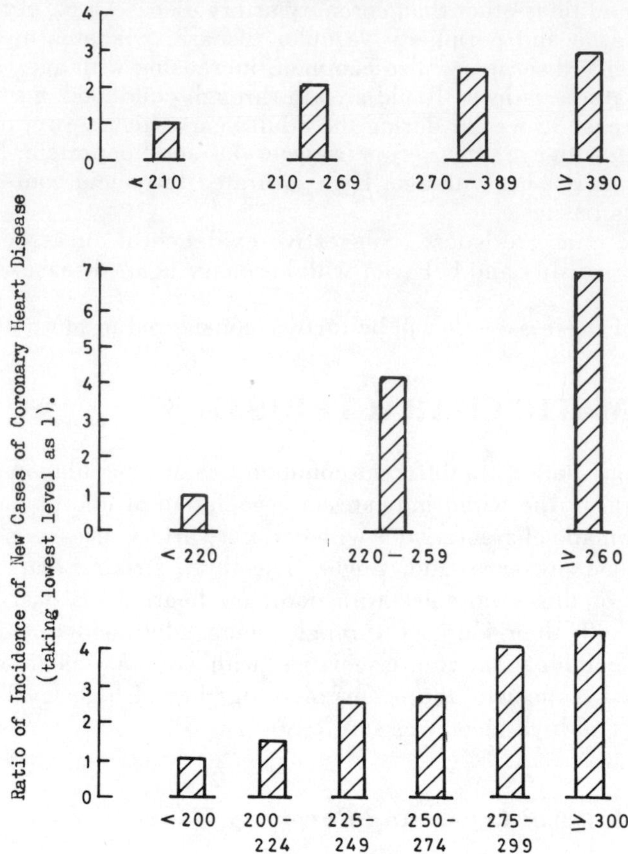

FIG. 21-1. Three studies showing the direct association of serum cholesterol level with incidence of subsequent clinical coronary heart disease. (Adapted from Chapman & Massey,[13] Kagan and associates,[14] and Stamler and associates.[15])

Blood Pressure Levels and Coronary Heart Disease

In communities in which coronary atherosclerosis and coronary occlusion with myocardial infarction are common, high blood pressure has been shown to be an important "risk" factor. However, the association between high blood pressure and coronary heart disease is not consistent. This is a well-established fact in hypertensive women of child-bearing age among whom coronary heart disease is uncommon. Occlusive coronary artery disease is less common among blacks (Afro-Americans) in the United States than among whites, although they have a high prevalence of hypertension which is associated with a relatively high incidence of hypertensive heart disease and cerebral vascular disease.[17] In Jamaica, where severe hypertension is common, myocardial infarction is rare.[18] Similarly, in postmortem studies of African hypertensive subjects in East Africa, myocardial infarction was seldom found.[19] Mortality from coronary heart disease in Japan has consistently been lower than that of countries such as the United States, United Kingdom, and those of Western Europe. A fact of importance to our present discussion is that this is true of areas in Japan in which hypertension and cerebral vascular disease are common, demonstrating that hypertension by itself is not necessarily associated with a high rate of coronary heart disease.

Blood pressure and cholesterol levels need not be associated and communities with high prevalence of hypertension may have very low blood cholesterol levels.[20] Thus low cholesterol levels may be indicative of a metabolism which does not result in high rates of coronary heart disease even in the presence of widespread hypertension. On the other hand, atherosclerosis which is induced by deposition of lipids may be accelerated by hypertension.[21]

Weight, Body Fat, and Coronary Heart Disease

The relation between overweight and mortality from cardiovascular diseases and from diabetes is well recognized. However, it has been difficult to establish an association between overweight as such and coronary heart disease.[6] While obesity has been shown to be associated with hypertension, and to a lesser extent with high serum cholesterol, its association with coronary heart disease has not been established.[22,23] More relevant than obesity per se may be the composition of the body fat, namely the proportions of polyunsaturated, monounsaturated, and saturated fats. Ways of determining obesity include weight : height ratios[24–27] and skin fold thickness.[28]

To summarize, in communities in which coronary artery disease is common, blood pressure and serum cholesterol levels are not only relatively high but are characterized by a rise with age especially through young and middle-aged adulthood. Obesity and increase in weight are not as clearly related to coronary heart disease, although they have been shown to be correlated with blood pressure and cholesterol levels.

Serum Triglycerides, Glucose Tolerance, and Serum Insulin

Less well-studied eqidemiologically but nevertheless holding much promise for the future understanding of the total systemic picture which finds expression in coronary artery disease, are serum triglyceride levels, glucose tolerance, and serum insulin. An association between these three variables has been demonstrated.[29,30]

Study of the association between the three variables—glyceride, glucose tolerance, and insulin levels—in a normal population may assist in understanding the findings of a number of studies of the relation between triglyceride levels and coronary heart disease; blood sugar levels, atherosclerosis, and coronary heart disease; and between these variables and others associated with coronary artery disease.

Since 1959 when Albrink and Man[31] pointed to an association between raised serum triglyceride levels and coronary heart disease, much attention has been given to this relationship. Albrink and her associates made several pertinent observations and suggestions arising from their various investigations. Triglyceride levels may be raised in diabetes[32] and men with a family history of diabetes had higher levels of serum triglycerides than men with a negative family history for this disease.[33] Also, study of the relation between obesity and serum triglyceride levels[34] provides evidence that men who have gained weight in adulthood, rather than all who are overweight, are the ones who have hypertriglyceridemia.

An association between coronary artery disease, elevation of serum triglycerides, and abnormal glucose tolerance has been suggested.[35,36]

Diabetes and Coronary Heart Disease

Clinicians have long recognized that diabetics have a high risk of acute ischemic heart disease. The extent of the risk has been measured in several studies.[37–39] In one such study 1,356 men employed in an industry were investigated over a period of 6 years. The incidence of new cases of acute myocardial infarction in diabetics was found to be 2.55 times higher than in nondiabetic controls.[39] In recent years interest in the association of coronary artery disease and blood sugar levels has gone beyond its occurrence in diabetes. Clinical studies have shown consistently that a high proportion of survivors of acute myocardial infarction have hyperglycemia. Their response to glucose tolerance tests resembles that of diabetics.[40]

Epidemiologic community studies of this association are still limited but the evidence of studies in Tecumseh, Michigan,[41–43] and Bedford, England[44] points in the same direction.

Information on incidence of myocardial infarctions in persons with different levels of glucose tolerance is even more limited than prevalence studies. Early evidence from the Tecumseh community health study, based on only a 4-year period of follow-up, indicates that death from coronary artery disease is markedly higher among those with initial hyperglycemia.[45]

The association between glucose tolerance and plasma insulin referred to above may have much relevance to an understanding of the relation between hyperglycemia and coronary artery disease. Raised levels of blood sugar are common among middle-aged and older people and the total amount of insulin output in response to a glucose load increases with age.[46] It has been suggested that this state of hyperinsulinemia is a cause of atherosclerosis and may thus be an important determinant of coronary disease.[41,47]

PSYCHOLOGIC FACTORS AND CORONARY HEART DISEASE

Psychologic factors associated with coronary artery disease have been studied in different contexts of theory as to the kind of relation that exists between them and the disease. There are situations, variously defined as stressful experiences or crisis situations, in which people with coronary artery disease may respond with an acute episode of angina pectoris or myocardial infarction. Pioneers in the field warned against equating the particular circumstances or situation with the emotional and behavioral response of the individual. Epidemiologically, both elements are important, i.e., the crisis situation and the response of individuals in such situations. Personality characteristics may be associated with the kind of response as well as being an immediate cause of the crisis situation itself.

A question which has been asked, to which epidemiology might usefully contribute some answers, is the following: Are there personality characteristics, as reflected in specific personality traits or "total" behavior types, which may be associated with one or more of the following aspects of coronary artery disease?—(1) The development of the foundation pathologic process of coronary artery disease. (2) The occurrence of acute attacks of angina pectoris or episodes of myocardial infarction. (3) Degree of disability following such episodes, or the prognosis for life.

The main studies performed to date have been in communities in which coronary artery disease is common, and hence the answers, if any, will be directed mainly to (2) and (3).

The most persistent investigations into relations between personality and coronary heart disease are those of Friedman and Rosenman.[48] The personality which they consider to be associated with coronary heart disease has been designated by them as "Behavior Pattern Type A." Men of this type are

> "characterized particularly by excessive drive, aggressiveness, and ambition, frequently in association with a relatively greater preoccupation with competitive activity, vocational deadlines, and similar pressures. An enhanced sense of time urgency . . . "

Persons in whom these characteristics were relatively absent are labelled "Behavior Pattern Type B." This person

> . . . is relaxed and more easy going, seldom becomes impatient and takes more time to enjoy a vocational pursuit. He is not easily irritated and works steadily, but without a feeling of being driven by a lack of time. He is not preoccupied with social achievement, and is less competitive in his occupational and vocational interests. He moves and speaks in a slower and more smoothly modulated style.[49]

There is not a sharp dichotomy between these two types of personality. They consider that the "A type" merely exhibits to an enhanced degree the characteristics outlined and they grade persons into four categories: at the extremes the fully developed A type is labelled A1, the extreme B type is B4, and those between the extremes are A2 and B3. Various methods have been used for the measurement of these behavior types.[49–52]

Behavior pattern type A, especially the fully developed Type A (A1), has been found to be associated with (1) an increased prevalence[53–55] and incidence[48] of coronary heart disease; (2) an increased level of serum cholesterol, triglyceride, and lipoproteins;[53,55–58] (3) postprandial prolonged hypertriglyceridemia and marked sludging of red blood cells as noted in examination of conjunctival vessels;[58,59] and (4) a faster clotting time.[56]

Reports of a long-term prospective study in which cohorts of men of different behavior types are being followed-up point to a strong association between behavior type and subsequent development of coronery heart disease.[48,50] Men of behavior type A have a considerable excess risk of developing the disease, and this risk is independent of other risk factors such as hypertension and hypercholesterolemia. This raises the possibility that type A behavior may be of more importance in development of coronary heart disease than has been generally accepted, and this may be especially so when the basic pathology, namely coronary atherosclerosis, is present.

There are a number of important difficulties obstructing investigation of consistent associations between personality characteristics and coronary heart disease. For example, very few prospective studies which have included personality appraisals in the initial examination have used different tests. They are thus not readily comparable and yet the evidence is sufficiently suggestive to warrant more extensive and intensive personality studies in epidemiologic investigation of coronary heart disease. Retrospective case studies will not make the contribution needed, especially in investigation of a condition like coronary heart disease. Not only do a high proportion of cases die in the first attack, but those that survive the traumatic experience of an acute episode of myocardial infarction may

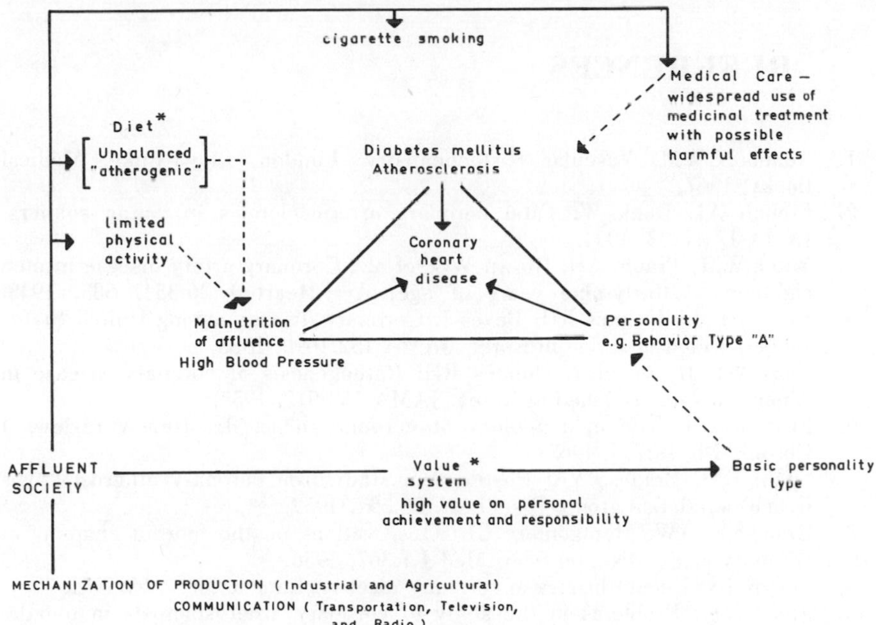

FIG. 21-2. The determinants of a community syndrome, in which coronary artery disease is the central feature in an affluent society. *These two determinants of coronary artery disease are discussed further in Chapters 22 and 23.

well evidence change in their personality profile.[60] Then, too, it has been suggested that personality factors may be associated with the outcome of an attack, those dying differing from those who survive.[60]

As knowledge of various features of the syndrome accumulates, coronary heart disease becomes better understood as a dramatic expression of a group of pathologic processes and disease entities associated with somatic and behavioral characteristics. The syndrome which emerges is now well recognized and has been demonstrated in a number of epidemiologic studies in different communities. Its varied features suggest its multiple causation. The community syndrome, of which coronary artery disease is a central feature, is common in the more affluent societies at the present time. It has been thought to be associated with particular attributes of these societies, such as particular dietary excesses, cigarette smoking, limited physical exercise, and high value-attitudes of society for individual achievement of success, especially by men (Fig. 21-2). The possible impact of value-attitudes and of dietary practices on the occurrence of coronary artery disease are considered in Chapters 22 and 23.

REFERENCES

1. Adams CWM: Vascular Histochemistry. London, Lloyd-Luke, Medical Books, 1967.
2. French AJ, Dock W: Fatal coronary arteriosclerosis in young soldiers. JAMA 124:1233, 1944.
3. Yater WM, Traum AH, Brown WG, et al.: Coronary artery disease in men eighteen to thirty-nine years of age. Am Heart J 36:334, 683, 1948.
4. Enos WF Jr, Holmes RH, Beyer J: Coronary disease among United States soldiers killed in action in Korea. JAMA 152:1090, 1953.
5. Enos WF Jr, Beyer J, Holmes RH: Pathogenesis of coronary disease in American soldiers killed in Korea. JAMA 158:912, 1955.
6. Epstein FH: The epidemiology of coronary heart disease. A review. J Chronic Dis 18:735, 1965.
7. Spain DM, Bradess VA: Postmortem studies on coronary atherosclerosis in one population group. Dis Chest, 36:397, 1959.
8. Branwood AW, Montgomery GL: Observations on the morbid anatomy of coronary artery disease. Scott Med J 1:367, 1956.
9. Morris JN: Recent history of coronary disease. Lancet 260:1, 69:1951.
10. Spain DM: Problems in the study of coronary atherosclerosis in population groups. Ann NY Acad Sci 84:816, 1960.
11. Morris JN, Kagan A, Pattison DC, et al.: Incidence and prediction of ischaemic heart disease in London busmen. Lancet 2:553, 1966.
12. Meade TW: The epidemiology of ischaemic heart disease. Trans Soc Occup Med 18:127, 1968.
13. Chapman JM, Massey FJ: The interrelationship of serum cholesterol, hypertension, body weight, and risk of coronary disease. Results of the first ten years' follow-up in the Los Angeles heart study. J Chronic Dis 17:933, 1964.
14. Kagan A, Kannel WB, Dawber TR, et al.: The coronary profile. Ann NY Acad Sci 97:883, 1963.
15. Stamler J, Berkson DM, Lindberg HA, et al.: Coronary risk factors. Their impact and their therapy in the prevention of coronary heart disease. Med Clin North Am 50:229, 1966.
16. Fejfar Z, Masironi R: Dietary factors and cardiovascular diseases—epidemiological studies in man. Third International Congress of Food, Science and Technology. Chicago, SOS/70, 1970.
17. McDonough JR, Hames CG, Stulb MS et al.: Coronary heart disease among Negroes and Whites in Evans County, Georgia, J Chronic Dis 18:443, 1965.
18. Fodor J, Miall WE, Standard KL, et al.: Myocardial disease in a rural population in Jamaica. Bull WHO 31:321, 1964.
19. Hutt MSR, Coles R: Postmortem findings in hypertensive subjects in Kampala, Uganda. East Afr Med J 46:342, 1969.
20. Kimura T, Ota M: Epidemiologic study of hypertension. Am J Clin Nutr 17:381, 1965.
21. Kannel WB, Gordon T, Schwartz MJ: Systolic versus diastolic blood pressure and risk of coronary heart disease. The Framingham Study. Am J Cardiol 27:335, 1971.

22. Epstein FH, Francis T Jr, Hayner NH, et al.: Prevalence of chronic diseases and distribution of selected physiological variables in a total community: Tecumseh, Michigan. Am J Epidemiol 81:307, 1965.
23. Montoye HJ, Epstein FH, Kjelsberg MO: Relationship between serum cholesterol and body fatness. Am J Clin Nutr 18:397, 1966.
24. Billewicz WZ, Kemsley WF, Thomson AM: Indices of adiposity. Brit J Prev Soc Med 16:183, 1962.
25. Khosla T, Lowe CR: Indices of obesity derived from body weight and height. Brit J Prev Soc Med 21:122, 1967.
26. Grimley Evans J, Prior IAM: Indices of obesity derived from height and weight in two Polynesian populations. Brit J Prev Soc Med 23:56, 1969.
27. Boe J, Humerfelt S, Wedervang F: The blood pressure in a population. Acta Med Scand (Suppl) 321:1, 1957.
28. Edwards DAW, Hammond WH, Healey MJR, et al.: Design and accuracy of calipers for measuring subcutaneous tissue thickness. Brit J Nutr 9: 133, 1955.
29. Abrams ME, Jarrett RJ, Keen H, et al.: Oral glucose tolerance and related factors in a normal population sample. II. Interrelationships of glycerides, cholesterol, and other factors with the glucose and insulin response. Brit Med J 1:599, 1969.
30. Boyns DR, Crossley JN, Abrams ME, et al.: Oral glucose tolerance and related factors in a normal population sample. I. Blood sugar, plasma insulin, glyceride, and cholesterol measurements and the effects of age and sex. Brit Med J 1:595, 1969.
31. Albrink MJ, Man EB: Serum triglycerides in coronary artery disease. Arch Intern Med 103:4, 1959.
32. Albrink MJ, Man EB: Serum triglycerides in health and diabetes. Diabetes 7:194, 1958.
33. Albrink MJ, Meigs JW, Granoff MA: Weight gain and serum triglycerides in normal men. New Engl J Med 266:484, 1962.
34. Albrink MJ, Meigs JW: Interrelationship between skinfold thickness, serum lipids, and blood sugar in normal men. Am J Clin Nutr 15:255 1964.
35. Albrink MJ: Tryglycerides, lipoproteins, and coronary artery disease. Arch Intern Med 109:345, 1962.
36. Brown DF, Kinch SH, Doyle JT: Serum triglycerides in health and in ischemic heart disease. New Engl J Med 273:947, 1965.
37. Clawson BJ, Bell ET: Incidence of fatal coronary heart disease in non-diabetic and in diabetic persons. Arch Pathol 48:105, 1949.
38. Czerkawski JW: Diabetes and vascular degeneration. In Hall DA (ed.): International Review of Connective Tissue Research, Vol. 1. New York, Academic Press, 1963.
39. Pell S, D'Alonzo CA: Acute myocardial infarction in a large industrial population. Report of six-year study of 1356 cases. JAMA 185:831, 1963.
40. Wahlberg F: Intravenous glucose tolerance in myocardial infarction, angina pectoris and intermittent claudication. Acta Med Scand (Suppl 453) 180:1, 1966.
41. Epstein FH: Hyperglycemia. A risk factor in coronary artery disease. Circulation 36:609, 1967.
42. Epstein FH, Ostrander LD Jr, Johnson BC, et al.: Epidemiological studies of cardiovascular disease in a total community: Tecumseh, Michigan. Ann Intern Med 62:1170, 1965.

43. Ostrander LD Jr, Francis T Jr, Hayner NS, et al.: The relationship of cardiovascular disease to hyperglycemia. Ann Intern Med 62:1188, 1965.
44. Keen H, Rose G, Pyke DA, et al.: Blood sugar and arterial disease. Lancet 2:505, 1965.
45. Epstein FH: Some uses of prospective observations in the Tecumseh Community Health Study. Proc R Soc Med 60:56, 1967.
46. Chlouverakis C, Jarrett RJ, Keen H: Glucose tolerance, age, and circulating insulin. Lancet 1:806, 1967.
47. Reaven GM, Olefsky J, Farquhar JW: Does hyperglycaemia or hyperinsulinaemia characterise the patient with chemical diabetes? Lancet 1: 1247, 1972.
48. Rosenman RH, Friedman M, Straus R, et al.: Coronary heart disease in the Western collaborative group study. JAMA 195:86, 1966.
49. Jenkins CD, Rosenman RH, Friedman M: Development of an objective psychological test for the determination of the coronary-prone behavior pattern in employed men. J Chronic Dis 20:371, 1967, p 371.
50. Caffrey B: Reliability and validity of personality and behavioral measures in a study of coronary heart disease. J Chronic Dis 21:191, 1968.
51. Bortner RW, Rosenman RH: The measurement of pattern A behavior. J Chronic Dis 20:525, 1967.
52. Bortner RW, A short rating scale as a potential measure of pattern A behavior. J Chronic Dis 22:87, 1969.
53. Friedman M, Rosenman RH: Association of specific overt behavior pattern with blood and cardiovascular findings. JAMA 169:1286, 1959.
54. Friedman M, Rosenman RH: Overt behavior pattern in coronary disease. Detection of overt behavior pattern A in patients with coronary disease by a new psychophysiological procedure. JAMA 173:1320, 1960.
55. Rosenman RH, Friedman M: Association of specific behavior pattern in women with blood and cardiovascular findings. Circulation 24:1173, 1961.
56. Friedman M, Rosenman RH, Carroll V: Changes in the serum cholesterol and blood clotting time in men subjected to cyclic variation of occupational stress. Circulation 17:852, 1958.
57. Rosenman RH, Friedman M: Behavior patterns, blood lipids, and coronary heart disease. JAMA 184:934, 1963.
58. Friedman M, Rosenman RH, Byers S: Serum lipids and conjunctival circulation after fat ingestion in men exhibiting type-A behavior pattern. Circulation 29:874, 1964.
59. Friedman M, Byers SO, Rosenman RH: Effect of unsaturated fats upon lipemia and conjunctival circulation. JAMA 193:882, 1965.
60. Lebovits BZ, Shekelle RB, Ostfeld AM, et al.: Prospective and retrospective psychological studies of coronary heart disease. Psychosom Med 29: 265, 1967.

22

Culture, Personality, and Coronary Heart Disease—An Hypothesis

It is important to consider the potential implications of the relation between culture and personality for the epidemiology of a common disease, such as coronary heart disease. An individual's life experience determines his phenotypic adult personality in the continuing interaction with his genotype. In this way, the shared life experience of a group will tend to produce personality characteristics which are shared by many members of the group, and which will be expressed in behavior in accord with group expectations and hence satisfying to the individual. This concept has been referred to by different workers as national character,[1] basic personality,[2] and group regularities in personality.[3] The following quotation from Linton is a clear presentation of the postulates involved in the concept of basic personality type.

1. That the individual's early experiences exert a lasting effect upon his personality, especially upon the development of his projective systems.
2. That similar experiences will tend to produce similar personality configurations in the individuals who are subjected to them.
3. That the techniques which the members of any society employ in the care and rearing of children are culturally patterned and will tend to be similar, although never identical, for various families within the society.
4. That the culturally patterned techniques for the care and rearing of children differ from one society to another.

If these postulates are correct, and they seem to be supported by a wealth of evidence, it follows:

1. That the members of any given society will have many elements of early experience in common.

2. That as a result of this they will have many elements of personality in common.
3. That since the early experience of individuals differs from one society to another, the personality norms for various societies will also differ.

The *basic personality type* for any society is that personality configuration which is shared by the bulk of the society's members as a result of the early experiences which they have in common. It does not correspond to the total personality of the individual but rather to the projective systems or, in different phraseology, the value-attitude systems which are basic to the individual's personality configuration. Thus the same basic personality type may be reflected in many different forms of behavior and may enter into many different total personality configurations.[4]

This concept of a determinant relationship between culture and some basic attributes of personality and behavior is of relevance to our present considerations of the causal role of cultural value-orientation in health An illustration of this is the following hypothetical discussion of the possible ways in which trends in the incidence of clinical episodes or deaths from myocardial infarction may be influenced by value-systems.

Among various countries in which coronary heart disease is common, high rates of death from this cause have been reported in the United States. It is probable that this has been associated with a relatively high standard of living expressed in changes in diet and hence in nutrition and metabolism, and in decreasing physical activity. However, the changes in standards of living characteristic of the United States were associated with, and possibly caused by, the values which were dominant among its people. Looking at this from the outside, it would seem that at the present the United States is undergoing radical social change, in which the dominant middle-class values are being rejected by large segments of the population. Not only is there revolt by those who were formerly excluded, especially the black Americans, but also by the new generation of young adults, more especially the young adults from middle-class families at colleges and universities. The present discussion is focused on the dominant value-system before this very recent explosive situation, over a period of time when the values were effective influences in the life experiences of the present generations of middle-aged to older persons.

A summary of some of the main behavior and personality characteristics which have been found to be associated with coronary artery disease in the United States has been presented in Chapters 5 and 21. The following discussion should be read together with that summary of psychologic factors and coronary heart disease.

A theoretical formulation of the possible causal role of the value-system of a community with respect to coronary heart disease might be outlined to include the following:

1. Men with the characteristics outlined, or particular combinations of

them, are likely to have a higher attack rate of myocardial infarction. Behavior which rated high in the value-system was "doing." This meant being active and striving.

2. Other things being equal, such as nutritional status, communities in which these personality-behavior characteristics are common are likely to have a relatively high attack rate of myocardial infarction.
3. The value-system of a community is likely to determine the frequency of this basic personality-behavior configuration as well as the intensity of its expression.

Writing in 1942, Parsons stated: "In a certain sense the most fundamental basis of the family's status is the occupational status of the husband and father. . . . This is a status occupied by an individual by virtue of his individual qualities and achievements."[5]

The emphasis on individual responsibility for achievement, together with the high value placed on striving and overcoming of obstacles, is not characteristic of all groups. Thus in the United States itself there are marked sex differences as well as ethnic group and social class variant value-orientations. Florence Kluckhohn[6] drew attention to the slow cultural assimilation of Spanish-Americans and Mexicans in the United States and their distinctive system of orientations. In contrast to the Anglo-American stress on individualism, the Spanish-American's emphasis is on group goals; the Anglo-Americans "set out to conquer, overcome, and exploit nature, they [the Spanish-Americans] accept the environment with a philosophical calm bordering on the fatalistic." The one's emphasis on doing and accomplishing is not usual behavior in the other. "That which is" is in large part taken for granted and considered as something to be enjoyed, rather than altered.

Such marked differences in cultural values, reflected in behavioral differences, may influence the biologic processes involved in coronary heart disease. Friedman suggests this in his discussion of the incidence of behavior pattern A which he and his associates have described and investigated in its relation to coronary heart disease. "The exact or even the approximate incidence of behavior pattern A is not known. Since the genesis of the pattern itself is so strongly dependent ipon the *interaction* of the personality with its environment, the nature of the latter probably plays a large part in determining the incidence of the pattern."[7]

In a system which places high value on achievement through personal endeavor, it might be expected that certain groups of individuals would be especially exposed to strain and stressful experiences. For example, there are those striving to improve their occupational status. Those who succeed will not only have had the strain of working toward their objective but the strain of the increased responsibility that accompanies their success. Those who fail will suffer frustration. Thus, a society in which upward social mobility through individual achievement is valued makes certain types of behavior more valued than others and taxes the individual, especially the man, to strive, compete, achieve, and overcome. There are also those who because of their family background and education should more readily be able to maintain high social status and yet fail to rise in the expected way.

The difficulty of testing hypotheses which relate these factors to the occurrence of acute myocardial infarction is well illustrated in the studies of Hinkle and his associates.[8–11] Their reports on a nationwide industrial organization in the United States, employing some 270,000 men, indicate a high rate of coronary heart disease consistent with the findings of other investigations in that country. Thus in examining the 30 years' experience of a sample of 1,160 men, almost 40 percent (65 of 166) of those who died before the age of 60 years had been certified as having died from coronary occlusion or myocardial infarction.

There were very marked differences between men who had begun working in the industry after they had completed their college education compared with those who had not. The death rate from coronary heart disease among the "college" men was 36.8 per 1,000 as compared with 62.5 per 1,000 for the "noncollege" men. This difference was not found for other major causes of death. This difference between "college" and "noncollege" men was, with occasional exceptions, a consistent finding throughout the industry. It was found for death rates from coronary heart disease, and for first and total events of various episodes of illness categorized as definite or probable coronary heart disease. The findings were consistent for various ages, different parts of the country, and men involved in different types of occupation. As the authors stress, these findings should not be generalized to other situations, in which quite different associations between education and coronary heart disease could readily be found. The vast majority of college men above 40 years of age had reached occupational levels of supervisors and managers, and relative to "college" men a much lower proportion of "noncollege" men attained these higher levels. This finding is associated with the fact that the rate of coronary artery disease was lower among higher occupational levels than it was among workmen and foremen. At all levels above foremen, "college" men had a lower rate of first events than did "noncollege" men. The high proportion of "college" men to "noncollege" men at the executive level (3.5:1) favorably influenced the rates as did their proportion among general area managers (2.3:1).

Upward mobility of the "noncollege" men was not found to be associated with an increased rate of coronary heart disease events. On the other hand, among "college" men at lower levels of occupation (workmen and foremen) there was a higher rate than among those who were supervisors or above. This high rate was comparable with that of "noncollege" men. Of the approximately 5,000 "college" men who were in the workmen or foremen category only 965 were in the age range 40 to 55, and these had a high coronary heart disease attack rate. This was thought to be caused by a larger number of men who were in a "high-risk" category because of chronic illness.

The difference between "college" and "noncollege" men might be considered in relation to the hypothesis outlined above. It is tempting to relate it to the greater striving of the one group compared with the other to reach higher levels but it must be noted that there was little difference in rates between noncollege men at various occupational levels. Mobility in itself was not shown to be associated with the rates of coronary heart disease attacks. Hinkle and his associates suggest that men who had a college education in the 1920s and 1930s in the United States, compared with those who did not, differ in important social and economic respects which go back to earlier life experience than the history of their employment status. Thus, they record that the "college" men were taller and slimmer, and fewer were cigarette smokers. In one sample studied they found that by age 55 years there were twice as many cigarette smokers among "noncollege" men as among "college" men. The association of differences in physique, in smoking habits, and personality characteristics of the kind discussed in Chapter 21 would be a further stage in investigation.

In a discussion of social stress and coronary heart disease, Matsumoto[12] contrasts the value-orientations and life situations of industrialized Japan and the United States. Noting the considerable difference between these two countries with respect to death rates from coronary artery disease, which is probably associated with the marked differences in their dietary habits and nutrition, he presents an hypothesis which adds another dimension to causal factors of coronary heart disease. In Japanese industry the individual functions within a different social system from that of his counterpart in the United States. It is a system in which the dominant value-orientations are toward the collectivity rather than the individual. Emphasis is on the group and in-group solidarity, the group being the work-group which has continuity over many years. At work and at leisure men tend to associate with their work friends, rather than with their wives and families. Matsumoto believes that despite the change in Japan from an agrarian to an urban-industrial society, collectivity orientations have been strongly maintained and he cites much evidence to this effect. Characteristics of work-groups in industry are their continuity in one company, high employment security, and very limited mobility from one job to another. There is stress on group welfare and group consensus. This is supported by an employment system in which seniority as much as competence determines promotion in occupational grade, and in which a number of facilities are provided by the company for the workers. Thus, while the nature of the group has changed from that of the agrarian kinship network to that of the work-group, feelings of dependence on the group are socially approved with less emphasis on individualism as the primary goal.

The hypothesis of a relation between social stress and coronary heart disease needs further discussion. The questions raised by this hypothesis go beyond the solution of reduced social stress through group dependence and security as factors in lower frequency of coronary heart disease. As we have noted, there is evidence from the United States that in communities in which coronary atherosclerosis is common, men with certain behavior and personality characteristics have higher-than-expected rates of acute episodes of myocardial infarction. The description of the features of Japanese industrial society raises several possibilities. For example, there is the possibility of personality being a product of the culture and social system. Do cultural value-orientations determine the prevalence of the behavior-personality types which have been found to be associated with myocardial infarction? This suggestion has been made and warrants investigation[7,13] Are the various characteristics which have been described differentially distributed in different communities and culture groups and are these differences reflected in different rates of myocardial infarction? An affirmative answer to these hypothetical questions would provide an important link in the causal chain of myocardial infarction. Another question related to, but different from the first, is that concerning the possible influence of the social system on the way in which particular personality characteristics influence health. If we were to assume that "Behavior Type A" individuals are found in groups such as those described by Matsumoto, does the group functioning and collective orientation modify the outcome in terms of myocardial infarction? These epidemiologic questions are indeed difficult to test, but in them lies a basic problem in understanding health, namely the relation between culture, personality, and health. There is obvious need for epidemiology to develop as a biosocial science in which health problems are answered by methods developed in the social sciences as well as in the biologic sciences.

REFERENCES

1. Gorer G: The concept of national character. Sci News 18:105, 1950.
2. Kardiner A, Linton R, Du Bois C, et al.: The Psychological Frontiers of Society. New York, Columbia Univ Press, 1945.
3. Inkeles A: Some sociological observations on culture and personality studies. In Kluckhohn C, Murray HA (eds.): Personality in Nature, Society and Culture, 2nd ed. New York, Knopf, 1953.
4. Linton R: Foreword. In Kardiner A, Linton R, Du Bois C, et al.: The Psychological Frontiers of Society. New York, Columbia Univ Press, 1945, p vi.
5. Parsons T: Age and sex in the social structure of the United States. Am

Sociol Rev 7:604, 1942. Reprinted in Kluckhohn C, Murray HA (eds.): Personality in Nature, Society and Culture, 2nd ed. New York, Knopf, 1953, p 368.

6. Kluckhohn FR: Dominant and variant value orientations. In Kluckhohn C, Murray HA (eds.): Personality in Nature, Society and Culture, 2nd ed. New York, Knopf, 1953, p 351.
7. Friedman M: Pathogenesis of Coronary Artery Disease. New York, McGraw-Hill, 1969, p 85.
8. Hinkle LE Jr: The use of a large industrial population to study the effects of social and behavioral factors on coronary heart disease. Am J Public Health 56:1470, 1966.
9. Hinkle LE Jr, Benjamin B, Christenson WN, et al.: Coronary heart disease. The 30-year experience of 1,160 men. Arch Environ Health 13:312, 1966.
10. Lehman EW, Schulman J, Hinkle LE Jr: Coronary deaths and organizational mobility: The 30-year experience of 1,160 men. Arch Environ Health 15:455, 1967.
11. Hinkle LE, Whitney LH, Lehman EW, et al.: Occupation, Education and Coronary Heart Disease Among Men in the Bell System. Mimeograph.
12. Matsumoto YS: Social stress and coronary heart disease in Japan. A hypothesis. Milbank Mem Fund Q 48:9, 1970.
13. Stewart IMG: Coronary disease and modern stress. Lancet 2:867, 1950.

23

Diet and Nutrition in the Epidemiology of Coronary Heart Disease

Comparison between people of economically better-developed countries of the world with those of less well-developed countries points to wide differences in rates of atherosclerosis and coronary heart disease. These differences are probably associated with diet as well as with other aspects of daily living. Among the noticeable differences in the food consumption of these communities are not only the total calories but their composition. Thus, in the better-off communities, total proteins and fats (especially those from animal sources) and refined sugar are main constituents of the diet. In contrast to this, cereals of various kinds (i.e., complex carbohydrates), or potatoes, yams, and even plantains form the subsistence diet of poorer communities. These differences are not only found between peoples of different countries, but in different communities or ethnic groups of the same country.

Which, if any, of these various dietary differences is relevant to our problem of explaining the differences in morbidity and mortality rates from coronary heart disease?

THE EVIDENCE FROM GEOGRAPHIC AND COMPARATIVE COMMUNITY STUDIES

The pioneer studies relating diet and coronary heart disease were of the following kind. Ancel Keys postulated a causal relationship between diet and atherosclerosis,[1] which he and his associates followed through in comparative studies in Italy[2] and South Africa,[3] with Japanese in Japan, Hawaii, and Los Angeles,[4] and in Finland.[5] This led to the inference of a causal relationship between diet, serum cholesterol level, and the incidence of coronary heart disease. Coronary artery disease was rare and the serum cholesterol level low in those communities in which there was little animal fat and cholesterol in the diet. It has been noted by many observers that there were probably other important differences between these communities and others in which coronary artery disease was common.

In a comparative geographic study of arteriosclerotic and degenerative heart disease (AHD) and dietary factors, Masironi[6] found high positive correlations between death rates from AHD and total caloric intake, and percentage calories from fats (especially saturated fats) and sucrose. He also found a high negative correlation between AHD death rates and consumption of complex carbohydrate foods. His analysis also demonstrated a high correlation between a number of these dietary constituents themselves.

While there have been reports of communities having a high-fat diet without a high rate of coronary heart disease or high serum cholesterol levels, there have *not* been reports of groups having a low fat diet, especially saturated fats, with a high serum cholesterol and a high coronary heart disease rate. This last fact suggests that diets with a high fat content, especially saturated fats, and a high cholesterol content, are needed for the development of coronary heart disease.[7]

Coronary Heart Disease in Seven Countries

Of the many comparative community studies which Keys and his associates have undertaken in various countries, one particular study was the most definitive in relating specific elements of diet to coronary heart disease and serum cholesterol levels.[8] Men aged 40 to 59 years were included in the investigation which involved areas in Japan, Yugoslavia, Finland, Italy, Greece, the Netherlands, and the United States. The methods of investigation were standardized and where they differed for any reason this has been reported. With the exception of four groups, those selected for study came from rural villages. In each country several contrasting rural areas were chosen, such as areas from both eastern and western Finland, a fishing village and an agricultural village in Japan, and villages in Corfu and in Crete. The aim was to examine all the men in the age groups required who were residents of the villages selected, and to follow them through for 10 years with subsequent examinations at 5-year intervals.

Individual diet investigations were conducted as part of the study and were repeated during different seasons. The average findings from these dietary studies in each group have been related to the incidence of coronary heart disease in the men during the first 5-year period of the investigation, as well as to the median serum cholesterol levels at the first examination.

There was a high correlation between the proportion of saturated fats in the diet and the 5-year incidence of new cases of coronary heart disease ($r = 0.84$). The coefficient of correlation between saturated fats in the diet and the median serum cholesterol level at first examination was equally high ($r = 0.89$). Other correlations between dietary factors and the disease were: mono-ene fatty acids ($r = -0.42$) and total fats ($r = 0.38$).

The absence of any correlation between dietary calories per kilogram of body weight and the incidence of coronary heart disease cases focuses attention on the importance of the composition of the diet rather than the caloric value in itself. The absence of any correlation between dietary calories as such and the incidence of coronary heart disease cases was also found in its lack of association with serum cholesterol level. A similar observation was made with respect to dietary proteins where their lack of association with incidence of coronary heart disease cases was also expressed in no correlation between dietary proteins and serum cholesterol levels.

DIRECT EVIDENCE FROM STUDIES IN RELATIVELY HOMOGENEOUS POPULATION GROUPS

Direct studies of the relation between diet and serum cholesterol involve comparative investigation between individuals who differ with respect to their diets to a degree that might be expected to be reflected in differences in serum cholesterol levels. Such direct studies are not readily achieved and the results of such investigations might rather reflect the limited difference in the dietary practices. Two studies with different results are presented to stress the importance of not assuming that a relation between diet and serum cholesterol level is readily demonstrable under varying circumstances.

A Study of Seventh-day Adventists

Seventh-day Adventists living in the same community but differing in their adherence to vegetarian diet practices offer an interesting contrast.[9] Two hundred and thirty-three vegetarian Seventh-day Adventists, living in a Washington, DC suburban area, were matched in pairs with nonvegetarians of the same church. The matching was conducted according to the following factors: the specific church attended which reflected the place of residence, sex, age within a 5-year age group, marital status, height, weight, and occupation. The nonvegetarians were further classified into four subgroups, according to the frequency with which they consumed meat, fish, or poultry. The vegetarian group was more homogeneous. The vast majority, 221 of the 233, were lacto-ovo-vegetarians, and only 12 were pure vegetarians. At all ages from 25 years to over 70, the vegetarians had consistently lower levels of serum cholesterol, the differences being more marked as the frequency of meat consumption increased in the nonvegetarians.

A Study of London Bank Employees

In contrast to the above findings of a direct association between serum cholesterol level and diet is the lack of association reported by Morris and co-workers in their investigation of bank employees.[10] The bank workers they investigated were aged 30 to 55 years and were managers, cashiers, and clerks in four different banks of London. They found wide differences in the diets of individual workers but despite these differences of dietary intake, no association was found between serum cholesterol levels and the various dietary fat intake indices, namely total fat, animal fat including dairy fat, dairy fat itself, marine and vegetable fat, the percentage of calories from fat, or the ratio of saturated to unsaturated fatty acids. Even at the extremes of food consumption there was no association with serum cholesterol levels.

EXPERIMENTAL EPIDEMIOLOGIC EVIDENCE

The nearest approach to experimental epidemiologic evidence which we have are various primary and secondary preventive trials. It is now some 20 years since the first observations were published on the effect of vegetable oils in lowering serum cholesterols.[11,12] That the level of serum cholesterol could be altered by changes in fat intake was soon confirmed in a number of relatively short-term experiments and it became clear that the following changes reduced serum cholesterol level:[13–16] (1) reduction of saturated fats in the diet reduced the serum cholesterol and their increase in the diet raised the serum cholesterol level; (2) increase of unsaturated fats reduced the serum cholesterol level; and (3) reduction of cholesterol itself in the diet reduced the level of serum cholesterol. Because of the association between ischemic heart disease and raised levels of serum cholesterol, it was expected that there would be long-term investigations of the effects of dietary change on serum cholesterol and coronary heart disease. Both primary and secondary prevention trials have been conducted.

Primary Prevention

Long-term trials aimed at the primary prevention of coronary artery disease and ischemic heart disease have been performed among volunteers and institutionalized men. They include the Anti-coronary Club of New York City, [17–20] the Chicago Coronary Prevention Evaluation Program,[21] the National Diet-heart Feasibility Study of the American Heart Society,[22] a study of ex-servicemen living in a special center for such men in Los Angeles,[23–25] and a study of patients in two mental hospitals not far from Helsinki, Finland.[26]

While differing from one another in many respects, their common features are of special interest. All aimed to encourage a diet which would moderate calorie intake, reduce saturated fats by substituting polyunsaturated fats, and reduce cholesterol. It was shown that it was feasible to achieve this among free-living men as well as among those in institutions. In general the results of these studies were in accordance, with the following effects in "treated" groups compared with the controls.

1. Loss of weight in those groups where it was considered desirable.
2. Sustained reduction in the serum cholesterol levels.
3. Subcutaneous fat composition was modified by increase in linoleic acid (polyunsaturated fatty acid) and reduction in saturated fatty acids.[20,26]
4. Suggestive evidence of a lower incidence of coronary events in two of the studies,[19,20,26] and in another study, lower combined incidence of myocardial infarction, sudden death, and cerebral infarction.[23–25]

This accumulating evidence concerning the importance of diet as a determinant of coronary artery disease is now impressive and for this reason several of these long-term primary prevention trials are reviewed here.

The Anti-coronary Club Study. The Anti-coronary Club of New York City Department of Health was initiated in 1957 by Jolliffe and his associates[17] with the objective of investigating the effects of diet change in preventing coronary heart disease. In doing this, they aimed to test the feasibility of a large group of free-living men continuing to have a "cholesterol-lowering" diet ("the prudent diet") over a long period of time. They established the feasibility of such a diet and its effectiveness in lowering serum cholesterol levels on 200 men over a period of 2 years. Having successfully done this, the group of men was expanded to include 600 active members, and a control group was recruited from men who had reported at three New York health department cancer detection clinics. In this way they hoped to have a control group of men who had, like the experimental group, shown an interest in their health.

This pioneering public health trial pointed the way to the practicability of developing community programs which might be used as research trials.

The men were placed on a "prudent diet,"[18] the features of which were that (1) it consisted of 30 to 33 percent of total calories as fat with a P/S ratio of 1.25 to 1.50 : 1 compared with a P/S ratio of 0.3 to 0.4 : 1 in a typical American diet; and (2) it provided approximately equal quantities of the three types of fats, namely saturated, polyunsaturated, and monounsaturated.

Comparison between the experimental group and the control group after a period of at least 4 years showed marked differences between the two groups.[19,20] The changes in the experimental group, which were not found in the control group, included reduction in the mean serum cholesterol level, with a considerable decline in the number of men who had serum cholesterol levels of 260 mg or more per 100 ml. There was also a marked reduction in the proportion of men with obesity, and of men with a diastolic blood pressure of 95 mm Hg or more. The fatty acid composition of subcutaneous fat showed an increase in linoleic acid with a decline in saturated and monounsaturated fatty acids. There was a lower incidence of new coronary events.

It was noted that of the eight new coronary events in the 814 active experimental subjects, seven occurred during the first 2 years of the individual's participation in the study. This rate is much the same as the expected rate, based on the experience of the control group. Only one of the eight new events occurred among active experimental subjects subsequent to the first 2 years of participation. The authors assumed that this was the result of the diet having had a greater opportunity to exert its effects over the longer period of time.

The Helsinki Study on Dietary Prevention of Coronary Heart Disease. Phase 1 of the Helsinki study[26] extended over the period January 1959 to February 1965. The observed population consisted of male patients, aged 34 to 64 at the beginning of the 6-year period, from two mental hospitals not far from Helsinki. The total number of patients studied in hospital N was 327 and in hospital K, 254. Beginning in January 1959 the diet of hospital N patients was changed, whereas that of K continued as before. The diet of the patients of hospital N compared with that of hospital K was lower in saturated fatty acid, higher in polyunsaturated fatty acid, lower in cholesterol content, and had less sugar, both before and during the trial period. While not part of the planned change this may have relevance for the findings.

At the end of the 6 years the following occurred: (1) The serum cholesterol level of the patients of hospital N was considerably reduced and was lower than that of hospital K. (2) The percent of fatty acids in adipose tissue differed between the two groups. The ratio between the patients of hospital N to those of hospital K was as shown in Table 23-1.

TABLE 23-1

FATTY ACID	RATIO OF AMOUNT OF FATTY ACID BETWEEN PATIENTS OF HOSPITALS N AND K
Lauric	0.49:1
Myristic	0.40:1
Palmitic	0.74:1
Oleic	0.89:1
Linoleic	2.62:1
Linolenic	2.51:1

(3) Combining two sets of data, there was a significant difference in the occurrence of coronary heart disease in the subjects of the two hospitals. The two sets of data combined were electrocardiographic evidence of probable coronary heart disease (classes I and II, Epstein et al.[27]) and deaths considered to be the result of coronary heart disease.

At the end of phase 1, the dietary program was switched over, the patients of hospital K becoming the trial group and those of hospital N, the control.

The Los Angeles ex-Servicemen Study. The Los Angeles ex-servicemen study[23–25] involved 846 volunteer ex-servicemen living in a center in Los Angeles (Veterans Administration Center). The group receiving the experimental diet consisted in 424 men selected at random, with a control group of 422. The feature of the experimental diet was the restriction of saturated fat with the substitution of vegetable oils. The result of the change in diet was that the cholesterol intake was decreased by half (365 mg per day compared with 653 mg per day in the control group), and the polyunsaturated fatty acids were more than tripled at the expense of saturated fatty acids (38 percent of the total fatty acid of the experimental group was in the form of linoleic acid compared with 10 percent in the control group). The maximum period of observation extended over 100 months but the total duration of study for each individual depended on his time of entry into the study. The combined incidence of myocardial infarction, sudden death, and cerebral infarction was significantly lower in the experimental group than in the control group. This difference was accompanied by a lowering of the serum cholesterol levels. The difficulties of establishing such a study and maintaining it over a long period of time have been discussed by Dayton and his associates as well as by others.[24,25]

The Chicago Coronary Prevention Evaluation Program. Stamler and his colleagues[21] initiated a long-term experimental study in men who were selected from volunteers, mainly from several industrial organizations in Chicago. The men, aged 40 to 59 years, were selected on the basis of high-risk for coronary artery disease in the absence of organic heart disease, clinical atherosclerotic disease in other major arterial beds, or diagnosed diabetes mellitus requiring drug treatment. The high-risk criteria included the following statistical elements:

Serum cholesterol level of 325 mg per 100 ml or higher as a single risk factor, or any two of the following risk factors:
Serum cholesterol 260 mg per 100 ml or higher
Weight 15 percent or more above desirable weight
Diastolic blood pressure 95 mm Hg or higher
Electrocardiogram: the presence of fixed minor nonspecific T-wave abnormalities (i.e., low-voltage, diphasic, or flat T-waves)
Cigarette smoking 10 or more per day

Matched groups with similar criteria for inclusion as were used for the experimental group were identified from seven large ongoing prospective epidemiologic studies in the United States.

In the first instance the objectives were to gain experience in management of known major coronary risk factors and to test the ability to maintain large numbers of free-living men in such a study for long periods of time. The second objective was to accumulate a sufficient number of men and follow them over a number of years in order to evaluate the program by measurement of end-points, such as mortality from coronary heart disease and from all causes. By 1966, 335 high-risk men had been enrolled in the study which began in 1957. The program aimed to change diet, smoking, and physical activity in order to modify the risk factors.

The major dietary change they wanted to induce was a moderation of the caloric intake, emphasizing certain features and deemphasizing others.

1. Dietary effects: They had considerable success in changing the men's diets in the desired direction, i.e., lowering caloric intake and total fats, especially saturated fats and cholesterol.
2. Smoking: Thirty percent of the smokers abandoned the habit either by stopping smoking or by switching to pipe or cigar smoking.
3. Health effects: There was a drop in the serum cholesterol level. In the men who had an associated hypertriglyceridemia, the serum triglyceride levels tended to decline along with the decrease in the hypercholesterolemia.
4. There was a moderate loss in weight.
5. Anti-hypertensive drugs were recommended if the men with hypertension did not show a reduction in blood pressure as a result of weight reduction or a moderate restriction of dietary salt. As a result, the majority of men with high blood pressure were controlled.
6. Mortality from coronary heart disease: The cumulative death rate of the 262 men remaining active in the program up to 1966 was as follows. Two died of coronary heart disease, a rate of 1.4 percent in the span of 6 years. Of the 73 men who dropped out, five died over the same period of time, a rate of 9.7 percent in the 6 years. It was noted by Stam-

ler and his colleagues that the dropouts were more heavily weighted with very high-risk men.

The Feasibility of a National Diet–Heart Study. Because of the considerable evidence of the effects of diet as an important causal factor of atherosclerosis, the American Heart Society conducted a research study to determine the feasibility of testing whether change in the fat content and cholesterol of the diet would reduce incidence of first attacks of clinical coronary heart disease in middle-aged American men.[22] The report indicated that the study was possible and in addition gave evidence of changes in the serum cholesterol levels in the expected direction. They also reported lowering of the serum triglycerides, especially in men whose initial levels were high. Of interest too, were the changes reported in other risk factors for coronary heart disease. Thus, the prevalence of smoking decreased markedly and the report discusses the importance of such changes as confounding variables in a study which was concerned with dietary change only. Motivation for participation by free-living persons in such a program suggests that they are likely to alter their behavior in ways over and above those planned for in a study.

Secondary Prevention

Trials to control reinfarction rates or death after a first myocardial infarction are no less difficult than primary prevention trials. In fact, the added risk of having had a recent myocardial infarction might itself nullify the effectiveness, for example, of lowering the fat content of a diet or of lowering the cholesterol. While such modification could be expected to lower the serum cholesterol level, whether this in itself is sufficient to counter the effects of a previous or recent infarction is much in doubt. The epidemiology of the outcome of myocardial infarction (MI) can be expected to be somewhat different from the epidemiology of the primary infarct and of the risk factors leading to the primary infarct. A number of studies have been conducted and two of these will be reviewed here. One was in Oslo, Norway, and the other in London, England.

The Oslo Study. The specific objective of this secondary prevention trial in Oslo[28,29] was to lower the blood cholesterol by diet in patients surviving a myocardial infarction and to judge the effects of this by the incidence of myocardial reinfarction, new cases of angina pectoris, and sudden unexpected death. The diet was one which was made rich in highly unsaturated fats by the use of soya oil; it was low in saturated fats and low in cholesterol. The time from the primary infarction to inclusion in the study was not less than 1 year and ranged from 13 to 24 months. The study included 412 men, aged 30 to 64 years, randomized into two equal groups, one on diet treatment and the other acting as a control. Two reports have been issued; one was a comprehensive report after 5 years of the study and the other, issued after 11 years, was concerned with mortality in the two groups.

The first objective of reducing the level of cholesterol was achieved quite early and maintained throughout the 5-year period. The end-point effects were judged by incidences of myocardial reinfarction, new cases of angina pectoris, and sudden unexpected death. Below the age of 60, the incidence of both myocardial reinfarction and new cases of angina pectoris was significantly lower in the diet group. There was no difference between the two groups in the occurrence of sudden death.

After 11 years, i.e., 6 years after the study itself had ended, the original diet group had a significantly reduced MI mortality—32 of the 206 in the diet group had died compared with 57 of the 206 in the control group. In the total number of probable coronary deaths, i.e., deaths from MI and sudden death, the difference was markedly less: 79 in the diet group and 94 in the control group.

The London Study. A research committee of the Medical Research Council conducted a trial[30] similar to that of the Oslo study. It was similar in that soya bean oil was the polyunsaturated fat given in the diet. Using four hospitals in London, the committee randomly selected 199 men under 60 years of age who had recently recovered from a first myocardial infarction and had been discharged from hospital. These men were given a diet low in saturated fats and including 85 g of soya bean oil daily. One hundred and ninety-four control patients continued with their normal diet. Both groups measured their diet regularly. As in the Oslo study, the test diet lowered the serum cholesterol from a mean initial figure of 272 to 213 mg per 100 ml after 6 months. This is in contrast to the level of controls, which fell from 273 to 259 mg per 100 ml.

This study differed from the Oslo study in the following respects:

1. The mean cholesterol level at the beginning of the trials in London was lower than that of Oslo, as shown in Table 23-2.
2. The time between the primary infarction and inclusion in the study was very much shorter in the London study, i.e., 12 to 90 days compared with not less than one year to 13 to 24 months in the Oslo study.
3. The trend of results was similar but none of the differences in relapse rates between the trial and control men were found to be significant. This may be due to differences in the initial cholesterol levels of the two populations and, even more likely, to the difference in time period that elapsed before patients were included in the studies.

TABLE 23-2

	LONDON	OSLO
Test diet	272	296
Control	273	296

SUCROSE, SERUM LIPIDS, AND CORONARY HEART DISEASE

High sugar intake as the chief dietary cause of ischemic heart disease was presented as an hypothesis by Yudkin in 1957.[31] This hypothesis was based on his analysis of the association between coronary heart disease incidence and sugar consumption in various countries. Yudkin and Roddy[32] followed this through in a limited investigation of men, aged 45 to 66, who comprised the following three groups. (1) Men who recently had myocardial infarcts and were interviewed within three weeks of the attack (20 patients). (2) Men attending a clinic with peripheral vascular disease (25 patients). (3) Men with orthopedic disorders or no health problems (25 patients). They assessed the sugar intake by using a questionnaire, paying particular attention to the use of sucrose in various forms, especially in tea and coffee. They found that the amount of sucrose in a typical day's diet of the two groups of men with atherosclerotic disease was about twice that of the control group.[32] Studies by others have not confirmed these findings.[33–35] Not only were there smaller differences in sucrose consumption between myocardial infarct cases and controls, but where found they were associated with other factors such as cigarette smoking. Paul and his associates[33] demonstrated the problem of a too-ready delineation of an association between two variables as a causal one. They reviewed the original diet records gathered in their study of men aged 40 to 55 years who worked for the Western Electric Company in Chicago. Men who subsequently developed myocardial infarctions had a higher mean intake of sucrose over a 28-day period than did a control group of men, who were followed-up for at least 7 years and selected at random from the men who had remained noncoronary cases.

Further analysis showed a positive association between high sucrose intake and high use of both cigarettes and coffee. When these factors were combined in the analysis, cigarette smoking showed a major independent association with subsequent coronary disease, and both sucrose intake and coffee drinking showed lesser independent association.

There is evidence that modifying dietary intake of sugar has effects on serum lipids. Differentiation of carbohydrate-induced lipemia and fat-induced lipemia was an important landmark in these early experimental approaches to study of the effects of diet on serum lipids.[36] Variation in the amount and ration of sugar (sucrose) and more complex carbohydrates in the diet has been demonstrated to have effects on serum triglyceride levels; in particular, a higher ratio of sugar has been associated with a higher level of serum triglyceride.[37,38] Reducing dietary sucrose is followed by a decrease in serum triglyceride levels as well as a loss in weight, which may itself be a factor in reduction of the serum triglyceride level. In these studies there was little change in the serum cholesterol level.[39-40] In several of these experiments[38,40] the fasting serum triglyceride level fell more in those who had higher initial levels.

While these studies may pioneer the way to greater understanding of the causes of different lipidemias, their relevance to the epidemiology of serum triglyceride levels in relation to coronary heart disease remains to be explored.

REFERENCES

1. Keys A: Human atherosclerosis and the diet. Circulation 5:115, 1952.
2. Keys A, Fidanza F, Scardi V, et al.: Studies on serum cholesterol and other characteristics of clinically healthy men in Naples. Arch Intern Med 93:328, 1954.
3. Bronte-Stewart B, Keys A, Brock JF: Serum-cholesterol, diet, and coronary heart disease. Lancet 2:1103, 1955.
4. Keys A, Kimura N, Kusukawa A, et al.: Lessons from serum cholesterol studies in Japan, Hawaii, and Los Angeles. Ann Intern Med 48:83, 1958.
5. Keys A, Karvonen MJ, Fidanza F: Serum cholesterol studies in Finland. Lancet 2:175, 1958.
6. Masironi R: Dietary factors and coronary heart disease. Bull WHO 42: 103, 1970.
7. Stamler J: Lectures on Preventive Cardiology. New York, Grune & Stratton, 1967.
8. Keys A (ed.): Coronary Heart Disease in Seven Countries, Monograph No. 29. New York, American Heart Association, 1970.
9. West RO, Hayes OB: Diet and serum cholesterol levels. A comparison between vegetarians and nonvegetarians in a Seventh-day Adventist group. Am J Clin Nutr 21:853, 1968.
10. Morris JN, Marr JW, Heady JA, et al.: Diet and plasma cholesterol in 99 bank men. Brit Med J 1:571, 1963.
11. Groen J, Tijong BK, Kanminga CE, et al.: The influence of nutrition, individuality, and some other factors, including various forms of stress, on the serum cholesterol. Voeding 13:556, 1952.
12. Kinsell LW, Partridge J, Boling L, et al.: Dietary modification of serum cholesterol and phospholipid levels. J Clin Endocrinol Metab 12:909, 1952.
13. Bronte-Stewart B, Antonis A, Eales A, et al.: Effect of feeding different fats on serum cholesterol level. Lancet 1:521, 1956.
14. Keys A, Anderson JT, Grande F: "Essential" fatty acids, degree of unsaturation, and effect of corn (maize) oil on serum-cholesterol level in men. Lancet 1:66, 1957.
15. Ahrens EH Jr, Hirsch J, Insull W, et al.: The influence of dietary fats on serum lipid levels in man. Lancet 1:943, 1957.
16. Gordon H, Brock JF: Studies on the regulation of the serum-cholesterol level in man. S Afr Med J 32:397, 1958.
17. Jolliffe N, Rinzler SH, Archer M: The anti-coronary club: including a discussion of the effects of a prudent diet on the serum cholesterol levels of middle-aged men. Am J Clin Nutr 7:451, 1959.

18. Christakis G, Rinzler SH, Archer M, et al.: Effect of the anti-coronary club program on coronary heart disease risk-factor status. JAMA 198:597, 1966.
19. Christakis G, Rinzler SH, Archer M, et al.: Summary of the research activities of the anti-coronary club. Public Health Rep 81:64, 1966.
20. Christakis G, Rinzler SH, Archer M, et al.: Effect of a serum cholesterol-lowering diet on composition of depot fat in man. Amer J Clin Nutr 16: 243, 1965.
21. Stamler J, Berkson DM, Levinson MJ, et al.: A long-term coronary prevention evaluation program. Ann NY Acad Sci 149:1022, 1968.
22. National Diet Heart Study Research Group. The National Diet-Heart Study Final Report, Monograph No. 18. New York, American Heart Association, 1968.
23. Dayton S, Pearce ML, Goldman H, et al.: Controlled trial of a diet high in unsaturated fat for prevention of atherosclerotic complications. Lancet 2:1060, 1968.
24. Dayton S, Pearce ML: Prevention of coronary heart disease and other complications of atherosclerosis by modified diet. Am J Med 46:751, 1969.
25. Editorial. Lancet 2:939, 1969.
26. Turpeinen O, Miettinen M, Karvonen JL, et al.: Dietary prevention of coronary heart disease. Longterm experiment. Am J Clin Nutr 21:255, 1968.
27. Epstein FH, Ostrander LO, Johnson BL, et al.: Epidemiological studies of cardiovascular disease in a total community—Tecumseh, Michigan. Ann Intern Med 62:1170, 1965.
28. Leren P: The effect of plasma cholesterol lowering diet in male survivors of myocardial infarction. Acta Med Scand (Suppl) 466:1, 1966. Also specially published by Norwegian Monographs on Medical Science. Oslo, Scandinavian Univ Books, 1966.
29. Leren P: The Oslo diet-heart study. Eleven-year report. Circulation 42:935, 1970.
30. Report of a Research Committee to the Medical Research Council: Controlled trial of soya-bean oil in myocardial infarction. Lancet 2:693, 1968.
31. Yudkin J: Diet and coronary disease. Hypothesis and fact. Lancet 2:155, 1957.
32. Yudkin J, Roddy J: Levels of dietary sucrose in patients with occlusive atherosclerotic disease. Lancet 2:6, 1964.
33. Paul O, MacMillan A, McKean H, et al.: Sucrose intake and coronary heart-disease. Lancet 2:1049, 1968.
34. Howell RW, Wilson DG: Dietary sugar and ischaemic heart disease. Brit Med J 3:145, 1969.
35. Report of Working-party to the Medical Research Council: Dietary sugar intake in men with myocardial infarction. Lancet 2:1265, 1970.
36. Ahrens EH Jr, Hirsch J, Oette K, et al.: Carbohydrate-induced lipemia. Trans Am Assoc Phys 74:134, 1961.
37. Antar MA, Ohlson MA: Effect of simple and complex carbohydrates upon total lipids, nonphospholipids, and different fractions of phospholipids of serum in young men and women. J Nutr 85:329, 1965.
38. Kaufman NA, Poznanski R, Blondheim SH, et al.: Changes in serum lipid levels of hyperlipemic patients following the feeding of starch, sucrose, and glucose. Am J Clin Nutr 18:261, 1966.
39. Rifkind BM, Lawson DH, Gale M: Effect of short-term sucrose restriction on serum-lipid levels. Lancet 2:1379, 1966.

40. Mann JI, Truswell AS, Hendricks DA, et al.: Effects on serum lipids in normal men of reducing dietary sucrose or starch for five months. Lancet 1:870, 1970.

SECTION 5

Community Medicine and Primary Health Care

In Chapter 1, brief reference was made to community medicine and personal health care. As used in the present context, community medicine is a practice which focuses on the community as a whole, aiming to change its state of health by intervention at the individual and group level. By developing these objectives it unites certain features of clinical practice with aspects of public health practice. At the present time there is in many countries a near-complete separation of clinical medicine and public health practice and, before considering ways of uniting them in community health care, it is expedient to define their distinctive features.

CLINICAL MEDICINE

Clinical medicine involves the care of a patient—a person who is ill or disabled and who turns to a medical practitioner or an institution for care. In all societies this is the dominant function of practitioners both in their self-perception of their roles as well as in the minds of the public. However, clinicians are also involved in care of well individuals who want protection against illness, such as immunization, health examinations of adults and children, advice on ways of promoting individual health, advice and technical help on family spacing and contraception, and so on. While some specialties of clinical practice focus much of their skill on the well person, as in obstetrics and pediatrics, in general, clinical medicine is essentially patient-oriented, with some limited extension to care of the well individual. It is the individual who is the center of attention with varying degrees of emphasis on the whole person as a patient. The skills of the clinician involve interview and examination of the individual, differential diagnosis, and treatment and continuing observation of the patient, both to evaluate his progress and for purposes of diagnosis. The scope and methods of history-taking, physical examination, and laboratory, roentgenologic, and other special investigations have been systematized in different specialties. The intending practitioner must develop skill through experience in the use of the various techniques that have evolved and in ways of relating with patients that promote the patient's care and his response to the treatment advised. Both with respect to understanding the background of the patient's illness and as a guide to his care, the history and interview often extend to more personal-social attributes. These usually include the family history and home circumstances, personal relationships, life situation and status, and various health-relevant habits. It is the exception rather than the general rule for the physician to have the same skill in this area of clinical practice as he has in physical examination and other special techniques.

Primary medical care, as usually understood, involves the doctor to whom a person first turns when ill or when seeking advice on personal health. Although oriented toward the needs of the individual, it often involves others who are closely associated with the patient, such as the family. This extension to the family has been a feature of European and American medicine, and the terms general practitioner (GP) and family physician are often used synonymously. It is not always realized that the GP-family physician is not the traditional doctor in many societies. Furthermore, primary medical care is undergoing considerable change, a change that is part of social change and also the product of specialization of medicine and the use of other professional health personnel. The community nurse is much involved in primary health care and many approaches to the doctor-nurse team in community practice have been reported. Specialization has raised the potential for health care and at the same time created problems in the provision of primary medical care. The more general specialties—pediatrics, psychiatry, and internal medicine—are well suited to provide primary medical care and such specialists working together in groups are to be found in community health centers and, as in the United States, in private group practice. Even more narrowly defined specialties are involved in primary medical care. This is especially noted in care of patients with long-term illness for whom it is not unusual for a cardiologist, neurologist, or other specialist to be in fact, if not in name, the personal physician.

PUBLIC HEALTH PRACTICE

In contrast to primary medical care, in which the individual patient is the unit of care, focus on the health of population groups such as the community is the feature of public health practice. The public health movement is one of the major elements of social action, aimed at transforming community behavior and the environment in order to promote the health and welfare of the society. Its origins lie deep in the traditions of all societies, but its scientific development is comparatively recent. It is linked with the technologic and industrial revolution, and with advances in scientific knowledge of the environment and of ourselves. Technology has made it possible to increase and improve material resources of food, communications, and housing, and advanced scientific knowledge has led to the application of biologic, psychologic, and social sciences to medicine, social planning, and public health.

Problem-solving is at the root of much social action aimed to improve conditions of living, including the public health. It is a fact that medical practice in the community is not usually oriented toward the community as a whole. The traditional public health team has usually been responsible for this. The medical care needs of individuals were, and often still are, met apart from the main stream of public health practice and even of hospital care.

The main objectives of public health practice are to prevent disease, promote health, and ensure the best possible distribution of health and medical care facilities. It aims to protect the community from preventable diseases; to promote health by actions which will result in, for example, improvements in diet and housing; and to draw attention to the health implications of social and economic planning. Its administrative functions not only include the organization and development of promotive and preventive services, but also making provision for care of the sick and rehabilitation of the disabled. Public health practice places greater emphasis on preventive than on curative care and hence more on modification of the environment and community activities than is customary in clinical medicine. However, its main distinguishing feature is its concern with *community* and it is in this respect that it differs markedly from clinical medicine in its history-taking, methods of examination of a problem, diagnosis, and action. Its history-taking is in reality a study of the community's history in relation to changing health trends. Its examination involves both the direct health examination of groups of individuals as well as the gathering of knowledge about the state of health of the community from various sources. These sources include death records, and the records of clinics, hospitals, and school health services. Analysis of this data provides the basis for diagnosis of the community's state of health (community diagnosis). This includes mortality rates and the rates of various disorders, their differential distribution, such indices of health of the community as the outcome of pregnancy, and differences in physical growth and mental and behavioral development of various groups of children. The unit of measurement in public health practice is the population group. Its etiologic and preventive orientation involves such activities as surveillance and improvement of the environment, of food production and the national or community food balance sheet, of ways of rearing children, and of facilities for health activities of elderly persons. Its treatment is directed toward modification of the environment and other factors relevant to the health of the community or those segments of it at special risk. In evaluation of progress it is concerned both with ensuring that what should be done is being done and that it is having the desired effects on the community. Thus, measurement of the proportion of the population immunized against various infectious diseases or the proportion of mothers and individuals using facilities for health care are important indices of the health services. These must be related to such indicators of a community's health as rates of diseases preventable by immunization, outcome of pregnancy, and infant growth, as well as to morbidity and mortality rates.

24

Meeting Points Between Primary Health Care and Community Medicine

The possibility of bringing together medical practice in the community and health care conducted by public health agencies must be examined with respect to a number of factors. The historical forces that led to their separate development might no longer be operating. The ways health and sickness are regarded, the ways in which services are organized and financed, and the kind of training of the various practitioners are all fundamental to our understanding of the various health services that are found in different communities. The acceptance by society that health is a right of all individuals leads to action which is thought to be of help in the attainment of maximum potential health. Realization by society that healthy individuals are economic and social assets and that sickness is not only disabling for the individual but costly for the group leads to similar action. The action taken will depend as much on the perception of what constitutes a desirable social order as it will on the body of knowledge available for application in the promotion of health, care of the sick, and rehabilitation of the disabled.

The potential for change in the state of community health is not matched by the action taken. There is considerable time-lag in the application of knowledge to the welfare of people and this is no less true in health and medical care than in many other fields. Insofar as community health care is concerned, we need answers to questions such as: Are there meeting points between apparently distinct types of health and welfare services such as public health practice, family practice or clinic systems, and social service departments? Do they have a greater contribution to make when jointly planned? Would their integration be helpful in promoting the community's health and at the same time improve the way the needs of individual patients are met? There are many answers to these questions, but few are based on careful, scientific study.

There are some who feel that the answer lies in modern development of the traditional practitioner of Europe, the general practitioner who used to be the village or neighborhood doctor and the family doctor. It should be appreciated that the social structure in which he fulfilled his role has changed considerably. The village life in which he was reared and practiced has itself been transformed, and present-day medical education is hospital-based and oriented toward the patient in hospital. Basing the future of community medical care on a nostalgia of the past, albeit one's childhood memories, is not helpful to communities that are now emerging. And yet, the failure to replace this kind of doctor or the medical care he represented is decried by most health professionals and by people who had experience of a personal or family doctor. Much attention and effort is being expended on this subject, while at the same time the role of general practitioners becomes less attractive to students and young graduates of medical schools.

There are others who see the hospital as the center of future health and medical care with detached clinics radiating into various localities in order to make services more readily available. Often the services are concentrated or centered in or at the hospital or clinic. People come to the center, converging on it from many directions, turning toward it for various health reasons. The limitations of such fixed-point services are that they are not readily available for use by all individuals who need the kind of care they provide. Distances and transportation facilities are important, as has been demonstrated in studies of the use of services in different rural communities, e.g., by Frederiksen in India[1] and by Jolly and King in Uganda.[2]

This is not meant to underestimate the importance of extending hospital facilities for care of the sick individual but rather to emphasize their differences from a very important feature of community health practice, namely that of extending health activities into the various groups of the community, in homes, schools, and workplaces. This ensures surveillance of health of different population groups associated with a policy of active intervention. Mobility of staff in such programs is in marked contrast to more clinic- or hospital-bound staff receiving the patients who initiate the contact. Both situations are needed. Very often it is the static service only that operates. Even a maternal and child health clinic that is a subclinic of a hospital might easily become a static service, restricting its activities to mothers who turn to it for care rather than extending its surveillance to the whole population of mothers and children. However, when a maternal and child health service is a component part of a public health program it is more usual for it to turn its attention to the needs of mothers and children in the community as a whole.

The importance of continuing personal health care, by a personal doctor, a family nurse, or other practitioner, is agreed upon by almost all students of health and medical care. Less clear is the potential scope of their functions in community health care and the training they would need to prepare them for such a role. Similarly, it is agreed that hospitals can have a most important function in community health care by having close links with community-based services. But something more is needed if community health care is to make the effective contribution to health of communities that is now possible.

Some years ago we thought

> when the families being cared for in a family practice constitute a neighborhood, the community implications of the service become immediately apparent. The family practice becomes directly concerned with community health and the role of the doctor as family physician and community health adviser provides a single foundation in practice for the association of preventive and curative responsibilities.[3]

We have since learned that this is only partly true. In fact, it is one of those half-truths which we so often make in our wishful thinking and which hinder clarity of thought on what is actually needed. Effective community medicine is as dependent on adequate training and experience as is any other aspect of medicine.

The features of individual, family, and community health care which community medicine can unite are especially those that are oriented toward the local community. It would bring together the following groups: (1) the clinician practicing in the community whether he is a general family physician, family pediatrician, or internist; (2) those involved in public health practice, such as maternal and infant care and school health services; and (3) those in rural villages, who are in the sanitation services and who control the village water supply and agricultural hygiene. Community medicine in this way combines the *in-community* personal or individual health services with those services concerned with the health of subgroups of the community or of the community as a whole, and is both a preventive and curative service. The clinical or individual care element of the practice is a central feature, but as a result of being conducted in a community-oriented framework is seen in a different perspective. It involves activities which are not confined to the individual patient who turns to it for care. It has a commitment to the health of the community as a whole and is therefore actively concerned with determining the health of the individuals in that community and involving them in programs of care before they become sick. Community medicine thus assumes the initiative, and in doing so changes the responsibility practitioners have traditionally had, namely that of helping patients who have turned to them for care. Changing the role of medical care in its daily functioning changes the orientation of doctors, nurses, and other practitioners and demands new kinds of practice.

Having these commitments, the practice needs to develop on foundations of community diagnosis, community health action, and evaluation of change in the community's health no less than with care of the individual. Community medicine is concerned with groups that are significant for health of the community, such as the family, friendship, and other primary groups; schools; and work-groups. The family becomes an important unit not only with respect to understanding the background and care of the individual patient, but also as a significant determinant of a community's health. The term *family and community medicine* might best be applied to this aspect of health care in a local community.

If community medicine and primary health care are to be brought together in the health care of *local* communities, we must ensure that doctors, nurses, and other members of the team are trained for this purpose. The team must have knowledge of epidemiology and community diagnosis no less than it has in examination and diagnosis of the individual. It must have the skills for action that will affect the health of the community as a whole, or its subgroups, no less than its skill in patient management. While not all members of the team can be expected to have the same kind or amount of knowledge in these various areas, the team as a whole must develop it and use it in its practice of community medicine.

Writing of the basic questions which confront a physician, the editors of a recently published medical textbook list the following: "What is the matter with the patient? What can I do for him? What will be the outcome?" They add, "A fourth question, Why did it happen? will also arise in the mind of the inquiring physician who feels that each patient affords an opportunity and imposes a responsibility to contribute to a better understanding of causation and prevention."[4]

The cardinal questions which face practitioners of community medicine are the following.

What is the state of health of the community?
What are the factors responsible for this state of health?—why and how did it happen?
What is being done about it by the community and, more specifically, by the health service system?
What can be done, and what is the expected outcome?
What measures are needed to continue health surveillance of the community and evaluate the changes taking place?

The usual training of medical, nursing, or social-work students does not prepare them to deal systematically with these questions.

The development of new forms of community medicine involves consideration of the possible complementary functions of clinical and epidemiologic skills and their application to the care of individuals and to group and community health action. In Table 24-1 are listed the corresponding components of clinical and epidemiologic approaches.

TABLE 24-1. Summary of the Complementary Functions of Clinical and Epidemiologic Skills in Development of Newer Forms of Community Medicine and Primary Health Care

CLINICAL Individual	EPIDEMIOLOGIC Population Group
Examination of a patient: Interview and examination of individuals by history-taking, physical and psychologic examinations, laboratory, x-ray, and other special techniques.	Survey: State of health of community and families, using questionnaires, physical and psychologic testing, and special facilities for mass investigation.
Diagnosis 1. Usually of a patient. Differential diagnosis to determine main cause of patient's complaint. 2. Appraisal of health status of a "well" person, such as a pregnant woman, well children, periodic health examinations of adults.	Community Diagnosis 1. Health status of the community as a whole or of defined segments of it, e.g., health of expectant mothers, outcome of pregnancy, birth and and death rates, and so on. 2. Usually problem-oriented. Differential distribution of a particular condition in the community and the causes of this distribution.
Treatment 1. According to diagnosis and depending on resources of patient and medical institutions. 2. Intervention, usually follows on the patient seeking care for illness or advice about health.	Treatment 1. According to the community diagnosis and depending on resources of the health service system. 2. Intervention on basis of survey findings often before any illness notified or recognized.
Continuing observation: Evaluation of patient's progress and sometimes for further diagnostic work-up.	Continuing surveillance: Surveillance of health state of community and ensuring continuing action. Newer methods of sampling and ongoing surveys have much to offer the future practice of community medicine and primary health care.

COMMUNITY HEALTH SURVEYS

Health surveys comprise the foundation for community diagnosis, action, and continuing surveillance. They include direct assessment of the state of health, examination of environmental and community determinants of health, and investigation of the health service system.

There are various ways of gathering data about the health of a community.

Mortality Records

Since 1662, when John Graunt, citizen of London, published his *Observations Made Upon the Bills of Mortality*, mortality data have been widely used in health indices and epidemiologic investigations.[5]

Age-specific mortality rates by sex and cause of death are a first-level objective in the use of mortality rates as indicators of a community's health. For this purpose the following data are required: (1) census of the population, by age and sex; (2) birth registration; and (3) death reporting by age, sex, and cause of death. In countries in which this information is routinely obtained, special arrangements need to be made to make it available for the "local community." There are many parts of the world where such records are not yet available, and the health program must develop its own system for gathering the data.

Additional desirable information includes differential mortality rates of various neighborhoods or villages, different social classes or ethnic groups, or any other demographic or social variables which may be of health relevance in the particular area. It is important to note that the information can be of use in calculating mortality rates only if the variable is determined for the denominator (the population as a whole), as well as for the numerator (recorded deaths).

Hospital Records

Hospital records are a useful source of information, more especially if the addresses of all patients are accurately recorded and relevant data are known about the population from which the patients are admitted. These records allow at least for analysis of hospitalization rates by age and sex according to cause. The usefulness of hospital records lies in the increased reliability of diagnosis compared with diagnosis in most ambulant services. Their main defect is that they do not reflect the greatest part of day-to-day illnesses in a community.

Records of Ambulant Care Facilities

The records of general practitioners, clinics, and health centers are being increasingly subjected to analysis. Again, if data on the population eligible for the service are known, these data provide much additional information on the community's health. They commonly include diagnoses of common illnesses, disabilities of various degrees and kinds, and measures of health such as the data that can be obtained from well-organized records of maternal and child health centers.

Special Surveys of Health and Disease

Surveys of health and disease which are specially designed have such important contributions to make to knowledge of the community's health that they are becoming a feature of modern medical care and public health practice.[6] The development of such surveys has been very rapid and has become a cause of concern to a number of workers. Both the public and the health professions themselves may expect more from such surveys than has yet been shown to be useful. From their overenthusiasm and extravagant use of resources, doubt and even rejection of the whole approach may result.

Mass health examinations have a relatively long history and well-rooted place in public health practice, and it is useful to briefly review some aspects of their development.

Communicable Diseases. Screening methods have been developed for finding cases of communicable diseases affecting large numbers of people. Such diseases include malaria, syphilis, yaws, tuberculosis, leprosy, smallpox, and trachoma. Initiated in the 19th century as part of the public health movement, these investigations have been extended to vast areas of the world. The methods of investigation have been simplified and refined by the use of laboratory and other special facilities. The purposes of these surveys include case-finding, surveillance of infection and its transmission, and epidemiologic research.

Nutrition and Growth. Surveys of growth and nutritional state also have a long history. It is now almost 100 years since Bowditch demonstrated a relation between the height and weight of Boston schoolchildren and socioeconomic status.[7,8] The physique and nutritional status of population groups are fundamental indicators of their health. Surveys assessing nutritional status are now widespread and the need to standardize methods of investigation was recognized by the Health Organization of the League of Nations and subsequently by the World Health Organization. The planning of surveys of malnutrition, including details of direct assessment—especially in early childhood—have been outlined by Jelliffe.[9] Such guides are not only needed for all age groups, but for assessment of nutritional status of all communities. The present focus of attention on atherosclerosis, diabetes, obesity, and their implications for coronary artery disease and cerebral vascular disease is stimulating further interest in the need for surveys of nutritional status in all communities. The purposes of nutrition surveys are similar in their basic aims to those referred to above in relation to infection and infectious disease.

MULTIPLE EXAMINATIONS

Health surveys geared to detect specific infections or infectious diseases, and more general but nevertheless defined nutritional surveys, have been developed as integral elements of public health practice. Another avenue for the development of mass health examinations has been the introduction of screening procedures for a number of conditions as a routine in the examination of hospital or clinic patients and of persons joining medical insurance programs. Often the primary orientation of these examinations is toward the individual and his treatment. However, when those examined represent a population group, the public health relevance of the findings can readily be explored by use of epidemiologic methods. In fact, the initial planning and carrying out of the program should include consideration of its potential effect on community health care as well as its value as a screening procedure for treatment of affected individuals.

There was a time in medical practice when laboratory and other special investigations were undertaken only when indicated by the history, interview, and physical examination. This practice, while sound in its insistence on thorough interview and examination and careful consideration of differential diagnosis, did not encourage realization of the full potential of technologic advance. This has made it possible to recognize an increasing number of disorders in their early stages in individuals, while at the same time measuring differential distribution of health-relevant variables in the community. Indeed, it is this particular feature which has so much potential for good, in the sense of promoting community health or the health of an individual, and yet causes misgivings. A doctor investigating a patient's complaint in order to help the patient who has turned to him for care is the model of traditional medical practice. By extending his investigations to include screening procedures for conditions other than that for which the patient turns to him for care, he is modifying his practice. The change is in the direction of public health practice, in which the practitioner rather than the patient takes the initiative in exploring the health condition. Implicit in such surveys is that the findings will be utilized for the good of the public's health and for the individuals concerned.

Multiple screening is growing very rapidly and becoming an integral part of medical care. The extent to which the practice of multiple screening should be encouraged and the problems involved in this kind of decision making have been reviewed by a number of workers.[10–15] Its extension is likely to change the nature of traditional medical care, bringing it much closer to public health practice.

The Purposes of Multiple Examinations in Primary Health Care

The place of multiple examinations in community medicine as practiced in primary health care needs further consideration as to the purpose and usefulness of each investigation. In general the purposes of multiple examinations may be for epidemiologic research, for action promotive of the community's health, and for treatment of the individuals who need it. At least one of these purposes must be served if a survey is to be justified scientifically and ethically, and if it is to be acceptable to the community and the individuals concerned.

Insofar as the individual is concerned, the very least he should expect is information about his state of health. The survey should include examination procedures which lead to primary or secondary prevention, such as immunization, feeding practices in infancy, change in dietary habits, and treatment of asymptomatic or neglected symptomatic disorders. If specific medicinal treatment is to be used to correct a disorder or what might be regarded as a high-risk factor for disease it should be based on evidence that the treatment is helpful, and at least not harmful.[16]

As an instrument of community medicine, multiple health examinations must provide information on which action to take to improve the health of the community as a whole or particular subgroups. This includes control of the environment in order to protect the community against conditions such as chronic bronchitis, dysentery, streptococcal infection, and so on. It also includes provision of information for action by more personal, group-oriented services such as maternal and child health centers.

The factors that must be considered when deciding on the tests to be conducted in any multiple screening survey are cost, validity, and reliability of the tests, and the facilities available for treatment of the conditions found.

EPIDEMIOLOGIC SURVEILLANCE OF THE HEALTH SERVICE SYSTEM

The distinctive approach of epidemiologic surveillance of a health service system is its focus on the implications of the system for the population's health. It may concern itself with one or more elements of the system or the system as a whole. It may focus on one defined segment of the population or compare different groups; it usually concerns itself with one or another specific aspect of health. This epidemiologic approach involves continuing surveillance of the health service system in relation to the changing state of health of the community. Its impact on the health of the community may be direct or indirect. Direct measures include the treatment of sick people, preventive measures such as immunization, or promotive measures such as prenatal, hospital obstetric, infant, and child services. Indirect measures involve changing the habits of a community or modifications of the environment. The importance of maintaining a view of the whole must not preclude focus on specific elements of the service and their implications for the community's health. In examining the impact of a service on community health each organization within the system may need study. Figure 24-1 summarizes an epidemiologic approach to study of the association between a health service system and

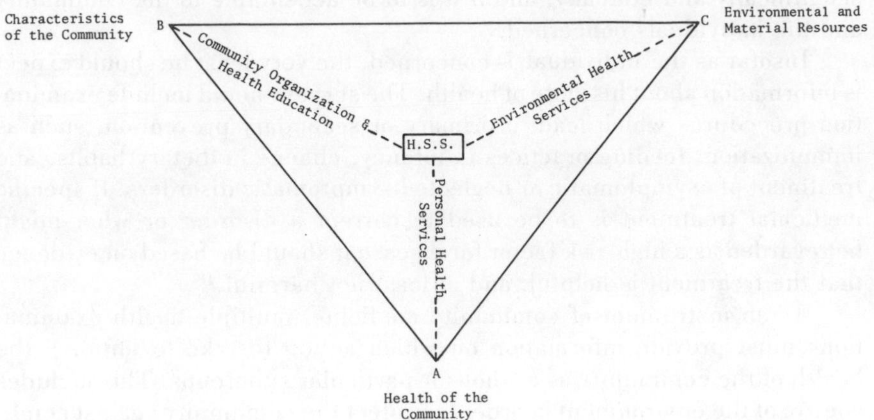

FIG. 24-1. Epidemiologic model for surveillance of the effects of a health service system (H.S.S.) on a community's health.

the health of the community. This approach to epidemiologic surveillance involves two broad areas.

1. Continuing surveillance of each of the three elements of the service, namely direct personal health services, environmental health services, and community organization and health education.
2. Continuing surveillance of the three areas of the epidemiologic triangle, namely the changing state of the health of the community, the characteristics of the community, and the environment and material resources.

REFERENCES

1. Frederiksen HS: Epidemiological surveillance. In Epidemographic Surveillance: A Symposium. Carolina Population Center, Monograph 13. Chapel Hill, Univ of North Carolina, 1971.
2. Jolly R, King M: The organization of health services. In King M (ed.): Medical Care in Developing Countries. London, Oxford Univ Press, 1966.
3. Kark SL, Kark E: A Practice of Social Medicine. In Kark SL, Steuart GW (eds.): A Practice of Social Medicine. Edinburgh and London, E & S Livingstone, 1962, p 8.
4. Harvey AM, Cluff LE, Johns RJ, et al.: The Principles and Practice of Medicine, 17th ed. New York, Appleton, 1968, p xxiii.
5. Graunt J: Natural and Political Observations Made Upon the Bills of Mortality. First published in London, 1662. Republished Baltimore, Johns Hopkins Press, 1939.
6. National Center for Health Statistics: Origin, Program, and Operation of the US National Health Survey. Public Health Service Publication No. 1,000,

Series 1, No. 1. Washington, DC, Department of Health, Education, and Welfare. Reprinted 1965.

7. Bowditch HP: The Growth of Children. Annual Reports of the Massachusetts State Board of Health, 1877 and 1879.
8. Roberts LJ: Nutrition Work with Children. Chicago, Univ of Chicago Press, 1935, Chapter 4.
9. Jelliffe DB: The assessment of the nutritional status of the community. WHO Monogr Ser 53:1, 1966.
10. Wilson JMG, Jungner G: Principles and practice of screening for disease. WHO Public Health Pap 34:1, 1968.
11. Benson ES, Strandjord PE: Multiple Laboratory Screening. New York, Academic Press, 1969.
12. Working Group of The Nuffield Provincial Hospitals Trust: Screening in Medical Care. London, Oxford Univ Press, 1968.
13. Ferrer HP: Screening for Health. London, Butterworths, 1968.
14. Technical Discussions at the World Health Assembly: Mass health examinations. WHO Public Health Pap 45:1, 1971.
15. Collen M: Multiphasic laboratory screening and health care in the outpatient clinic. In Benson ES, Strandjord PE (eds.): Multiple Laboratory Screening. New York, Academic Press, 1969.
16. Cochrane AL: Effectiveness and Efficiency. London, Nuffield Provincial Hospitals Trust, 1972.

25

The Development of Community Medicine and Primary Health Care in a Neighborhood

Kiryat Harim is a neighborhood of west Jerusalem with a population of about 21,000. Building activity is a sign that it is still growing. It has some of the finest houses in Jerusalem, built along the hills overlooking the valleys below to Ein Karem, a town of monasteries and churches with deep historic meaning for religious Christians, where John the Baptist was born and Mary stopped to refresh herself at the spring which still flows.

Here also are some of the worst homes of Jerusalem, in which live overcrowded, poor, and uneducated families. The houses are temporary structures built of asbestos, and are spread across a whole valley of the neighborhood. The best homes do not have this valley as their view, nor do the asbestos homes look up to the hills where the better-off families live.

Between these two extremes of Kiryat Harim is a wide range of housing. Buildings of two stories with four to eight apartments predominate, and single family homes or "villot" (villas), as they are called, are also to be found. Larger multistoried units are now being built and the density of population in the neighborhood is increasing. It is a growing area of a city that is itself becoming a bustling, active capital of the country. It is traversed by asphalt roads which not only link various parts of the neighborhood with the city center, but along which buses and other traffic pass beyond Kiryat Harim to still further areas of the city. Shopping centers, schools, a variety of public services, university student residences, and a well-built reception center for new immigrants all add to the active, if not beautiful, setting of this district of Jerusalem. It is in this neighborhood that a new form of community and family health care was initiated when the Kiryat Harim community health center was established in 1953.[1]

The present practices of the health center are different and more varied than those which were initiated 20 years ago. There has been a growth in ideas and a widening of the concept of the potential of community medicine and primary health care when united in a community health center. Most important perhaps has been the learning experience this center has provided regarding the problem of translating concepts into the reality of practice. The development of our present-day practices has been the product of changes in emphasis and orientation, changes we hope will continue as part of the progress of growth toward newer and improved health care of people as individuals and in their various groups. The phases through which the health center has passed are not sharply defined, but we need to focus our present discussion on the initiation of the center, the effects of its subsequent integration into a university department of social medicine, its move toward community medicine and primary health care, and the use of epidemiology as an important element in decision making in the policy of the various practices of the health center today.

INITIATING THE PRACTICE

The health services of Jerusalem at that time (1953) did not constitute a system of interdependent elements. There was some interaction in the care of individual patients but there was no single coordinating body of the many agencies involved, nor was there a strong central direction. The Ministry of Health had itself only recently been established and like other fields of public administration, it lacked experienced public health personnel. Prime Minister Ben Gurion recognized this in these words:

> Never was so vital and so precious a charge entrusted to Jewry's public servants, as the Israel Civil Service now assumes. . . . into their care are given security and absorption, development and reconstruction, education and health . . . Let us be frank. This is a calling we knew not formerly or, at least, have not followed for centuries past. We have to ply a new craft, create something out of nothing, almost.[2]

Personal health services in Jerusalem were separately provided by a number of different agencies. There were three general hospitals—Hadassah, Bikur Holim, and Sha'are Tzedek—run by separate voluntary organizations. The Ministry of Health, the Municipal Council, and the Kupat Holim of the Histadrut (the Sick Fund of the General Federation of Labor Unions) did not run any general hospitals in Jerusalem, although it was and still is usual for at least one or more of them to do so in other cities of the country.

On the other hand, personal health services which were community based reflected the nationwide tradition of separation between preventive and curative care; e.g., maternal and child health stations and ambulant curative clinics were housed separately, often considerable distances apart. They were conducted by different agencies, Hadassah being responsible for the preventive services in the community and Kupat Holim for the curative clinics. Welfare services were developed independently of both these health services.

Separate units were responsible for different aspects of the mother and child services, namely the mother–infant–young-child clinics and the school health services. In the mother-infant clinics, public health nurses had the main administrative professional responsibility. With the clinics as their base they carried out intensive home visiting in their preventive and educational functions. Prenatal care was supervised by obstetricians from the Hadassah Hospital. During regular visits by pediatricians to the various child health stations the public health nurses were able to refer cases about whom they had some concern. The school health service department was staffed by specially trained school physicians, working with public health nurses whose base of operations was in the schools. The latter also visited the homes of schoolchildren when necessary. This school doctor-nurse team was a well-developed service providing physical and psychiatric care since several of the doctors had had special training in schoolchild psychiatry.

In contrast to the considerable development of home visiting by public health nurses of the mother and child services, the curative clinics of the Kupat Holim were static services to which the members turned for care when they felt the need for treatment. There was, and still is, very limited care of the sick and disabled at home. In certain cases a doctor would visit a patient at home, but care of home-bound patients by a nursing service had not been developed by the Kupat Holim clinic system in Jerusalem.

This was the background of the personal aspects of public health practice and of medical care at the time the health center was initiated in Kiryat Harim.

In 1951 Kiryat Harim was not yet incorporated in Jerusalem. It lay to the west of the growing city, a sparsely populated area on the urban periphery. Then the first of the new housing projects (shikunim) were built and immigrant families were settled in them before they were completed and before community facilities such as roads and transportation had been developed. The need for settlement of immigrants was very great, with pressures to settle the masses who were arriving in the country.

At the time the health center commenced its activities in January 1953, the diversity of ethnic groups was a striking feature of the neighborhood; a modern Babel had emerged in but a few years. Families living as neighbors had very limited communication. In many buildings there were families of different origin, with different culture and behavior, speaking different languages.

The present social class differences of neighborhoods within the area were already evident in 1953. There were different housing projects, one for new immigrants, another for veteran members of the General Federation of Labor Unions (Histadrut), and yet another for public servants of the newly-established public service system which was being centered in Jerusalem. The projects housing these different groups were readily distinguishable. Not only was each project geographically defined, but the social distance was readily observed by such differences as the general appearance of the homes, the state of their immediate environs, and the kind and standard of dress of adults and children.

Families originating from more than 25 countries were settled in the first immigrant housing project, and it was to these families that much attention was initially given, based on the decision that the health center was an agency that could assist the process of assimilating an immigrant population. This was not a latent function of a medical service, as described by Judith Shuval in her study of the functions of medical practice.[3] It was an explicit objective of the program, even if not perceived to be so by the communities involved.

Our early endeavors in involving the community in the development of this health center were better described by Ross than by any of those who were involved. Ross, whose interest as a professor of social work was in theory and principles of community organization, wrote the following in 1954.

> Two elements combine to make this work of special interest: (1) The composition of the population of the village. This community has about 800 inhabitants. They come from many parts of the world, have a great variety of ideas about health and physical care, and have a multitude of diet and health practices, many of them unknown in the Western world. Their attitude to modern medicine and its practitioners also varies greatly, many groups being quite superstitious and regarding doctors and nurses with a good deal of suspicion. Some groups have deep-rooted traditions which make no provision for modern medicine and its directives. (2) Kark's philosophy of work is similar to Rene Sand's dictum, "Health cannot be given to people, it demands their participation." Thus the purpose is not to impose a health scheme on the community but to attempt to have the community participate in developing its own health program.
>
> The interesting problem which [the team] faces is how to implement such a philosophy in a setting as unfavorable as this appears to be.
>
> To begin with, an attempt is made to clarify philosophy so that all the staff are agreed on fundamental objectives and methods. For those on the staff who had no more than orthodox medical training, this is often a difficult learning process. [The director] does not direct, impose,

> or lead his staff in the traditional sense. There are frequent staff meetings in which village practices are discussed and in which [he] questions many of the assumptions and value-judgments of staff members. This, as suggested, is difficult for some staff persons—all their lives they have been taught what was "right" and what was "wrong." They see many "wrong" practices in the village and feel that their duty is to correct them. This is their job as they conceive it. To have a director who not only does not support their efforts at reform but questions their authority for judging "right" and "wrong" makes for a difficult period of adjustment. But [his] philosophy with staff is approximately the same as with the villagers. Roughly it might be summarized thus: "As a rule of thumb, one should never attack the fundamental types of belief directly. If erroneous and incompatible with reality, the fundamental beliefs will themselves dissolve in the course of time, but nothing gives them life like a direct attack upon them. Their untruth has to be discovered slowly by the people, and at the same rate at which the people are finding new sources of security. A belief upon which a person's security depends cannot simply be wiped out. Disillusion from the belief has to be accompanied by a shift to dependence upon a new kind of support."
>
> [The] work begins, then, not with lectures, moving pictures or distribution of literature on how to be healthy (the Western way) but with an attempt to understand the health practices of various national groups in the community and how these practices fit in with their whole culture. This is done with considerable objectivity, with a recognition that these practices have meaning for these people, and may in fact have absolute value which has not hitherto been recognized in Western society.
>
> Secondly, there is no attempt to impose new standards on these people—to challenge existing beliefs and practices. Rather an attempt is made to create a situation (or a social climate) in which free interaction of medical staff and villagers will take place. This interaction will lead to exchange of ideas and it is hoped to a feeling of need on the part of the villagers for change in some practices. Here again it is recognized that people will change only when they feel ready for change. The objective, therefore, is to create readiness for movement.[4]

It can only be added that even at this time some 20 years later, we are still seeking ways to make this a reality. For in truth, the degree of community involvement is not what we hoped for. Those responsible for medical care—doctors, nurses, and social workers—are not yet being trained toward these objectives. It is now clear that new approaches cannot always emerge from the old. More than minor modifications of basic curricula of training of health service personnel is needed. New approaches need new forms. New kinds of institutions, such as our health center, need new types of personnel. To the question, whether the present traditional schools provide this training, the answer is no. The hospital-based training of doctors and of nurses is an unsuitable foundation.

The approach to practice at this health center differed in several important respects from traditional practice. It differed in ways of combining curative and preventive care, in the home and at the health center itself. In addition, it was interested in establishing a practice which would provide for care of the individuals in the setting of their family and community groups. Also, a health team was established as the most desirable way of developing this approach to practice.

This early phase of the health center program was described in a report in 1957, which is reproduced here with some modifications.[5]

Among the distinctive features of the practice of the center was the allotment of a neighborhood of homes to a team of a family doctor and nurses. The same doctor and nurses attended to individual family members during health and illness. The combination of these preventive and curative functions by a doctor and nurse team required considerable preparation and planning if high standards of practice in both fields were to be developed. The task of the family nurse of combining traditional public health nursing functions with those of care of the sick is a considerable challenge. It is often spoken of as if it were a simple and easy task of integration. In fact, we found it to be a very difficult process. This particular approach in comprehensive family nursing was associated with the development of a new form of family medicine. The medical aspects were performed by family physicians who aimed to combine curative and preventive functions in the care of their families. This too demands much of the individuals directly concerned. The development of doctor-nurse teams was a process in which both the doctors and the nurses were involved in a learning function regarding their own as well as their reciprocal roles as members of a team.

Continuity of care of families by a physician and nurse introduces a personal relationship between staff and family in which the roles of doctor and nurse are of a complex kind. It is within the framework of a relatively enduring relationship between doctor and family, nurse and family, and doctor and nurse that family diagnosis and care proceed.

Family diagnosis resembles traditional clinical diagnosis in that it requires similar personal and intimate relations with individuals. The study of a family needs to expand beyond the immediate intrafamilial processes of interaction which are of significance to health. Because of the very significant role the family has in the epidemiology of health and disease, and because of the implications which epidemiology as a discipline has for family diagnosis, the family physician's diagnostic work is of an epidemiologic nature. Being at the same time clinical and epidemiologic, family diagnosis is best regarded as a study in clinical epidemiology.

Exploring methods of clinical epidemiologic study in family diagnosis was thus a distinctive feature of the practice by such a family and community health center. To this end we spent much time on the methodologic problems involved, and a series of practical seminars on the subject of family diagnosis was conducted.

The development of community medicine within the framework of individual and family medical care requires much interest on the part of the practitioners concerned. It also needs education additional to that which the average doctor and nurse receive in their schools of medicine and nursing.

One of the earliest stated objectives of the center was that of promoting community health, and since its inception it has been concerned with finding ways of doing this. Early on, the health center attempted to promote health through community action. While doctors, nurses, and other "casework-oriented" professional staff have a most important role in such community development work, the field extends beyond the main areas of experience of such personnel. The process involved in community action concerned with the promotion of its own health is community organization and health education. Before the establishment of this health center, Israel had no experience with such personnel. Despite this lack of experience it was agreed that the center should initiate a program of health education and for this purpose several posts of "community health educator" were created, but the early experience of the center in the field of community health education was difficult.

The center's concern with the social, cultural, and emotional aspects of health led to a decision to include special staff who would ensure satisfactory progress in these areas. A clinical psychologist, a social anthropologist, and a psychiatric social worker were appointed for this purpose. This was a bold decision in that there was little, if any, precedent in the country for associating such personnel with a general medical service or public health agency. There were many difficulties in integrating this specialized staff in the health center's team.

The processes by which professional workers of different disciplines grow together as a team are most complex, and the inevitability of gradual progress should be accepted. Providing that the difficulties, and the occasional failures, constitute a learning experience for those concerned with pioneering this approach to medical care, each difficulty will have served a most useful function in testing various approaches.

THE PRESENT PRACTICE

We have focused the present-day practice of the Department of Social Medicine in Kiryat Harim on the development of a unified practice of community medicine and primary health care. By this we are testing the practicability of developing this approach in different kinds of practice.

One type is the family practice described above, in which curative and preventive care are provided by the same doctor-nurse team units to approximately 1,000 families, 750 of which live in well-defined housing projects. The second type of practice in which we are testing our approach is in the two maternal and child health centers which provide preventive services, namely pre- and postnatal care of women, and care for mothers with their babies and young children. These services are more in line with the traditional system of medical care organization in the country as a whole in that they are not responsible for delivery of curative services. Also, we have instituted a program concerned with surveillance of long-term illness in the community in addition to initiating and assuming responsibility for a home-care service of home-bound patients and patients discharged from hospital and needing continuation of care.

Epidemiologic methods of community diagnosis are the basic tools for describing the community's state of health and its determinants. Based on these foundations we are aiming to provide a health care service that is directed toward changing the trends of health of the community in desirable directions, and meeting the needs of sick or well individuals who turn to the center for their personal care. In the steady development toward community medicine, individual care is being increasingly undertaken in the framework of various problem-oriented programs which are widening to involve the community as a whole.

To perform these functions various methods have been used, and it is important to emphasize that they are methods rather than objectives in themselves. They include a defined area of practice, a health team such as a doctor-nurse team combining curative and preventive health care, community participation in the program, and so on. Different methods will need to be used in different settings. These may be related to the wide variation between communities, such as their cultures and economic situations, their traditions in medical and health care systems, or the kind and numbers of health personnel.

Changes which have been made in the practice of the health center include the product of experience in its operations over the 20 years since its inception, changes in Kiryat Harim itself, the growth of Jerusalem and its health services, and the development of the center's role in the teaching and demonstration functions of the University Department of Social Medicine.

The population of Kiryat Harim has grown from several hundred families to well over 20,000 people since the area was settled 20 years ago. While Kiryat Harim itself was then beyond the western boundaries of Jerusalem, it is now well within the city limits. Not only has the population grown, but the demographic characteristics of the different neighborhoods and housing projects have changed. Selective immigration and emigration have resulted in changes in the ethnic and social class composition, and there has been a change in the age-sex pyramid of some neighborhoods. This demographic change is of direct consequence to the nature of the family practice in these neighborhoods and to the problems confronting community medicine (Fig. 25-1).

As residents of Jerusalem, with transportation readily available to

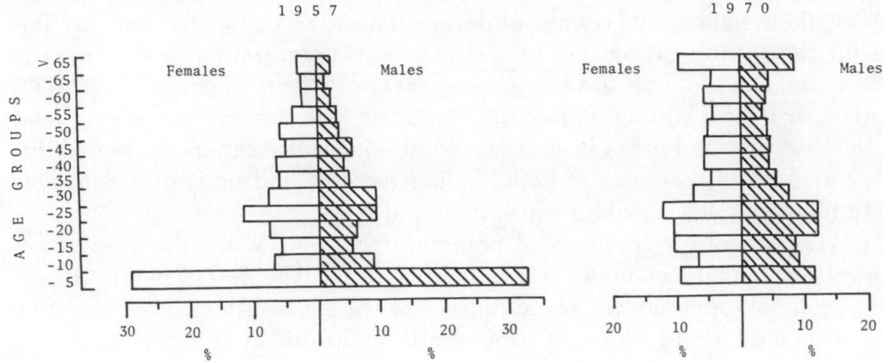

FIG. 25-1. The changing composition of the population in a family practice of Kiryat Harim. Age-sex pyramid.

various parts of the city, the people of Kiryat Harim have access to, and use, various health services in the city. The services include a number of hospitals, curative and preventive clinics throughout the city, and various special facilities.

Viewing the hospital and clinic services as a whole it is clear that they do not constitute a health care system. They are not a set of connected things or parts, nor do the services together make a complex whole. They are a complexity of nonrelated pieces rather than a mosaic, which although diversified comprises a whole. How does this affect the health center program we are aiming to develop in Kiryat Harim?

Services in Kiryat Harim

Both curative and preventive clinics are situated in various parts of the district, within relatively easy walking distance of most homes. The curative and preventive clinics are separately administered, separately staffed, and usually separately housed. This applies to all but our departmental health center. Not only are the curative and preventive health services separated, but the welfare services in the area are the responsibility of a special department of the municipality and are housed separately from the health services.

There is an assumption that continuity of care is in the interests of the well and the sick, of families and their individual members. As indicated above, one of the methods we aimed to use in developing an integrated practice of community medicine and primary health care was that of continuity of care by a health team, especially the family doctor-nurse team. The health services of Jerusalem and the way their facilities are organized do not encourage continuity of care. The following is a summary of the situation and the potential impact on continuity of care of the Jerusalem health services for patients in Kiryat Harim.

1. Services in Kiryat Harim itself
   a. Attendance at different clinics in the area when sick and when well
   b. Attendance at different offices for "welfare" and for "health" needs
   c. Separate night and holiday call service from day-time routine
2. Hospitals
   a. General hospitals are not area-oriented
   b. Emergency room and in-patient facilities of the three hospitals are arranged on a rotational system of intake on different days of the week

There is thus limited continuity of care in the full meaning of the term. Patients are attended by different physicians and these physicians are not members of the same team. There is also discontinuity of care for patients needing repeated hospitalization, as they are often admitted to different hospitals for recurrence of acute episodes of a single illness. One of the roles of our health center is to reduce the discontinuity as much as possible. The aim is to reduce the sense of discontinuity felt by patients and to ensure continuity in treatments by maintaining contact with families and providing for home care regardless of the particular clinic, emergency service, or hospital attended by the patient.

Yet another product of the lack of a unified health care system is the public health problem which is created by the limited relationship between the various services and by the ready access which people have to so many medical and health care facilities. This lack of coordination manifests itself in the orientation of the various services. With the possible exception of the citywide maternal and child health services, a main feature of the personal services is that the initiative for care comes from patient or family. The service does not go out into the community, exploring and investigating health problems and initiating care. In contrast to this static type of service is traditional public health practice, in which mobility is a feature. This is one of the main aspects of our health center's approach, namely conducting investigations into the community's health and its health attitudes and practices of relevance to health. On the basis of the findings, action is initiated by the health center.

The association between the Community Health Center of Kiryat Harim and the Department of Social Medicine had many mutual effects. For the university department, it meant the addition of community health care to its teaching and research functions. This department is in effect a small graduate school of community medicine and public health, and a social medicine research unit. To this end it is composed of a number of divisions which have responsibilities in all three of its functions, and hence in the health center. The orientation of its research has thus been toward community health research. The main studies have included epidemiologic investigation of various diseases, growth and development of children, studies in medical care and rehabilitation, and a comprehensive health survey of a total community. By focusing much of its research on the local community or neighborhood, scientific foundations have been provided for development of the practice of community medicine with primary health care. Thus epidemiologic investigations into the hemoglobin distribution in pregnant and parturient women of Jerusalem, including those of Kiryat Harim, led to a control program, which is described in Chapter 29. Studies of differential rates in growth and development of children have been the foundation community diagnosis for a program focusing attention on specific problems in the community through maternal and child health centers (PROD Program, Chapter 30). A health survey of the total community has provided the basic epidemiologic information for the primary and secondary prevention of the main causes of death in this community, namely heart disease and cerebral vascular disease. This program, which is being conducted through a family practice, is described in Chapter 31.

In a setting in which there are a multiplicity of agencies offering individual care in different institutions, there is likely to be much overlap and discontinuity in the services a patient receives. There are also likely to be gaps in his care. An illustrative example of the influence of investigations into medical care on the practice of the health center is provided by the community studies of hospitalization and the development of a community-based home-care service (Chapter 26).

The health center functions which have been described as those of community medicine and primary health care now include the following.

1. Individual care and family health maintenance
   a. A family practice
   b. Maternal and child health care, including schoolchildren
   c. A community-based home care service
2. Community health surveillance and special programs
   a. Community health survey
   b. Special programs of surveillance, action, and evaluation

This development needs new health teams, expanding on the doctor-nurse team which constitutes the nucleus of each family health maintenance unit. The specialties of the clinical teams have expanded to include psychiatry, pediatrics, and clinical nutrition. The integration of community medicine with primary health care has meant active involvement of epidemiologists and statisticians as well as newer approaches to community organization and health education. It has also led to an increasing amount

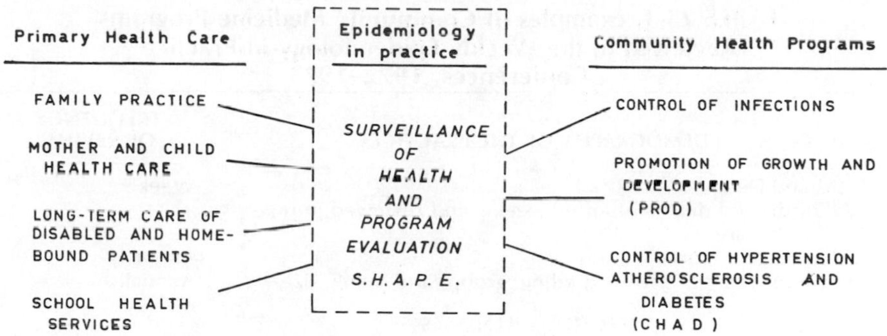

FIG. 25-2. Epidemiology in practice. The use of epidemiology in developing community medicine within, and through, primary health care.

of participation of graduate students in social medicine and public health, and of physicians and others in the activities of the center.

One of the central questions that may be raised concerns the role of epidemiology as a basic and applied science bonding community medicine to primary health care. Its role needs definition in exploring problems that require attention by the community health center, in continuing surveillance and evaluation of action taken. It is not merely a question as to whether epidemiologic research can be conducted in the framework of a family practice or other type of primary health care. It is rather whether epidemiology can be usefully applied in day-to-day practice, thereby extending primary medical care to a combined practice with community medicine. A diagrammatic representation of this combined practice is shown in Figure 25-2.

To this end, epidemiology is being developed as an integral feature of the practice. A weekly conference, "Epidemiology in Practice," is the nearest approach we have to the traditional ward rounds of clinicians. It involves systematic reviews and evaluation of progress of the practice and the community's health by a team of epidemiologists, family physicians, pediatricians, nurses, statisticians, resident physicians specializing in public health, and students of the university's Master of Public Health classes. It is both a practice and teaching session. The objective is that each participant, i.e., the majority of senior faculty and staff of the health center, has an active role to fulfill in this session and is concerned with one or more aspects of the community's health and the "treatment" being provided. It is at this session that decisions are made regarding necessary changes in health action.

The different facets of the practice are reviewed each week and decisions are made regarding ways of gathering the data and methods of record-

TABLE 25-1. Examples of Community Medicine Programs Reviewed in the Weekly Epidemiology-In-Practice Conferences, 1972–1973

DEMOGRAPHY OF THE PRACTICES	FREQUENCY OF REVIEW
Births and Deaths	Weekly
All births and deaths reported weekly and reviewed in relation to care	
Birth rates and mortality rates	Annually
Population change: age, sex, ethnic group, and family size	Annually
INFECTIOUS ILLNESSES	
Review of all acute infectious illnesses diagnosed in the family practice (Pickles-type chart used)	Weekly Three time a year cumulative
Rheumatic fever, rheumatic heart disease, and acute streptococcal disease. Treatment and prophylactic program	Three times a year
Immunization (triple vaccine: smallpox, poliomyelitis, measles)	Annually
Bacteriologic investigations and viral surveillance	Annually
THE "28TH DAY" REVIEW	
All births analyzed 28 days after delivery as normal or for classified abnormalities in pregnancy, labor, child at birth, and neonatal period to 28th day	Five times a year with each of the different programs being reviewed annually
Report on action programs and investigations re:	
Anemia in pregnancy	
Smoking in pregnancy	
Height of mothers, weight change during pregnancy, and outcome of pregnancy	
Management of major abnormalities in pregnancy and delivery	
Work during pregnancy	
PROD	
(Promotion of development and growth during infancy, with special regard to needs of children born to poor families with uneducated mothers and otherwise disadvantaged)	
Cumulative measurement of growth and development trends	Monthly
Physical growth	Four times a year
Behavior development	Four times a year
Report on action programs and investigations re:	Each of the programs is reviewed annually
Feeding practices	
Family spacing	
Anemia in infancy	
Family functioning	
Infections in infancy	
Questionnaire on various practices (pretest and initiation)	
Growth and development of disabled and chronic ill children	
Verbal stimulation	

TABLE 25-1. Examples of Community Medicine Programs Reviewed in the Weekly Epidemiology-In-Practice Conferences, 1972–1973 (cont.)

CHAD	FREQUENCY OF REVIEW
(Community program for control and treatment of risk factors for coronary heart disease, cerebrovascular disease, and peripheral arterial vascular disease, more especially hypertension, hyperlipidemia, hyperglycemia and obesity)	Monthly with each of the different programs being reviewed annually
Report on action programs and investigations, re:	
Risk factors	
Blood pressure and hypertension	
Serum lipids and hypercholesterolemia	
Diabetes	
Ischemic heart disease, cerebrovascular disease, and peripheral vascular disease	
Behavior related factors	
Diet	
Smoking	
Use of services	
Facilities for change and treatment	
CHAD clinics	
Community Organization and health education.	
COMMUNITY MENTAL HEALTH	Twice a year
LONG-TERM CARE, REVIEW OF PROGRAM	Annually
RURAL COMMUNITY HEALTH CENTER	
(Affiliated with the Department of Social Medicine, this rural health center provides a service for five rural settlements. The doctor attends these weekly "Epidemiology-in-Practice" sessions and participates in several activities)	
Reviews of infectious illnesses	Weekly
Special subjects presented for discussion	Three times a year

ing the community's health in relation to care; methods of analysis and presentation of the data for the regular reviews; and decisions on programs which need to be initiated, as well as modification of on-going programs.

A number of special teams made up of members of the staff, who work up the material and carry out the different aspects of community medicine in the practice, support the epidemiologic conferences. In each of these teams there is a group concerned with Surveillance of Health and Program Evaluation (SHAPE). The different elements of the practice and the frequency with which they are reviewed are decided upon by the conference group. The weekly conference takes place in the health center conference room, in which data of on-going activities are charted and mapped on the walls, providing visual aids for the conference. Table 25-1 illustrates the various subjects discussed and their frequency of review during the course of a year. A revised schedule is prepared for each year.

REFERENCES

1. Mann KJ, Medalie JH, Lieber E, et al: Visits to Doctors. Jerusalem, Academic Press, 1970.
2. Ben Gurion D: The Call of Spirit in Israel. In Rebirth and Destiny of Israel. New York, Philosophical Library, 1954.
3. Shuval J, in collaboration with Antonovsky A, Davies AM: Social Functions of Medical Practice. San Francisco, Jossey-Bass, 1970.
4. Ross MG: Community Organization: Theory and Experience. New York, Harper & Brothers, 1955, pp 30–32.
5. Kark SL, Kark E: Medicine in Community Development: Some Aspects of Health and Medical Care in Israel, 1952–1957. Mimeograph report, 1957. Department of Social Medicine, Hebrew University-Hadassah Medical School, Jerusalem.

26

Disabled and Home-Bound Patients: The Introduction of a Community-Based Home Care Program

THE CASE FOR ACTION

The care of patients at home as well as in clinics of the health center has been a function of the center since its inception. Family physicians have responded to calls to visit the sick at home and daily home-rounds remain a feature of the present-day family practice. Similarly, the public health nurses of the family practice team have a continuing responsibility for regular home visiting, such as the regular visits to mothers of new-born children on their return from hospital obstetric units and to patients in need of nursing care at home.

The special program to be reviewed here differs from this primary health care function of family medicine and nursing care. It is concerned with care and surveillance of home-bound patients, the after-care of patients discharged from hospital, and persons with chronic disabilities who are in need of care. It extends throughout the whole area of Kiryat Harim and is available to all regardless of the various agencies, hospitals, or clinics which the patients have attended. The institution of this home-care service resulted from the findings of a number of investigations into hospitalization and the care of patients after their return home from hospital. These studies were first conducted during the period 1954–1957 among some 2,000 people in the area.[1] Later, in 1962, a community study of hospitalization was conducted among the population of 17,590 who lived in the area in that year.[2] This was followed by a special study of patients, 6 weeks and 1 year after their discharge from hospital, during a 2-year period.[3,4] On the completion of this investigation it was decided to establish the home-care program. It was initiated in 1966, and an evaluation of one aspect was carried out over a 9-month period, beginning in September 1968.[5]

The crude hospitalization rate in 1962 was 72 per 1,000 persons at risk, which was similar to the earlier findings over the period 1954–1957, namely an average of 69 per 1,000 per year. The rate was not exceptional when compared with other countries such as the United Kingdom and the United States, and was somewhat lower than those for Jerusalem and for the Jewish population of Israel in that year (102 per 1,000).

The highest rate for hospitalization was in infancy, the rate for babies under the age of 1 year being 192 per 1,000. Although lower than the rate for Israel as a whole, it was very much higher than the rates in the United Kingdom and the United States at that period. Eighty percent of the hospitalization in infancy was for acute respiratory infections and gastroenteritis.

The basic cause of hospitalization was often a chronic disease which led to several episodes of hospitalization in a number of cases. The frequency of cases requiring long-term care was assessed to be 37 percent of the hospitalized men, 34 percent of the women aged 15 years and over, and 11 percent of the children. In the 1-year period of 1962 there were 253 such patients (112 men, 94 women, and 47 children) who were discharged from the three general hospitals and who lived in this area. Further study of this problem and the extent to which it was being met was therefore carried out.

A follow-up study was made of all patients living in Kiryat Harim who were hospitalized in the Hadassah University Hospital.[3] This investiga-

TABLE 26-1. Medical and Nursing Care One Year After Discharge From Hospital

AGE GROUP	TOTAL PATIENTS	NOT RECOVERED AND ASSESSED TO BE IN NEED OF CONTINUING CARE		NUMBER AND PERCENTAGE RECEIVING CARE OF THOSE IN NEED			
				By Physician		By Nurse	
		No.	Percent	No.	Percent	No.	Percent
0– 4	95	34	35.8	27	79.4	15	44.1
5–14	99	52	52.5	38	73.1	6	11.5
15–24	63	38	60.3	33	86.8	7	18.4
25–44	180	107	59.4	81	75.7	17	15.9
45–64	128	103	80.5	81	78.6	9	8.7
65 and over	36	30	83.3	24	80.0	5	16.7
Total	601	364	60.6	284	78.0	59	16.2

(From Kark and Hopp.[3])

TABLE 26-2. The Care Status of Adult Patients Followed-up One Year After Discharge from Hospital According to Length of Residence in the Country and Standard of Education

	IN NEED OF CONTINUING CARE		RECEIVING MEDICAL CARE
LENGTH OF RESIDENCE IN ISRAEL	No. of Patients	Percentage of Total Patients in Category	Percentage of Those in Need of Care
Recent immigrants (<5 years preceding hospitalization)	129	79	77
Immigrated 5 to 15 years preceding hospitalization	179	66	77
Born in Israel or immigrated more than 15 years preceding hospitalization	99	62	85
EDUCATION			
Less than 8 years of schooling	219	74	85
Nine years or more of schooling	178	61	76

(Adapted from Kark and Hopp.[3])

tion extended over a 2-year period, May 1963 to April 1965. Its objectives included assessment of the patients' progress at defined periods after hospital discharge with particular reference to their need for continuity of medical and nursing care, and whether those in need of care received it during the study period. Seven hundred and eighteen patients were originally included in this study. They were interviewed in hospital by a public health nurse on the staff of the Department of Social Medicine and were followed-up in their homes 6 weeks and again 1 year after discharge from hospital. At this latter time there were 601 patients seen. A considerable proportion of these patients were assessed to be in need of continuing care 1 year after being discharged (Table 26-1). This confirmed the findings of the earlier study. As expected, more older persons were in need of such care than were younger patients. Among the adult patients there was a larger proportion of recent immigrants and the less educated in need of care than there was of the patients who were more settled and more educated (Table 26-2). There were no differences according to sex, country of origin of immigrants, social class rated by occupation of head of household, marital status, family size, or crowding index. Also among children under age 15, none of these variables was found to be related to the need for care.

Of the patients considered to be in need of care there were no differences according to various personal and family characteristics in the proportion of those who were receiving medical care. Thus, social class, standard of education, and other variables, which might have been expected to have an important influence were not found to do so in this investigation. This should not be interpreted as relating to quality of medical care as no attempt was made to investigate this aspect of the problem of care. The investigation focused on the proportion of patients considered to be in need of care and, of these, what percentage were being attended by a doctor or nurse.

The proportion of those in need of care and who were receiving it from a physician was 78 percent as compared with only 16 percent who were receiving nursing care (Table 26-1).

Nursing Care

The lack of nursing care was an important gap in the service. Among the adults who did not have nursing care were cases with such conditions as malignant neoplasm, postcerebrovascular accident, and chronic heart disease. These patients were in need of direct nursing care, and the patients and their families were in need of the intensive education which can be provided by public health nurses trained in care of chronic sick patients at home. There were many patients who needed the advice and education which such family nurses can provide; they included men and women with a wide range of conditions beyond those already mentioned, such as psychosis and psychoneurosis, and eye disorders including glaucoma, cataract, and detached retina for which they had been treated in hospital. There were women who had had complications of pregnancy and childbirth, women with other gynecologic conditions, and patients with chronic lung disease, peptic ulcer, essential hypertension, chronic renal disease, chronic arthritis, and posttrauma.

TABLE 26-3

DIAGNOSIS	ADULTS	CHILDREN
Malignant neoplasm	3	1
Heart disease	59	1 (rheumatic heart disease)
Essential hypertension	2	—
Respiratory diseases	2 (chronic)	2 (recurrent severe acute upper respiratory infection
Digestive diseases	9 (3 peptic ulcer)	3 (recurrent gastroenteritis)
Inguinal hernia	3	1
Complications of pregnancy and other gynecological conditions	10	—
Posttrauma	3	1

Among the children who were not receiving nursing care were a number with recurrent gastroenteritis and bronchopneumonia, rheumatic fever with heart involvement, and chronic osteomyelitis.

A special study of the community nursing services as perceived by these patients indicated that the low use of nursing services was not only because they did not recognize their need for nursing care; it was also because a large proportion of the patients had little appreciation of the scope of nursing care and were not aware of the educational role of the nurse.[4] This was probably related to the fact that until recently the public health nurse's role had been predominantly associated with maternal and child health care.

Care by a Physician

While the situation with respect to physician care was much better than that regarding nursing, there were 22 percent of patients regarded as being in need of medical care who were not receiving it. They included a number of patients who were in need of active treatment as well as those who required continuing surveillance. There was no particular disease that was more neglected than others. Psychologic and social components of the illness or the patient's life situation as a whole were of importance. The diagnosis of the cases not under care at the time are illustrated in Table 26-3.[3]

At the 1-year follow-up the reasons given by the various patients for not attending medical care included the following: the patient did not feel the need because he "felt well," the patient had a feeling of hopelessness about recovery; the patient was dissatisfied with the care received; the patient lives alone, is disabled, and has nobody to take her to the doctor; there was no time to go for treatment; the patient was not given any instructions about care after discharge, or no suitable arrangements were made for continuity of care.

At that time, except for some special projects, the health care system of Israel did not ensure ongoing care and surveillance of patients discharged from hospital. The same is true for chronic disease in general. The system does not include primary or secondary preventive service as an integral part of the preventive or curative services. In a country in which hospital services are not area-oriented or regionalized in coordination with other health services, it is difficult, if not impossible, to ensure the development of such a program. In Jerusalem especially, where there are so many different agencies responsible for hospitalization, the need for community-based, long-term programs is imperative.

It was decided to test the feasibility of a community-based program in Kiryat Harim, which would ensure more continuity of care where needed.

THE COMMUNITY-BASED HOME CARE PROGRAM

This program was initiated in 1966 as a special part of a more broadly based project concerned with surveillance of long-term illness. It is directed toward the needs of the chronically sick and others with recurrent illness or any conditions requiring long-term care in the various neighborhoods served by the department's community health center in Kiryat Harim. These neighborhoods include the whole of the Kiryat Harim area with a population of approximately 20,000 persons.

General Objectives

1. To assess the care needs of patients and their families where there is long-term illness.
2. To assist in ensuring continuity of medical care and surveillance where required.
3. To help patients achieve the highest possible level of functioning within the limits of their conditions.

Specific Objectives

Case Finding. Identification of all index cases and their families by all available resources. Among the index conditions to be included in the first instance are the following:

Cardiovascular disease, e.g., coronary heart disease, cerebrovascular disease, peripheral vascular disease
Rheumatic fever and rheumatic heart disease
Severe anemias and other blood diseases, e.g., purpura
Chronic respiratory disease, e.g., chronic bronchitis, emphysema, bronchiectasis, asthma, tuberculosis
Chronic renal disease
Diabetes
Cancer (all types)
Arthritis, neurologic, surgical, and orthopedic conditions with marked physical disability
Other severe disabilities, e.g., blindness or other visual conditions
Selected mental diseases
Selected cases of recurrent illness such as recurrent abortion, gastrointestinal and respiratory infections.

The sources for case finding include hospitals and their outpatient departments, our departmental health center and its clinics, Kupat Holim clinics in the area, ministry of health—mental and chronic disease sections, and social welfare and voluntary health agencies.

Verification of diagnosis is achieved through comparison of reports of hospitals and other records, treating doctors, and special diagnostic clinics.

Registration of Cases and Maintenance of Records. Registration of cases and maintenance of records are aided by notification systems, card indexes, nurses' notebooks, and visual aids (e.g., wall pin maps).

Programming for Care Needs. Attempts are made to meet medical, nursing, and other care needs. Specific needs for certain diseases, e.g., diabetes, hypertension, atherosclerosis (Chapter 31), and rheumatic fever (Chapter 27), are also met. General medicine and nursing care are provided, as well as social case work, physiotherapy, occupational therapy, and special equipment. Consultation with experts in each field is also a part of the program.

Evaluation. Evaluations of the program as a whole and of patients' progress are conducted regularly.

Initiating the Project

At the time this special program was initiated there were already several services provided by the Department of Social Medicine that were concerned with the care needs of residents of Kiryat Harim with chronic disease or disability. These included the family practice, maternal and child health clinics, school health services, and old peoples' and diabetics' clubs. The various services provided needed coordination in order to obtain an overall community picture of the prevalence of chronic disease and the extent to which patients were being cared for.

The initial program of home-care included after-care of patients discharged from hospitals and care of home-bound patients. In the first instance the patients discharged from the Hadassah University Hospital were included and the system of patient identification and follow-up in hospital and home was worked out. Because of the large number of patients from Kiryat Harim who are admitted to this hospital, one nurse was assigned to part-time functions in the hospital and, with clerical help, she identified the area patients and obtained preliminary data about them. Their eligibility for home-care is then considered after she has visited the wards and seen the patient. Eligibility is based on disease and age categories, and degree of disability. The patients are then referred to the particular community nurse who is responsible for further care by herself as well as facilitating care by the family, or medical, welfare, educational, and other agencies.

The program was subsequently extended to Kiryat Harim patients discharged from other hospitals of Jerusalem, including patients discharged from mental hospitals.

Despite the obvious need for a service to care for home-bound patients, there is often very limited effective care provided by health service systems. The evidence of this gap in essential services in Kiryat Harim has been reviewed. In this Kiryat Harim was no exception. Thus, what seems to be a self-evident need is not necessarily seen to be so by various health agencies. About 2 years after the initiation of the program an evaluation study was undertaken.[5] The evaluation was based on a comparison between two groups of patients as assessed 3 months after their discharge from hospital. One group, namely the treatment group to which the after-care program was provided, consisted of all the patients from Kiryat Harim who were hospitalized in the Hadassah University Hospital over a 4-month period in 1968. The other group, the control group, included all the patients from a neighboring area of Jerusalem who had been admitted to the same hospital over the same period of time. No significant differences were found between the two groups of patients with respect to sex and age distribution, ethnic group, social class, or the disease categories for which the patients were treated in hospital; the proportions admitted to different major departments of the hospital were essentially the same. The details of the program being tested were as follows.

1. Each person was interviewed in hospital by a public health nurse as soon as possible after admission, to obtain information of relevance to the planning of the care program.
2. The physician on the team obtained details of the patients' diagnosis and prognosis. At the time of discharge the treating doctor was asked what his medical instructions were and his view on the patient's prognosis for return to his major activity.
3. The planning of the care program began soon after admission to hospital, especially in relation to referral to other services, e.g., social welfare. The program was finalized at the time of discharge and each program item was recorded together with the team's expectation of the outcome.
4. The program as recorded was conducted by the nurse and a routine interview was conducted 3 months after discharge, following a visit by the nurse to the patient's home where questions were asked about the patient's progress.
5. Following the interview, a reassessment was made of the needs for care and, if necessary, a further program was planned.

The patients living in the control area were not contacted during their stay in hospital so as not to influence their progress after discharge. The physician on the team obtained details of the prognosis and discharge instructions from the treating doctor at the time of discharge, using the same standard schedules as for the treatment group. The only contact with the members of the control group was 3 months after discharge when they were visited and interviewed.

Results. The differences were analyzed with respect to patients' compliance with discharge instructions, their feeling of well-being, return to major activities, and rehospitalization.

COMPLIANCE WITH DISCHARGE INSTRUCTIONS. Compliance with discharge instructions was measured for taking of drugs, adherence to diet, follow-up visit to the hospital, and visits to the treating community physician. Highly significant differences were found for all four areas in adult patients. Compared with the control group, a high proportion of adults of the treatment group complied with instructions in taking drugs prescribed (94 percent compliance versus 72 percent); in adherence to diet (91 percent versus 58 percent); in follow-up visit to hospital (93 percent versus 84 percent); and in recommended visits to community physician (66 percent versus 43 percent).

In contrast to the marked differences between the two groups of adult patients, there was a high rate of compliance for the children of both groups.

FEELING OF WELL-BEING. The feeling of well-being was measured by asking each patient to grade his own state of health at the 3-months-after-discharge visit. Significantly more patients of the treatment group rated themselves on the scale as "well" or "almost well" than did the control group.

Patients were also asked about the help they felt they needed and had received from other, i.e., nonmedical, agencies. The vast majority of the expressed needs were for social welfare assistance. Seventy-nine percent of the "treatment group" stated they had received the aid they needed, compared with only 20 percent of the control group.

RETURN TO MAJOR ACTIVITY. There were no significant differences in return to major activity between the two groups. Full return to major activity up to 3 months after discharge from hospital was recorded by 78 percent of patients in the treated group and 77 percent in the control group.

REHOSPITALIZATION. There was also little difference between the two groups with respect to rehospitalization. Thirteen percent of the "treatment" group and 11 percent of the "control" group were readmitted to hospital within the 3-month period following their discharge.

Summary and Inferences. The differences in compliance with instructions and in feeling of well-being or recovery from illness between the "treatment" and "control" groups was thought to be due to the after-care carried out by the public health nurses. The specific functions which seemed to be of importance included the following.

1. Educational—the nurses' explanations of the method of carrying out the instructions, such as taking of medicines and diet, as well as explaining the patient's condition.
2. Assistance—helping the patient and family to obtain satisfaction from other agencies when there was need.
3. Care and reassurance—interest in the patient and continuity of relationship with the patients and their families seem to have been important in the patient's feeling of well-being.

The fact that no differences in compliance were found between the children of the two groups is probably the result of several causes. First, the vast majority of children were admitted for acute illness and, second, adults in the family may tend to be more compliant in caring for their children than for themselves. Last, and perhaps most important, is the widespread distribution of maternal and child health centers in Israel as a whole. Both the treatment and control areas have such services. The public health nurses of these centers receive information on all pediatric cases in hospital and they review the problems of each case at regular meetings with hospital staff.

The absence of any difference between the two groups of adult patients with respect to return to major activities and rates of readmission to hospital suggests the need for further investigation. These investigations should include more refined measurements and differentiation between various disability groups of patients. One must also realize that there are many patients who recover without treatment and others who get worse even with it. Compliance with instructions may, therefore, not necessarily be associated with end-point results and there is need for differentiation of cases with varying prognosis in analysis of results of treatment.

Features of the Home-Bound Patients in Kiryat Harim

The program has been ongoing since its inception in 1966 and a considerable number of patients have been cared for. Children are not included in this special program which focuses its attention on long-term home-bound patients which, as expected, is much concerned with the elderly. It is reviewed at the Epidemiology-in-practice sessions of the Department of Social Medicine (Chap. 25). Features of the patients under active care at any one time are summarized in the figures for January 1971, given in Table 26-4.

TABLE 26-4

CATEGORIES OF HOME-BOUND PATIENTS	NO. OF PATIENTS
Total home-bound patients in care program during the month	80 (56 women, 24 men)
Age distribution	
<60	8
60–69	17
≥70	55
Length of time in program	
>1 year	56
<1 year	24
Status	
Bedridden	9
Chairbound	4
Homebound but neither of the above	66
Not essentially homebound	1

The distribution of patients in the program, according to an Index of Independence in Activities of Daily Living,[6] was as follows:

Independent in feeding, continence, transferring, going to toilet, dressing, and bathing (A)	41
Independent in all but one of these functions (B)	8
Independent in all but bathing and one additional function (C)	8
Independent in all but bathing, dressing, and one additional function (D)	3
Independent in all but bathing, dressing, going to toilet, and one additional function (E)	4
Independent in all but bathing, dressing, going to toilet, transferring, and one additional function (F)	5
Dependent in all six functions (G)	7
Dependent in at least two functions, but not classifiable as C, D, E, or F (other)	4

The expected age distribution led to further analysis of the use of medical services by older persons in the family practice of the Community Health Center in Kiryat Harim. Sixty-three percent of all persons 60 years and over attended the Center at least once during the month. The conditions for which they attend are analyzed and consideration given to ways of meeting their health needs beyond that of clinic and home-care. An older persons' club closely associated with the health center's activities has thus been formed.

In a city in which the hospital services are not regionalized, community-based services must of necessity carry considerable responsibility for continuity of care of hospitalized patients. This is true for the immediate after-care of patients discharged from various hospitals as well as for the patients with long-term disabilities. Close association with the various hospitals and the treating teams in these hospitals is needed but is difficult. However, it can be developed by an active public health nursing service based in the community which extends its service to the hospitals.

REFERENCES

1. Terespolsky LS, Yofe J: Epidemiological study of hospital admissions in a community of new immigrants. Brit J Prev Soc Med 19:30, 1965.
2. Kark E: A community study of hospitalization in Jerusalem, Israel. Med Care 5:401, 1967.
3. Kark E, Hopp C: A follow-up study of patients discharged from a Jerusalem hospital. Med Care 8:510, 1970.
4. Bergman R, Hellman G: Community nursing services as perceived by post-hospitalized patients. Am J Public Health 59:2168, 1969.
5. Epstein LM, Avni A, Hopp C, et al.: Evaluation of a program of after-care for patients discharged from hospital. Med Care 11:320, 1973.
6. Katz S, Ford AB, Moskowitz RW, et al.: Studies of illness in the aged. The index of ADL: A standardized measure of biological and psychosocial function. JAMA 185:914, 1963.

27

Infections in a Family Practice

Recording infectious illnesses in a medical practice was popularized by the ingenious and simple charts used by Pickles[1,2] in his rural practice among the villages of Wensleydale, Yorkshire, England. Using a Pickles-type chart and other more detailed records, the infectious illnesses in the family practice in Kiryat Harim are reviewed in the weekly Epidemiology-in-practice sessions. The review includes the daily incidence of new cases and discussion on the action which should be taken. The more common illnesses, and those against which we immunize, are recorded. The interest and importance given them in a practice will obviously vary in different communities. In this practice the absence of a record of new cases of tuberculosis and other important diseases is not due to a lack of interest in them. It is in fact a reflection of the absence of these diseases.

THE COMMUNITY PROGRAM

Objectives

The objectives of the recording and the weekly conferences about infectious illnesses include (1) ongoing description of the occurrence of infectious illnesses in the practice and their differential distribution; (2) early recognition of an epidemic; (3) expression and biologic gradient of infections, with measure of severity of illness; (4) prediction of changes in demand on service; (5) detection of diseases that are the later effects of an infectious illness; and (6) evaluation of immunization programs.

Methods

Each doctor in the family practice has a set of "contact sheets" (Appendix A) on his consulting room desk. He completes one of these for each patient he sees. The information listed includes data on diagnosis, date of onset of the illness, and, in the case of a respiratory infection, a list of symptoms and signs. This contact sheet also includes demographic data on the patient.

As far as possible, diagnoses are made in terms of the International Classification of Diseases. A list of the infectious diseases of relevance to this practice is available in each doctor's office. A partial list is given in Table 27-1.

Data Processing. All contact sheets are checked daily for completeness and accuracy by the family physician responsible for the program. Any doubtful recordings are thus discussed with the physician involved while the case is still fresh in his mind. The checked contact sheets are then processed by the records office as follows.

1. All infectious illnesses are charted by day of onset, and classified according to diagnosis. The data are then transferred to a Pickles-type chart

TABLE 27-1

INTERNATIONAL LIST NUMBER (After 8th Revision)	DISEASE
001–003	Typhoid fever, paratyphoid fever, and salmonella infections
004	Bacillary dysentery
006	Amoebiasis
005–007	Other intestinal infectious diseases
008–009	Enteritis and other diarrhoeal diseases
032	Diphtheria
033	Whooping cough
034	Streptococcal sore throat and scarlet fever
035	Erysipelas
052	Chickenpox
055	Measles
056	Rubella
070	Infectious hepatitis
072	Mumps
079	Other viral disease (i.e., viral infection unspecified)
120–129	Helminthiases
360–369	Inflammatory diseases of the eye
460–465	Acute (upper) respiratory infections
466	Acute bronchitis and bronchiolitis
470–474	Influenza
480–486	Pneumonia
680–686	Infections of skin and subcutaneous tissue

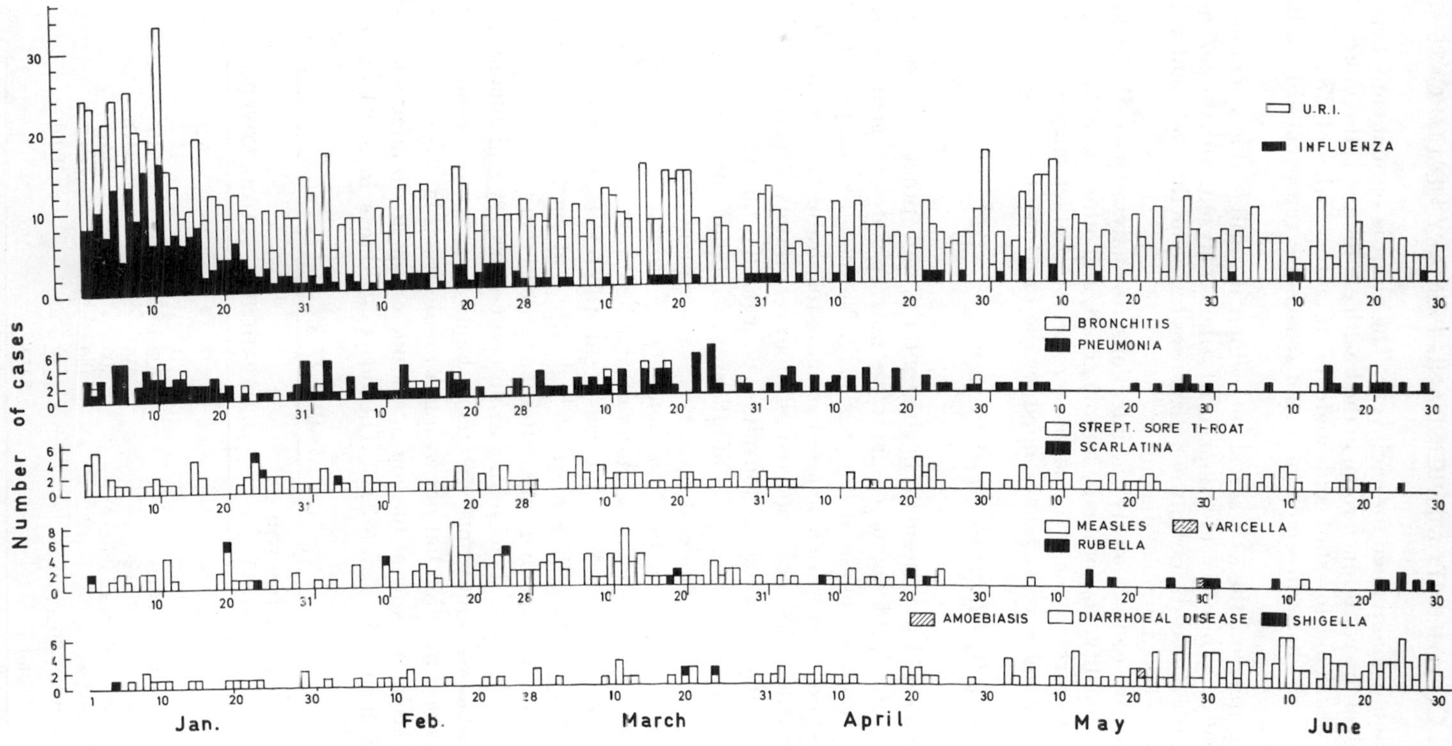

FIG. 27-1. Infectious illnesses diagnosed in a family practice, January–June 1972. This Pickles-type chart is maintained as a wall-chart, with each disease shown in a different color.

which is maintained for each year. The chart is permanently kept on a wall of the conference room in the health center and is therefore a readily visual aid for staff and students. (Figures 27-1 and 27-2 illustrate the wall-charts in which various diseases are represented by different colors.)

2. The data on the contact sheet, which describes the symptoms and signs of respiratory infections, are further analyzed, with the goal of testing the concordance between diagnoses based on this coded information and detailed clinical diagnoses.
3. From the contact sheets, the infections are analyzed periodically by age, sex, locality, size of family, ethnic group, and other variables of interest by cross-reference of the case record on the contact sheet with the basic demographic record maintained for the families of the practice.

The Epidemiological Picture

In four housing projects of the health center's family practice (2,463 persons) there were 3,114 doctor contacts for new episodes of acute infectious illnesses in the course of the year 1970. No less than 66 percent (2,062) of these contacts were diagnosed as acute respiratory infections, of which 51 percent (1,053) were reported as upper respiratory infection (URI) only; 25 percent (520) as acute tonsillitis, pharyngitis, laryngitis or tracheitis; and 24 percent (489) as cases of influenza, which occurred in an epidemic. The only other common diagnoses were gastroenteritic conditions in 339 cases, 11 percent of the total contacts recorded. Of these, 87 percent (298) had a nonspecific diagnosis of diarrheal disease, mainly in infants and children. There were no consistent differences between the sexes, other than a generally somewhat higher use of service by adult women than men. As expected, age differences were marked, as shown by the figures in Table 27-2 comparing combined respiratory and influenzal infections with gastrointestinal infections. Family size was associated with the respiratory infection but not with gastroenteritis (Fig. 27-3).

The immediacy of turning to the doctor for acute infection is shown by the figures in Table 27-3. The onset of illness in 3,114 episodes of

TABLE 27-3

TIME OF DOCTOR CONTACT	NO. OF PATIENTS	CUMULATIVE (%)
1st day of illness	193	6.2
2nd day of illness	1151	43.2
3rd day of illness	826	69.7
4th day of illness	454	84.3
5th–7th day of illness	300	93.9
2nd week	180	99.7
3rd week	10	100.0
Total	3114	

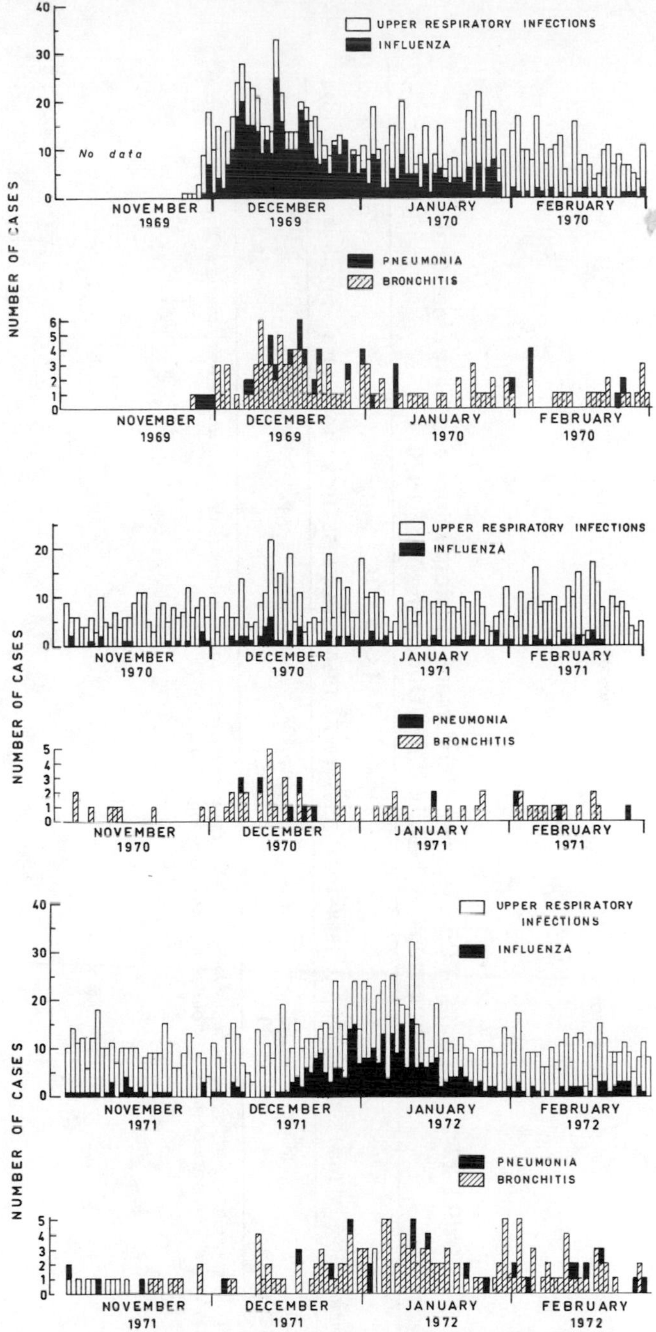

FIG. 27-2. Acute respiratory illnesses treated in a family practice during three successive winter seasons: November 1969–February 1970, November 1970–February 1971, and November 1971–February 1972.

TABLE 27-2. The Rate of Contacts per 100 Persons for Respiratory and Gastrointestinal Infections by Year of Birth, During the Year 1970

		YEAR OF BIRTH							
Infection	**Total**	**1970**	**1968–1969**	**1965–1967**	**1960–1964**	**1955–1959**	**1945–1954**	**1925–1944**	**1905–1924**
Respiratory	108	265	361	181	151	63	72	66	41
Gastrointestinal	14	39	33	16	14	8	6	11	9

When these data were analyzed by size of family there was a direct positive correlation between size of family and rate of infectious illness diagnosed as respiratory infection. This was not so for gastrointestinal infections (Fig. 27-3).

illness is seen in relation to attendance at the clinic or calling a doctor at home.

Influenza. Through the daily recording of infectious diseases early recognition of an epidemic becomes possible. In the early winter of 1969–1970 a number of cases were seen which were recognized to be clinical influenza by the family physicians. The criteria used for clinical diagnosis of influenza were then decided upon by the doctors of the family practice, and were as follows: patient suffers from acute malaise and fever, sore throat, and body pains (myalgia, joint pains, and abdominal pains). He may or may not show other signs of respiratory infection. There were 13 such cases recorded over the period October 22nd through November 28th, at which time there was a sudden rise in incidence of cases seen in the practice (Fig. 27-4). This epidemic was part of a countrywide epidemic of influenza, in which both A2 Hong Kong virus and B virus were reported by the Ministry of Health's epidemiology unit in December 1969.

Including the early cases, the period of the epidemic was 18 weeks, from October 22, 1969 to February 21, 1970, during which time there was a total of 467 cases of influenza and 596 cases diagnosed as upper respiratory infection only (URI). Of the 467 cases of influenza, 434 occurred from week 7 to week 15 (November 30, 1969 to January 31, 1970). Figure 27-4 shows the decline in number of diagnoses of URI as the epidemic of influenza dominates the epidemiologic picture and then an increase of URI as the epidemic of influenza abates. This trend was characteristic

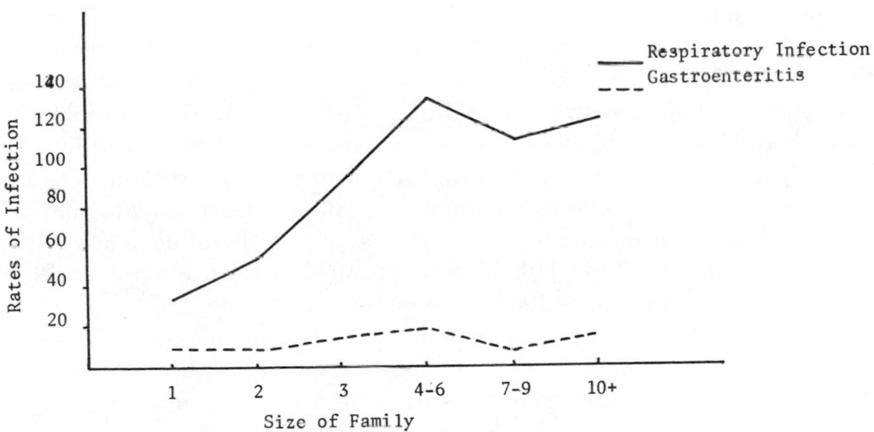

FIG. 27-3. Rates of diagnosed infectious illnesses per 100 persons in the year 1970, by size of family.

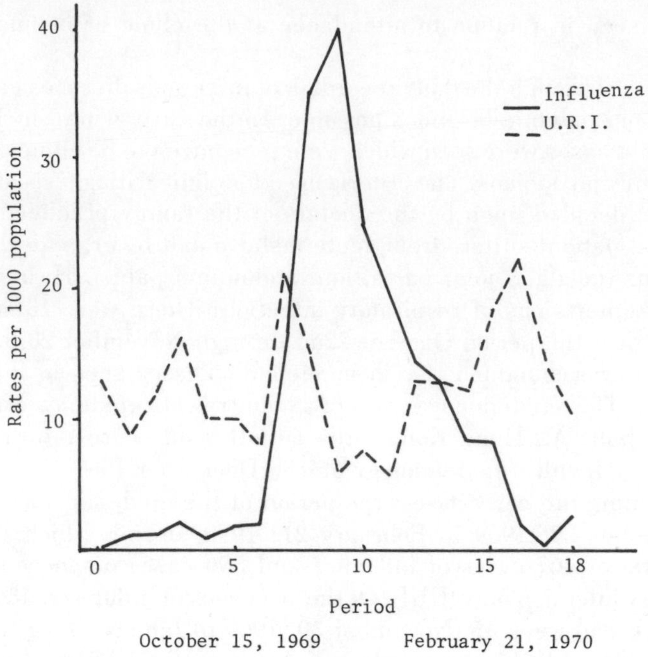

FIG. 27-4. Rates of diagnosed cases of influenza and URI per 1,000 of the family practice population. Kiryat Harim Health Center, October 15, 1969 to February 21, 1970.

of the population as a whole, but when analyzed for age groups there were two age groups which differed from the rest of the population. In those born between 1965 and 1969, the rates of URI were very high, higher than the rates of influenza, even during the epidemic (Fig. 27-5A). In those born before 1900, there was a comparatively low rate of influenza throughout the epidemic (Fig. 27-5B). Fifty percent of these older persons who had influenza developed complications, bronchitis or pneumonia, as compared to much lower rates of complications in the other age groups (those born from 1900 to 1919, 15 percent; 1920 to 1949, 5 percent; 1950 to 1954, 4.6 percent; 1955 to 1964, 6.5 percent; and 1965 to 1969, 2 percent).

The severity of the illness can be measured by the incidence of acute bronchitis and pneumonia during the epidemic. The contrast between the daily occurrence of these conditions over the same season, namely November through February, is shown for three successive years, in two of which epidemics of influenza occurred (Fig. 27-2).

At the Epidemiology-in-practice sessions the need for influenza immunization and early treatment of cases was discussed. Two aspects of immunization were emphasized. The first aspect emphasized the desir-

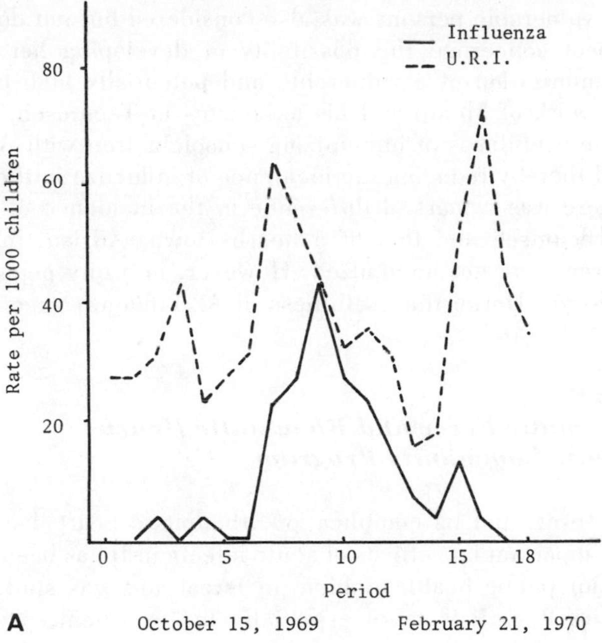

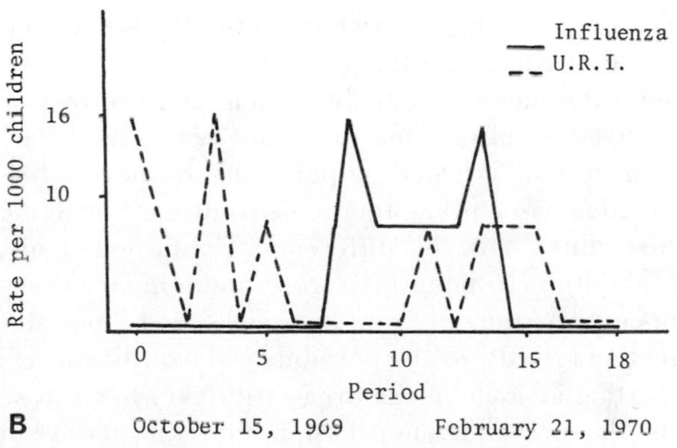

FIG. 27-5. A: Rates of diagnosed cases of influenza and URI per 1,000 of children born in 1965–1969. B: Rates of diagnosed cases of influenza and URI per 1,000 of the cohort born before 1900.

ability of immunizing elderly and chronically sick persons as well as those who were heavily exposed to infection. This was done with polyvalent vaccine available at that time, which did not include A2 influenza vaccine. The possibilities of using the drug amantidine in the early treatment of these more vulnerable persons was also considered but not done.[3,11] The second aspect concerned the possibility of developing herd immunity through immunization of a vulnerable and potentially high transmitting group. The work of Monto and his associates in Tecumseh, Michigan,[3] indicated the usefulness of immunizing schoolchildren with A2 influenza vaccine and thereby reducing the incidence of influenza in the total community. There was a marked difference in the incidence of respiratory illness in Tecumseh and that of a nearby town, Adrian, in which the schoolchildren were not immunized. However, in a city population such as that of Kiryat Harim the usefulness of A2 influenza vaccine requires testing.

Rheumatic Fever and Rheumatic Heart Disease Community Program

Rheumatic fever, and its complication, rheumatic heart disease, is one of the most important late effects of acute infection. It has been considered to be a major public health problem in Isreal and was studied in some detail (Figure 27-6),[12,13] more especially in Jerusalem, where special hospital provision for care of such cases was made and a Voluntary Rheumatic Fever Society was established to promote the well-being of cases and their families. This society influenced the authorities to house a number of families in new homes which were built in the 1950s in the newly developing neighborhood of Kiryat Harim.

A marked difference between Jerusalem and the rest of the country has been perceived by physicians for many years. In the period of 1967 to 1969, the registers maintained by public health nurses for all "known" cases of rheumatic fever and rheumatic heart disease in elementary school children of the country show this difference. Confirmed or suspected cases in Jerusalem children (16 per 1,000) were much higher than in any other district of the country, ranging from between 2 and 7 per 1,000 in various places. A question raised was the possibility of overdiagnosis in Jerusalem and underreporting in some of the areas with very low rates.

Owing to the prevailing impression that there were high rates of rheumatic fever and rheumatic heart disease, a special program was instituted by our health center in 1959 for detection, for primary and secondary prevention, and treatment of cases in Kiryat Harim.

Since the first prophylactic trials it has been repeatedly demonstrated that the initial attack rate of rheumatic fever can be reduced if the preceding streptococcal infection is effectively treated with penicillin for 10 days in doses sufficient to eradicate the streptococcus.[14–16] This is thought to be true even if treatment is started after the acute infection has subsided

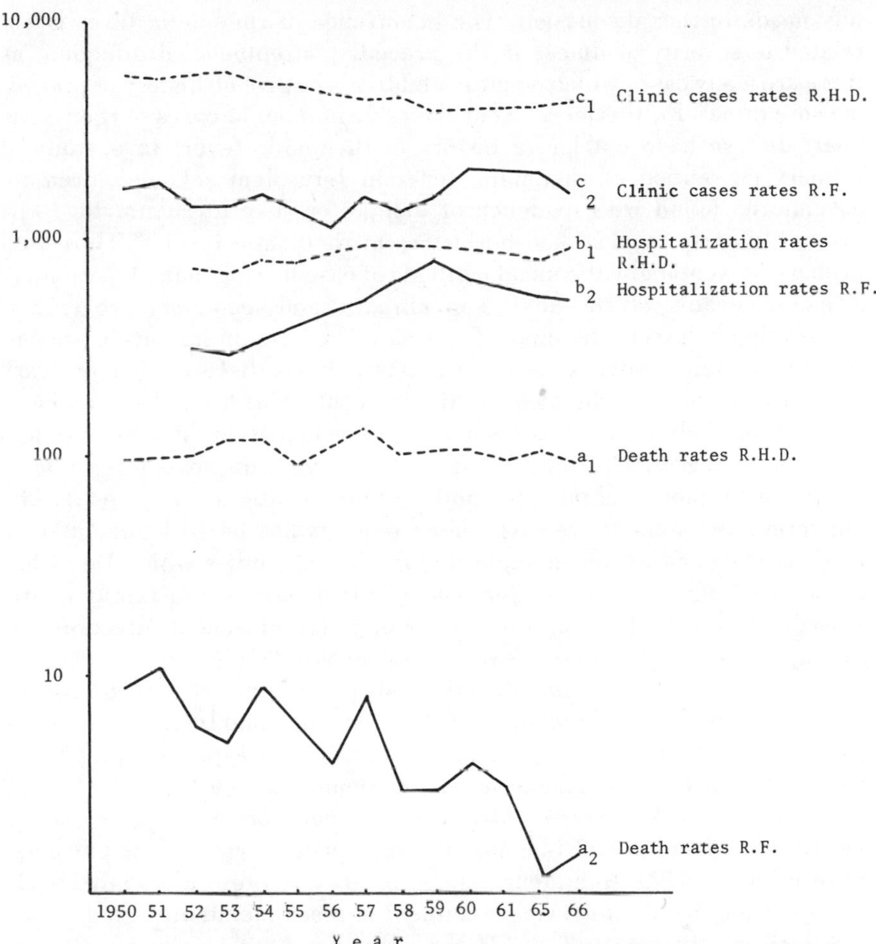

FIG. 27-6. Rheumatic fever (RF) and rheumatic heart disease (RH)—frequency of diagnosis in Jews of Israel, 1950–1966. (Adapted from Cohen.[12,13])

and patients are free of symptoms, since the latent period for rheumatic fever following the preceding streptococcal infection varies considerably. Fifty percent of 127 cases of rheumatic fever studied by Rammelkamp and Stolzer had a latent period between almost 3 and 5 weeks or more.[17,18]

While primary prevention of this kind is now a well-established procedure, and prophylactic care of known rheumatic patients is also generally accepted, the contribution which such programs can make to the overall attack rates of rheumatic fever and rheumatic heart disease in the community needs further discussion. The occurrence of rheumatic fever is not related to severity of illness in the preceding streptococcal infection, as there are many cases which occur in children who give no history of preceding sore throat. Furthermore, a considerable number of cases of rheumatic heart disease have not had a history of rheumatic fever. In a study of primary prevention of rheumatic fever in Jerusalem schoolchildren, of 56 children found with evidence of definite or suspect rheumatic heart disease, no less than 28 had no history of rheumatic fever.[19] Thus both primary prevention by the usual methods of case finding, namely attending a doctor because of an "acute sore throat," and secondary prevention, namely prophylaxis of rheumatic fever patients, have limitations in preventing the overall incidence rate of rheumatic heart disease. Primary care physicians or nurses who have continuing contact with families in a community are likely to overcome some of these limitations if they maintain community registers of individuals and families who are susceptible to recurring streptococcal infection and acute rheumatic fever episodes. The clustering of rheumatic fever in some families has been documented in many studies and has been supported in clinical studies which Davis has presented from his clinic in Jerusalem.[20] Paul introduced family charts in order to record the pattern of spread of streptococcal infection and the occurrence of rheumatic fever in households.[21]

The Program. The specific objectives of the program at present are: (1) primary prevention of rheumatic fever by detection and treatment of acute β-hemolytic streptococcal type A illness, and (2) care, especially prophylactic care, of cases of rheumatic fever and rheumatic heart disease.

PRIMARY PREVENTION. All cases with acute sore throat have a throat swab taken for culture of β-hemolytic streptococcus type A. The physician may order penicillin treatment before results of culture are available. In all positive cases the following treatment is recommended:

Infancy (1st year)—3 × 125 mg penicillin V oral daily for 10 days
Over one year of age—6 × 125 mg penicillin V oral daily for 10 days

In cases of penicillin sensitivity, erythromycin is used.

Children—50 mg per kg body weight per day for 10 days
Adults—4 × 250 mg per day for 10 days

Family contacts of cases are requested to have throat swabs taken for culture.

SECONDARY PREVENTION. Secondary prevention relates to prophylactic care of cases known to have had an episode of rheumatic fever or who have rheumatic heart disease.

Prophylaxis:
(1) Penicillin V 2 × 125 mg per day, or if penicillin sensitive, erythromycin 250 mg per day or
(2) Penicillin G injection 1.2 million units monthly for children, and every 3 weeks for adults

Cases requiring prophylaxis: (1) Every individual who had an episode of rheumatic fever or probable rheumatic fever should receive prophylaxis to age 18 years, or at least 5 years after the last episode
(2) Every patient with inactive rheumatic heart disease should receive prophylaxis to age 18 years or at least 5 years after the last episode.

REPORTING AND REVIEW OF PROGRAM. The program is reviewed at regular intervals at the Epidemiology-in-practice sessions. The review is based upon a report, which is abstracted from data of registers maintained for all cases and for cases requiring prophylaxis. There is one physician responsible for ensuring that the program is carried out. He maintains a register of all cases, which includes the following data:

1. Family and first name, date of birth, sex, country of birth, address, year of first diagnosis of rheumatic fever or year when first treated at the community health center.
2. Diagnosis: rheumatic fever, with signs according to Jones' criteria,[22] extracted from the patient's file as well as diagnosis of rheumatic heart disease and indications for prophylaxis.

In addition, he has a register of cases needing prophylaxis. This register is kept in the pharmacy of the health center, ensuring a check by the pharmacist of issues of prophylactic penicillin to individual cases. This enables the physician or nurse responsible to review compliance with the program.

Copies of the records used in the case register, the prophylaxis register, and the regular report of the program appear in the appendixes to this chapter.

A feature of the program at present is the fact that there have been no new cases of acute rheumatic fever or rheumatic heart disease for some time and recurrences are very rare. The program is being continued with less frequent reviews of its progress. Originally it was reviewed at monthly intervals. In 1971 this was changed to bi-monthly intervals. If the present favorable trend continues, quarterly reviews at the Epidemiology-in-practice sessions will suffice to ensure that the program is being effectively carried out.

Immunization

By examining the record of infectious illnesses in the practice it is possible to obtain a picture of the incidence of those diseases against which the community has been immunized. In the past two years the number of such cases has been negligible. There were only two cases of measles and none of the other conditions, e.g., diptheria, whooping cough, and poliomyelitis. The Ministry of Health has outlined a program of immunization for the country as a whole and this is carried out also by the Health Center in the Kiryat Harim area. The target population of this program comprises all children up to the age of 14 years. There are two parts to the program, one directed to children aged 0 to 2 years, and the other to elementary school children, aged 6 to 14.

Program for Children Aged 0 to 2 Years. There are two basic sources from which information on the target population is obtained: (1) The health center receives information from the hospitals of Jerusalem about all babies delivered by women who live in Kiryat Harim. It also receives confirmatory information from another source. The District Health Office of Jerusalem sends to all maternal and child health centers immunization booklets with a list of all new babies in the areas they serve. (2) A further source of information is the public health nurse of the health center itself who may know of pregnant women in the area who were delivered elsewhere and about whom the center has not received any information.

The information received is maintained in a general register at the health center, from which each nurse receives a list of all births belonging to her area. These she lists in her own special field book, which provides for the following data on each baby: number of the family's file at the health center, name of baby, date of birth, sex, and address. On the same printed page provision is made for the nurse to record the immunizations each baby is given.

The immunizations and the age at which they are recommended to be given to this group of children are listed below.[23]

2 months—oral polio
3 months—triple vaccine (diptheria, pertussis, and tetanus)
4 months—2nd oral polio and 2nd triple vaccine
5 months—3rd triple vaccine
6 months—3rd oral polio
13 months—4th oral polio and oral measles
15 months—smallpox vaccination
18 months—booster triple vaccine

The procedure is for each public health nurse to maintain ongoing surveillance of all newborns in her area. She checks whether the baby has been brought to the clinic within the first month and if not she invites the mother to do so. As part of the first examination and consultation, the mother is given the Ministry of Health booklet for the child's record of immunizations. The booklet makes provision for recording the immunizations listed above and additional procedures such as BCG vaccination. In addition it provides for recording of findings on tuberculin testing, blood group, and administration of transfusions and serum. The mother keeps this booklet and brings it to the clinic each time the baby is due for immunization, where the nurse records what was done. Mothers who do not attend at the required time are invited by the nurse by telephone, letter, or personal contact on a home visit.

Programs for Children Aged 6 to 14 Years. This program is conducted in the public schools by the nurse responsible for the school. The procedure is to inform parents that children will be immunized on a certain day at school and to ask them to indicate if they have any objection. The children are then immunized on the specified day. This is recorded in the immunization booklet which the children were asked to bring with them on that day. Absentees are followed-up by the nurse who then immunizes them. The immunizations given to this age group are the following.

Grade 1 (age 6 years) —booster: diptheria and tetanus
Grade 2 (age 7 years) —smallpox revaccination
Grade 7 (age 13 years) —Mantoux tuberculin test: if negative, BCG is given
Grade 8 (age 14 years) —tetanus booster

The immunization against rubella is under review. A decision has been made to immunize all 12-year-old girls.

Review of the Program. The program is reviewed once a year at an Epidemiology-in-practice session. There are two aspects to this review, the extent to which the immunization program itself has been carried out, and the incidence of cases of the relevant diseases.

Table 27-4 lists the figures for those babies (total: 502) who should have completed their schedule of immunizations by the end of 1970. The

TABLE 27-4. The Percentage of 502 Babies Who Completed the Required Immunizations by the End of 1970

VACCINATION	TYPE	PERCENTAGE OF CHILDREN IMMUNIZED
Triple vaccine (diptheria, pertussis, and tetanus)	Basic	100.0
	Booster	99.8 (one child had not yet received his booster dose)
Smallpox		96.6 (17 children not recorded as vaccinated)
Poliomyelitis	Basic	100.0
	Booster	95.8 (21 children had not yet received booster)
Measles		98.4 (eight not recorded as having had oral measles vaccine)

reason the program is reviewed annually, and not more frequently, is because of the very high rate of immunization which continues to be maintained. The annual review is to ensure that what we think is happening is in fact happening.

REFERENCES

1. Pickles WN: Epidemiology in Country Practice. Bristol, John Wright, 1939.
2. Pemberton J: Will Pickles of Wensleydale: The Life of a Country Doctor. London, Geoffrey Bles, 1970.
3. Monto AS, Davenport FM, Napier, JA, et al.: Effect of vaccination of a school-age population upon the course of an A2/Hong Kong influenza epidemic. Bull WHO 41:537, 1969.
4. Hornick RB, Togo Y, Mahler S, et al.: Evaluation of amantadine hydrochloride in the treatment of A2 influenzal disease. Bull WHO 41:671, 1969.
5. Dawkins AT, Gallager LR, Togo Y, et al.: Studies on induced influenza in man. II. Double-blind study designed to assess the prophylactic efficacy of an analogue of amantadine hydrochloride. JAMA 203:1095, 1968.
6. Finklea JF, Hennessy AV, Davenport FM: A field trial of amantadine prophylaxis in naturally-occurring acute respiratory illness. Am J Epidemiol 85:403, 1967.
7. Galbraith AW, Oxford JS, Schild GC, et al.: Protective effect of l-adamantanamine hydrochloride on influenza A2 infections in the family environment. Lancet 2:1026, 1969.
8. Togo Y, Hornick RB, Dawkins AT Jr: Studies on induced influenza in man. I. Double-blind studies designed to assess prophylactic efficacy of amantadine hydrochloride against A2/Rockville/1/65 strain. JAMA 203:1089, 1968.
9. Togo Y, Hornick RB, Felitti VJ, et al.: Evaluation of therapeutic efficacy of amantadine in patients with naturally occurring A2 influenza. JAMA 211: 1149, 1970.
10. Wingfield WI, Pollack D, Grunert R: Therapeutic efficacy of amantadine HCl and rimantadine HCl in naturally occurring influenza A2 respiratory illness in man. New Engl J Med 281:579, 1969.
11. Galbraith AW, Oxford JS, Schild GC et al.: Amantadine treatment in influenza A2/Hong Kong infection. Lancet 2:113, 1971.
12. Cohen J: Rheumatic fever and rheumatic heart disease. Problems of incidence, seriousness, and prevention in Israel (in Hebrew). Harefuah 45: 243, 1963.
13. Cohen J: Rheumatic fever and rheumatic heart disease (RF, RHD). Follow-up in elementary schools 1967–1969. Briuth Hatsibur year 13: 2:93, 1970.
14. Denny FS Jr, Wannamaker LW, Brink WR, et al.: Prevention of rheumatic fever. Treatment of the preceding streptococcal infection. JAMA 143:151, 1950.
15. Wannamaker LW, Rammelkamp CH Jr, Denny FW Jr, et al.: Prophylaxis of acute rheumatic fever by treatment of the preceding streptococcal infection with various amounts of depot penicillin. Am J Med 10:673, 1951.
16. Catanzaro FJ, Stetson CA, Morris AJ, et al.: The role of the streptococcus in the pathogenesis of rheumatic fever. Am J Med 17:749, 1954.

17. Rammelkamp CH Jr, Stolzer BL: The latent period before the onset of acute rheumatic fever. Yale J Biol Med 34:386, 1961/1962.
18. Rammelkamp CH Jr: Streptococcal infections. In Sartwell PE (ed.) Maxcy-Rosenau Preventive Medicine and Public Health, 9th ed. New York, Appleton, 1965.
19. Halfon ST, Brand-Auraban A, Szabo AM, et al.: Primary prevention of rheumatic fever in Jerusalem schoolchildren. III. Screening for heart disease by means of the PhonoCardioScan. Isr J Med Sci 6:584, 1970.
20. Davis E: Rheumatic Fever: Clinical, Ecological, and Familial Aspects. Springfield, Ill, Thomas, 1969.
21. Paul JR: Clinical Epidemiology. Chicago, Univ of Chicago Press, 1958.
22. Report of the Committee on Standards and Criteria for Programs of Care: Jones Criteria (modified) for guidance in the diagnosis of rheumatic fever. Circulation 13:617, 1956.
23. Department of Epidemiology, Ministry of Health: Immunization Manual. Translated into English from the Hebrew version. Jerusalem, 1971.

APPENDIX A

Physicians' Contact Sheet

(size of original: 15 × 10 cms)

Name ....

Address ....

Date of birth .... Sex M/F ....

If not resident of family practice area patient is: welfare case/personnel/other

Name of physician .... Date ....

Place of contact: Clinic/Home

Contact: New case (episode of illness)/reattendance (for same episode)

Routine mother and child health session

For certificate only

Diagnosis: ....

Date of onset of symptoms ....
(only for new contact for infectious illness)

In cases of acute diseases of the respiratory system please indicate:

Positive (+) or negative (−) next to each of the following:

	Signs of lower respiratory infection
	Stuffy or running nose
	Pyrexia or history of fever
	Myalgia
	Prostration
	Signs or symptoms of acute throat infection
	Follicles on tonsils
	Signs of otitis media
	Signs of sinusitis
	Evidence of tracheitis

APPENDIX B

The Rheumatic Fever and Rheumatic Heart Disease Program in Kiryat Harim

Copies of records used in the case register, the prophylaxis register, and the regular report of this program.

Extract from Prophylaxis Register, Department of Social Medicine, Community Health Center

Prophylaxis taken +
Prophylaxis not taken –

SURNAME	NAME	YEAR OF BIRTH	ONSET OF DISEASE	ADDRESS	1971 Feb	Mar	Apr
Angel	Orit	1961	1968	Olim 4	–	+	+
Bucher	Sh.	1954	1961	Amidar 5	–	–	+
Bonim	Dani	1961	1964	Olim 18	+	+	+
Cohen	Moshe	1953	1964	Amidar 4	+	+	+
Deutsch	Roni	1960	1966	Olim 3	–	–	+

APPENDIX C

Prophylactic Card

Clinic No. ________

Surname: Cohen   Name: Moshe   Age: 1953   Sex: M

Address: Amidar 6

Diagnosis: RF and RHD

Treatment advised: Durabiotic (Penicillin G)   Dose: 2 tabs per day

Changes in treatment: Rafapen (Penicillin V)

NO.	DATE	TREATMENT	SIGNATURE	REMARKS
1	8. 6.1970	60 Penicillin G Tab.		
2	5.10.1970	60 Penicillin G Tab.		
3	25.12.1970	60 Penicillin V Tab		
4	29. 1.1971	60 Penicillin V Tab		
5	5. 2.1971	60 Penicillin V Tab		
6	2. 3.1971	60 Penicillin V Tab		
7	2. 4.1971	60 Penicillin V Tab		
8	3. 5.1971	60 Penicillin V Tab		

APPENDIX D

Rheumatic Disease and Streptococcal Infections Program

Monthly Report

Month November 1971

(A) Rheumatic disease (cases with history of rheumatic fever and/or rheumatic heart disease)

1. No. of cases on register at end of month 65
2. No. of new cases during month 0 (detailed case reports overleaf)
3. No. of recurrences during month 1 (detailed case reports overleaf)
4. No. of cases requiring prophylaxis 18[1]
5. No. receiving prophylaxis during month:

   Rafapen (oral) 12

   Durabiotic (inj.) ____

   Sulphodiazine (oral) ____

   Erythromycin (oral) ____

6. No. requiring prophylaxis but not receiving it during month 6 (2)

   Of these, no. with recorded contact with Health Center during month 1

7. No. of rheumatic patients with acute throat infections during month:

					PROPHYLAXIS			
			TREATMENT			Not Received		
DIAGNOSIS	SWAB	NO.	Adeq.	Inadeq.	Received	Required	Not Required	?
Follicular tonsillitis	Pos.							
	Neg.							
	?Result							
	Not done	1				1		
	Total	1						
Other acute throat infections	Pos.							
	Neg.	1	1		1			
	?Result							
	Not done	1	1		1			
	Total	2	2		2	1		

(1) There was an additional case whose last episode was in January 1971 (information from another physician).

(2) One patient left Jerusalem for a short time after subacute bacterial endocarditis.

(B) Streptococcal throat infections

1. No. of new episodes of throat infection during month

DIAGNOSIS	NO.	SWAB			
		Pos.	Neg.	?Result	Not done
Follicular tonsillitis	38	2	14		22
Other acute throat infections	118	1	50		67
Total	156	3	64		89

2. Treatment of cases with positive swabs:

   Adequate 3 Inadequate 0 ? 0

3. Investigation of family contacts of cases with positive swabs.

   No. of family contacts 10

   No. swabbed 10

   Results of swabs: Pos. 0

   Neg. 10

   ? 0

28

The 28th Day Review —Progress Through Pregnancy to the 28th Day After Birth

There has been a considerable decline in infant mortality rates in Israel from 1950 to 1970. In the Jewish population the decline has been from 46.2 to 18.9 per 1,000 livebirths. In the Arab and other minority groups it declined from 62.5 in 1955 to 38.1 in 1970. The favorable changes in Israel are as good, and often better, than in many other countries. However, when compared with advanced countries such as the Netherlands and Sweden, which have high infant survival rates, Israel still has much preventable waste of life. The slope of the secular decline in Israel has also been relatively good, but there are other places such as Japan and Finland where the decline has been steeper, as shown in Table 28-1.

The decline in Israel is mainly a result of the sharp drop in infant deaths from gastroenteritis, pneumonia, and acute bronchitis. Associated with this has been the differential decline in mortality at different ages in the first year, the most marked changes having taken place in the postneonatal period (21.9 to 5.1). The net effect has been that 75 percent of all infant deaths in 1970 occurred as stillbirths or in the first week of life and 72 percent of all infant deaths took place during the first month. For this reason we are focusing these reviews on pregnancy, the perinatal, and neonatal periods. Infancy as a whole is reviewed in the PROD program in Chapter 30.

The "28th day" report is a review of progress of pregnancy and its outcome until approximately one month after birth. The objective of these reviews is surveillance of health of a specific population group of the community. It includes analysis of the state of health of women during pregnancy and delivery, and of their babies at birth until approximately 28

TABLE 28-1. The Decline in Infant Mortality Rates per 1000 Live Births in Several Countries

	INFANT MORTALITY RATE 1951–1955	1966–1967	DECREASE IN RATE	PERCENTAGE DECREASE
Israel	36.2	21.2	15.0	41.4
Sweden	19.3	12.7	6.6	34.2
Netherlands	22.1	14.1	8.0	36.2
Japan	48.5	17.1	31.4	64.7
Finland	32.4	14.9	17.5	54.0

days old. It is a continuing surveillance of a population for whom there is a special service, part of a highly developed health service system directed toward promoting maternal and child health. In this community the maternal and child health centers are part of the program of the health center which has been described in Chapter 25.

METHOD OF DATA GATHERING

There are two main sources for the information that is needed for this review, the prenatal and postnatal records of the maternal and child health clinics of the health center, and a report from the hospital in which the delivery took place. Notifications of deliveries by women living in the area are sent by each hospital to the records unit of the health center. These notifications include summary information on the course of labor and the state of mother and baby after delivery. At regular intervals the case reports of the health center with respect to these mothers and their babies are summarized together with the hospital information on a special record card. Appendix A is a reproduction of the record card used for this purpose.

These records are analyzed with the goal of classifying pregnancy, delivery, state of the new-born at birth, and the neonate (first 28 days) within one of the following categories:

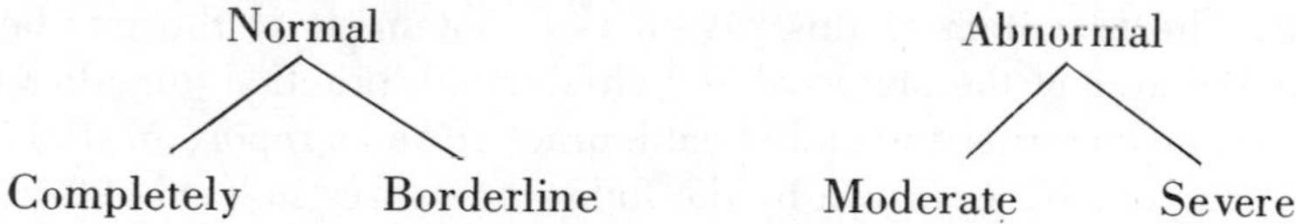

Criteria for the classification were determined following a series of pretests of their application to cases. The general guide is stated as follows:

Normal (N): Well, physically and emotionally.

Borderline normal (BN): Any condition which in itself is not normal, but is considered generally to have no unfavorable consequences for the future state of health, functional capacity, or social adjustment of mother or child, and to require no special treatment or follow-up.
Abnormal: Severe (SA): Any condition which in general or in the specific case is considered to constitute serious danger to the life or the functional capacity of mother or child, or an increased risk of congenital abnormalities or premature birth.
Moderate (MA): All other conditions.

The diagnoses relating to pregnancy are listed separately for specific disturbances of pregnancy and disturbances of general health occurring during pregnancy. The latter are classified in a simplified manner into "severe" and "nonsevere" only, and contribute to the overall pregnancy score as shown in Table 28-2.

TABLE 28-2. Pregnancy Score

SPECIFIC TO PREGNANCY		PREGNANCY SCORE		GENERAL HEALTH
Normal	→	completely normal	←	Normal
Borderline normal	→	borderline normal	←	Nonsevere abnormality
Moderate abnormality	→	moderately abnormal	←	
Severe abnormality	→	severely abnormal	←	Severe abnormality

Detailed lists of conditions used in the classification are shown in Appendix B to this chapter.

THE PERIODIC REVIEW

The 28th day review is presented quarterly at the Epidemiology-in-practice sessions. The first item of this review is a statement of the number of births in the area of the maternal and child health practice, together with a report of the maternal and child health practice and a report on stillbirths and neonatal deaths as shown by the following figures in Table 28-3.

The findings are then reviewed for each period, dealing with conditions pertinent to pregnancy, delivery, new-born, and neonatal period separately (Table 28-4A). Each case is also given a summarized score ranging from cases where all four stages are normal (4N) to cases where all stages are abnormal (4A). The in-between combinations, that do not specify during

TABLE 28-3. Births, Stillbirths, and Neonatal Mortality, 1971

Total births	416, of which 5 were twin births
Live births	409
Stillbirths	7
Neonatal deaths	6
Neonatal mortality rate	14.7 per 1,000 live births

which stage the abnormalities occurred, are 3N + 1A, 2N + 2A, and 1N + 3A. However, they may readily be classified to show the periods in which various abnormalities were found (Table 28-4B). Table 28-4 is an illustrative example of the data accumulated over a 6-month period. The cases shown in this table are further analyzed and those with severe abnormalities are reviewed individually.

Of the 206 pregnancies, 15 were classified as having had a severe abnormality, and 19 had severe complications during delivery. Twenty-two (10.5 percent) of the 209 babies born were classified as having a severe abnormality. The details of these various cases are outlined in Table 28-5.

Of the 15 cases with severe abnormality during pregnancy, there were 10 normal deliveries, and nine babies normal at birth and at 28 days. Further details of the outcome are considered at the review. These cases (Table 28-6) are reviewed in relation to progress during pregnancy and the condition of the baby at birth and at 28 days.

The 22 cases scored as having a severe abnormality at birth or at 28 days included the following:

4 deaths—2 stillbirths and 2 neonatal deaths
4 congenital abnormalities or birth injuries
9 low birth weight (2,250 g or below)
1 high birth weight (5,000 g and over)
3 fetal distress
1 severe icterus

The details of these cases, indicating the condition of the mother during pregnancy and the delivery, are considered.

The interest and usefulness of this kind of detailed consideration of the community distribution of normal and abnormal pregnancies and their outcome is itself under review.

Review of the Use of Services

In addition to consideration of the state of health of the woman and baby, the 28th day review includes the use of services during pregnancy. The

TABLE 28-4. The "28th Day" Cumulative Report July 1 to December 21, 1971

A. The Condition of the Mother During Pregnancy, the Delivery Itself, the Condition of the Baby at Birth and During the Neonatal Period

CONDITION	PREGNANCY		DELIVERY		BABY AT BIRTH		THE BABY DURING NEONATAL PERIOD	
	Single Birth	Twin Birth	Single Birth	Twin Birth	Single Birth	Twin Birth	Single Birth	Twin Birth
Normal (N)	134		132		148	1	134	3
Borderline normal	7	2	4	3	2		29	
Abnormal (A)—moderate	29	1	41	3	21	3	10	
—severe	17		22(2*)		24(2*)	2	10(2†)	1
Not recorded	16		4		8		18	2
Total	203	3	203	6	203	6	201	6

*Stillbirths
†Neonatal deaths

B. The Condition of Mothers and Babies During the Four Periods

THE DISTRIBUTION OF THE ABNORMALITIES: LIVE INFANTS ONLY

CONDITION	No. of Cases	Pregnancy	Delivery	Birth	Neonatal	Total Abnormalities
4N	74	—	—	—	—	—
3N + 1A	60	20	30	8	2	60
2N + 2A	30*	11	18	19	8	56
1N + 3A	14*	9	11	11	5	36
4A	2	2	2	2	2	8
Information not complete	29	—	—	—	—	—
Total	209					

*Including one stillbirth and one neonatal death in each category.

TABLE 28-5. Abnormalities of Pregnancy

ABNORMALITY	NO. OF CASES FROM A TOTAL OF 15
Severe abnormality during pregnancy	15
Specific disturbances of pregnancy	10
Bleeding	4
Toxemia	4
Infections of genital tract	1
Placental insufficiency	1
Disturbances of general health (during pregnancy)	5
Heart disease	2 (1 congenital heart disease; 1 rheumatic heart disease, mitral insufficiency)
Diabetes mellitus	1
Myopia	2

TABLE 28-6. Severe Complications of Delivery

ABNORMALITY	NO. OF CASES FROM A TOTAL OF 19
Severe complications of delivery	19
Cesarian section	7
Malpresentation	10
Breech	8
Brow	1
Occipitoposterior	1
Disproportion-cephalopelvis	1
Miscellaneous	3
"Revisio uteri" and postpartum bleeding	1
Induction and myomectomy	1
Abruptio placentae and fetal distress	1

regular procedure is for a woman who suspects pregnancy to visit the gynecologist or family doctor of the agency with which she is insured. Following diagnosis she is referred for prenatal care to the maternal and child health clinic, if abnormal to hospital or other specialty service, or she may prefer to attend an obstetrician of her choice. Of the 206 women delivered during July 1st to December 31st, 1971, 146 (71 percent) had prenatal care at one of the maternal and child health centers and 37 used another doctor (an obstetrician) in addition. There were 60 women (29 percent) who did not use the departmental service during their pregnancy, of whom 50 (24 percent) were recorded as having attended hospitals, obstetricians, or other municipal mother and child clinics. The care of ten women (5 percent) was not recorded.

TABLE 28-7. The Use of Prenatal Services Provided by Maternal and Child Health Centers of the Department of Social Medicine

	ATTENDANCES AFTER FIRST DIAGNOSIS OF PREGNANCY							
	Contacts with Doctor				Contacts with Nurse Only			
No. of Contacts	Trimester 1	Trimester 2	Trimester 3	Total Pregnancies	Trimester 1	Trimester 2	Trimester 3	Total Pregnancies
0	123	24	4	3	110	37	16	6
1–2	23	115	69	24	36	95	56	40
3–4		7	65	76		12	41	47
5–6			8	36		2	21	31
7–8				6			10	15
9–10				1			2	6
11–12				—				1
Total women				146				146

Analysis of attendances of the 146 women who used the maternal and child health services is summarized in Table 28-7. The 146 women had a total of 1,117 attendances at the center during their pregnancy, an average of about eight visits per woman, of which almost 50 percent were to nurses alone (550). As indicated in the table, the majority of the attendances were during the third trimester.

More detailed investigation is being undertaken into the use of services by cases known to have an abnormality. Anemia in pregnancy was a common condition in this community and is dealt with separately in the next chapter.

APPENDIX A

Record Card Used for "28th Day" Review

This card has two sides, reproduced here and on the following page

HADASSAH MEDICAL ORGANIZATION AND HEBREW UNIVERSITY
HADASSAH MEDICAL SCHOOL
DEPARTMENT OF SOCIAL MEDICINE

Notification of Pregnancy and Delivery

Mother's name________________ Address________________ Serial No. ________

Identity No.__|__|__|__|__|__|__|

Mother

Permanent resident yes/no

Year of birth ______|__|__|__|

Country of birth __________

Country of birth of mother's father ________________

Marital status __________

Year of Immigration__|__|__|

Years of education__|__|__|

No. of live births__|__|__|

No. of stillbirths__|__|__|

No. of miscarriages and abortions __________

Father

Country of birth__________

Country of birth of father's father ________________

Years of schooling __|__|__|

Occupation ____________

Occupational rating ______

Women Registered in M & Ch Center

Date of registration ______|__|__|__|__|__| Lived in area until end pregnancy Yes/no

Date of last menstruation |__|__|__|__|__|__| Estimated date of delivery______|__|__|__|__|

Condition requiring special treatment ________________________________

Treatment for disorders given by ________________________________

Trimester	I	II	III
No. of doctor contacts			
No. of nurse contacts only			

Women Not Registered in M & Ch Center

1. Lived in area till end pregnancy yes/no
2. Left area during pregnancy yes/no

APPENDIX A (cont.)

Trimester	I	II	III
Lowest Hemoglobin level			
Cigarette smoking	yes/no	yes/no	yes/no
Work	yes/no	yes/no	yes/no

Women Not Registered in M & Ch Center

3. Did not live in area

Care during pregnancy given by___

No. of visits to dr. |_|_|_|

Disturbances during pregnancy yes/no

Specify___________________

Bacteriuria: definite, probable, possible, none, not tested

Disorders during pregnancy yes/no

Hospitalization yes/no

Specify:___________________

Reverse Side of Record Card Used for "28th Day" Review

Delivery and condition of newborn

Date of delivery________ Length of gestation__________

Place of birth: Hadassah, Sha'are Zedek, Bikur Cholim, Mizgav Ladach, other hospital, other

Delivery complications: yes/no Specify: (summary)

____

Newborn

Live Birth Still Birth

Single Birth Multiple Birth

Identity No. |_|_|_|_|_|_|_|

Sex: F/M

Birth Weight___________

APGAR___________

Disorders in newborn yes/no

Specify: (summary)________

____

Neonatal Period

No. contacts per week:	1	2	3	4	5	6
Doctor						
Nurse only						

Hospitalizations: yes/no Specify_______________

Disturbances during first 28 days yes/no

Specify:______________________________

Abnormal condition at 28 days examination yes/no

Specify: (summary)____________________

Score

Pregnancy	
Delivery	
Newborn	
28th day	

APPENDIX B

The "28th Day" Program

Classification of Abnormalities in Pregnancy, Delivery, and Puerperium, and in the Newborn and Neonatal Period

I. Specific disturbances of pregnancy
Includes items 630–645 of ICD (eighth revision)
with the exception of 634.0—"Malposition of foetus"—to be classified under Delivery—Malpresentation of foetus, 656
with the addition of "Significant bacteriuria," 789.1, and "Benign tumors of genital tract"

A. Severe
Infection of genital tract during pregnancy
Ectopic pregnancy
Hemorrhage of pregnancy (except for hemorrhage as under "Moderate")
Rupture of pregnant uterus
Hydatidiform mole
Placental abnormalities
Air embolism
Molar pregnancy
Other complications as under 634.9
Renal disease
Preeclampsia, eclampsia, and toxemia
Other toxemias
Hypertension arising during pregnancy: systolic 160 + and/or diastolic 95 +
Rh sensitization
Abortion
Anemia of pregnancy—Hb under 8 g percent

B. Moderate
Hypertension—Systolic 140–159 and/or diastolic 90–94
Anemia of pregnancy—Hb 8–9.9 g percent
Premature rupture of membranes
Hemorrhage, not due to causes as under 632.0–632.5 and not requiring hospitalization
Urinary infections
Significant bacteriuria
Hydramnios
Hyperemesis gravidarum
Benign tumor of genital tract

C. Borderline Normal
Anemia—Hb 10.0–10.9 g percent
Multiple pregnancy
Vomiting other than hyperemesis gravidarum
Edema, without renal disease or toxemia
Rh-negative mother, Rh-positive father

II. Disturbances of General Health During Pregnancy
Diagnoses are classified according to criteria as in "I". The following is a list of diagnoses relating to pregnancies reported up to December 31, 1970

A. Severe
Hereditary hemolytic anemias

APPENDIX B (cont.)

A. Severe (cont.)
   Gonorrhea, not adequately treated
   Rheumatic heart disease
   Congenital heart disease
   Diabetes mellitus
   Schizophrenia
   Myopia, 6 + diopters
   Congential dislocation of hip
   Rubella
   Toxoplasmosis
   Mental retardation

B. Nonsevere*
   Emotional disturbances
   Dermatitis
   Benign tumor other than genital tract
   Cardiac arrhythmia
   Gonorrhea, adequately treated
   Trichomonas } vaginalis
   Moniliasis }
   Upper or lower respiratory infections
   Gastroenteritis
   Cholecystitis
   Influenza (during an epidemic, list as "severe")
   Obesity
   Varicose veins
   Myopia, under 6 diopters

III. Complications of Delivery and Puerperium
(items 650–678 ICD)

A. Severe
   Placenta previa
   Antepartum hemorrhage
   Retained placenta
   Other postpartum hemorrhage
   Abnormality of bony pelvis
   Fetopelvic disproportion
   Malpresentation of fetus
   Laceration of perineum (extensive, sphincter, third degree)
   Rupture of uterus
   Other obstetrical trauma
   Diseased placenta
   Obstetric shock
   Precipitate labor
   Anesthetic death
   Sepsis—as under 670, except for "postpartum fever"
   Puerperal phlebitis, thrombosis
   Puerperal pulmonary embolism
   Puerperal cerebral hemorrhage
   Puerperal blood dyscrasias
   Anemia of puerperium under 8 g percent Hb
   Sudden death in puerperium
   Abscess of breast
   Fistula of breast

Interventions
Forceps, mid and high
Cesarean section
Other surgical or instrumental intervention except for episiotomy and those interventions listed under "moderate" below

B. Moderate
Prolonged labor of origin other than under "Severe"
Laceration of perineum, slight
Pyrexia of unknown origin during puerperium
Anemia of the puerperium –8-9.9 g percent Hb
Placental polyp
Other and unspecified complications of puerperium
Mastitis puerperalis
Postmaturity
Postpartum fever
Interventions
Manipulation without instruments
Forceps, low
Forceps, unspecified
Vacuum extractor

C. Borderline Normal
Multiple birth
Premature birth
Anemia—10-10.9 g percent Hb

IV. Conditions of Newborn at Birth
To include all conditions originating from prenatal factors or from the birth process, observed at birth or during the hospital stay after birth; all postnatal events, e.g., infections, feeding difficulties, to be included in "neonatal period (28 days)"

A. Severe
Birth injury (except for cephalhematoma and hematoma of sternocleidomastoid)
Hemolytic disease of newborn
Jaundice of other origin, with bilirubin over 20 g percent and/or requiring exchange transfusion or other special treatment
Anoxic and hypoxic conditions:
Aspiration, hyaline membrane disease,
Respiratory distress syndrome, fetal distress,
Intrauterine anoxia, asphyxia of newborn
Immaturity—gestation period under 36 weeks
Low birth weight—2250 g or less
Fetal blood loss before birth
Hemorrhagic disease of newborn
Cold injury syndrome
Cardiac failure
Kernicterus
Hydrops
Fetal death (stillbirth)
Congenital anomalies
Congenital disorders of metabolism
Postmaturity—gestation over 43 weeks
Birth weight over 5,000 g

B. Moderate
Conditions of umbilical cord:compression, prolapse

APPENDIX B (cont.)

B. Moderate (cont.)
Cephalhematoma
Hematoma of sternocleidomastoid
Prematurity—gestation 36 to 37 weeks
Low birth weight—2,251 to 2,500 g
Postmaturity—gestation 42 to 43 weeks
Birth weight 4,000 to 5,000 g
Bleeding from umbilical cord
Meconium plug syndrome
Congenital anomalies*

C. Borderline Normal
Conditions of umbilical cord, other than above (771.9)
Congenital anomalies*—f.i. cryptorchism hydrocele

V. Neonatal Period (28 days)

A. Severe
Any condition which in general or in the specific case is considered to constitute serious danger to the life or the functional capacity of mother or child, or an increased risk of congenital abnormalities or premature birth

B. Moderate
All other conditions

C. Borderline Normal
Any condition considered generally to have no unfavorable consequences for the future state of health, functional capacity, or social adjustment of mother or child, and to require no special treatment or follow-up

Any condition listed here may also be classified under "severe" if occurring in individual cases of special severity.

29
Anemia in Pregnancy

THE CASE FOR ACTION

Anemia in pregnancy is a common problem, especially in underdeveloped parts of the world. It was recognized as a prevalent condition in parturient women in Jerusalem in the 1950s. Rachmilewitz et al. reported hypochromic iron deficiency anemia and "dimorphic," or mixed, anemia, as well as "pure" macrocytic anemia.[1–3] Low serum iron levels, low serum vitamin B_{12}, and low levels of folic acid in whole blood and serum were commonly found as a combined deficiency. The occurrence of anemia in women of Jerusalem during the years 1946 to 1962 in shown in Table 29-1.

This problem was also recognized in other parts of Israel, as is shown in Table 29-2. The problem was further explored in Jerusalem. In 1960 to 1961 a program to treat anemia in pregnancy was instituted in the whole of Jerusalem by the Department of Social Medicine. This was carried out by all the maternal and child health centers of Jerusalem and all the obstetrics and gynecologic clinics of Kupat Holim in the city (Kupat Holim—Sick Fund of the General Federation of Labor Unions). The exploration of the problem included an analysis of hospital records of women who gave birth in Jerusalem in 1958 to 1959. Table 29-3 shows the records of 3,578 normal cases analyzed by country of birth of husband.[7]

Occupational Rating and Hemoglobin Levels

The same records were analyzed for social class determined by occupational rating of husband (Table 29-4). This table shows an association between social class and hemoglobin level. The higher the social class, the higher the level of hemoglobin and consequently the lower the percentage of anemia. Nevertheless, there was an unexpectedly high proportion of upper-social-class women with hemoglobin levels below 10 g per 100 ml.

TABLE 29-1. A Summary of Reported Investigations on the Occurrence of Anemia* in Pregnant and Parturient Women of Jerusalem

YEAR OF STUDY	TIME OF EXAMINATION	NO. OF CASES	PERCENTAGE OF CASES WITH HEMOGLOBIN BELOW 10 g/100 ml
1946[5]	Prenatal second and third trimester	432	1.3
1953–1954[6]	Prenatal second and third trimester	848	16.6
1955–1956[1]	Prenatal second and third trimester	500	11.2
	Following birth	2,000	11.0
1958[2]	Following birth	1,100	28.0
1958–1959[7]	Following birth	3,578	18.6
1959–1960[8]	Prenatal	2,498	6.9
1961–1962[4]	Prenatal second trimester	2,459	8.1
1961–1962[4]	Prenatal third trimester	2,006	12.3
	Following birth	1,843	16.7

**Anemia was defined as a hemoglobin level of less than 10 g/100 ml. (From Kark.[4])*

TABLE 29-2. Occurrence of Anemia in Pregnant and Parturient Women in Areas of Israel Other than Jerusalem

YEAR OF STUDY	TIME OF EXAMINATION	NO. OF CASES	PERCENTAGE OF CASES WITH HEMOGLOBIN BELOW 10 g/100 ml	AREA
1955[10]	Prenatal	6,950	17.6	Petah Tikva
1965[10]	Prenatal	7,502	16.8	Petah Tikva
1960[11]	During pregnancy	57	17.5	Kafrit
1960[12]	During pregnancy	154	19.0	Shderot
1963–1965[13]	During pregnancy	890	22.2 (below 10.1)	Kiryat Shemona
1965–1966[14]	During pregnancy	403	45.6 (below 10.1)	Kiryat Shemona
	After birth	403	37.0 (below 10.1)	Kiryat Shemona

(From Gitlin et al.[9])

TABLE 29-3. Mean Hemoglobin Level and Anemia Rate in Parturient Women, Jerusalem 1958–1959, By Husband's Place of Birth

HUSBAND'S PLACE OF BIRTH	NO. OF CASES	HEMOGLOBIN (g/100 ml)	PERCENTAGE ANEMIA
Asia			
Israel	717	11.39	14.1
Yemen-Aden	203	11.24	22.2
Rest of Asia	977	10.97	23.2
Europe and other communities of European origin	439	11.24	16.2
North Africa	805	11.16	17.5
Not recorded	437	11.20	18.8

(From Kark et al.[7])

TABLE 29-4. Mean Hemoglobin Level and Anemia Rate in Parturient Women, Jerusalem 1958–1959, By Husband's Occupational Rating

OCCUPATIONAL RATING OF HUSBAND	NO. OF CASES	HEMOGLOBIN (g/100 ml)		PERCENTAGE ANEMIA
Class I	158	11.53	11.52	10.8
Class II	137	11.49		
Class III	1,285	11.22		17.4
Class IV	151	11.17	11.07	21.0
Class V	1,080	11.06		

(From Kark et al.[7])

Neighborhood and Hemoglobin Levels

A similar trend was found when the above records were analyzed by neighborhood. The various neighborhoods of Jerusalem City are rated by the Jerusalem Municipality for taxation purposes. A combination of several neighborhood attributes is used in assessing the grade of the particular neighborhood.

The nature and extent of roads, available municipal services, transport services, schools, and synagogues
Type of housing construction
The distance of the neighborhood from the business center of the city
The composition of the population in an arbitrary assessment of social stratification by occupation and standards of living (well-off or poorer neighborhoods)

Each neighborhood is given a numerical rating between 1 and 6, rating 1 being the highest. Table 29-5 shows the distribution of hemoglobin levels according to these municipal ratings.

Municipal rating is closely related to social class in that the people living in the higher-rated neighborhoods tend to be from the upper social classes and those in lower-rated neighborhoods are predominantly from the lower social classes. The exception to this is Kiryat Harim which is rated as 5 but has a higher proportion of social classes I, II, and III than do other neighborhoods rated 5 and 6. This is reflected in the higher level of hemoglobin but, as will be noted in Figure 29-1, even when controlling for social class, the women of this area (shown as 5a) have a higher hemoglobin level than in any other area of the city. Further analysis of the hemoglobin levels by occupational rating and areas of residence

TABLE 29-5. Mean Hemoglobin Level and Anemia Rate by Municipal Rating of Neighborhood

MUNICIPAL RATING	NO. OF CASES	HEMOGLOBIN (g/100 ml)	PERCENTAGE ANEMIA
1	175	11.63	8.6
2	351	11.35	14.8
3	533	11.14	18.4
4	484	11.09	20.2
5	521	11.01	23.2
5a	166	11.60	12.0
6	134	10.93	20.1

(From Kark et al.[7])

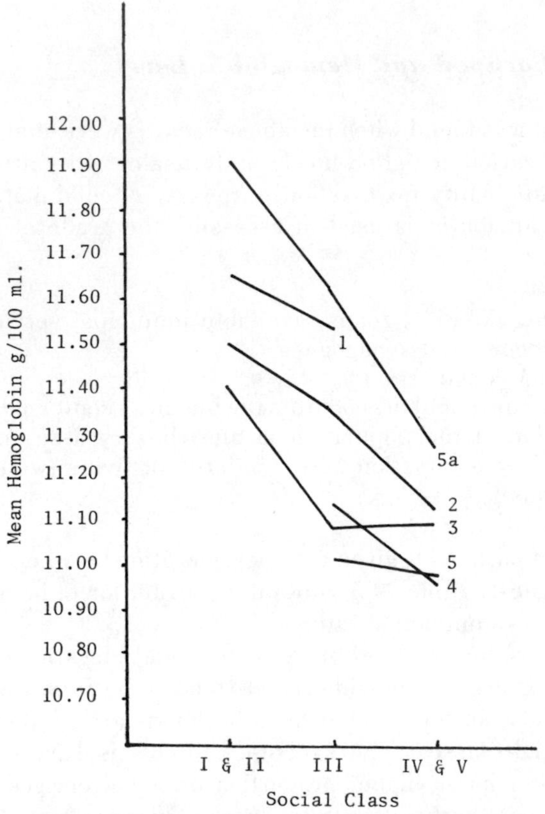

FIG. 29-1. Mean hemoglobin levels of women by area of living according to municipal rating and social class. (Adapted from Kark and associates.[7])

TABLE 29-6. Mean Hemoglobin and Anemia Rate by Husband's Occupational Rating and Municipal Rating

MUNICIPAL RATING	OCCUPATIONAL RATING								
	I AND II			III			IV AND V		
	No.	Mean Hemoglobin	Anemia (%)	No.	Mean Hemoglobin	Anemia (%)	No.	Mean Hemoglobin	Anemia (%)
1	59	11.64	6.8	90	11.52	10.0	3	(12.83)	(0.0)
2	78	11.50	11.5	175	11.34	15.4	34	11.12	14.7
3	62	11.40	12.3	280	11.09	19.3	127	11.09	19.7
4	25	11.66	8.0	233	11.14	19.3	154	10.97	22.1
5	21	10.71	38.1	204	11.02	20.1	257	10.98	25.3
5a	30	11.90	0.0	91	11.61	14.3	31	11.27	16.1
6	—	—	—	47	11.00	14.9	74	10.80	25.7

(From Kark et al.[7])

TABLE 29-7. Anemia in Relation to Social Class and Area Rating

SOCIAL CLASS AND AREA RATING		ANEMIA (%)
Social class I and II;	Area rating 1	6.8
	Area rating 3	12.3
Social class III;	Area rating 1	10.0
	Area rating 5	20.1
Social class IV and V;	Area rating 2	14.7
	Area rating 5	25.3
	Area rating 6	25.7

indicates the independent effects of each of these variables (Table 29-6).

Within each social class, the lower the municipal rating the higher the percentage of anemia as shown in Table 29-7.

Ethnic Group and Hemoglobin Levels

The birthplace of the husband was used as an indicator of ethnic group in the analysis in order to relate it directly to his occupational rating. A separate analysis was performed showing very high concordance between region of birth of wife and husband. Table 29-8 and Figure 29-2 show

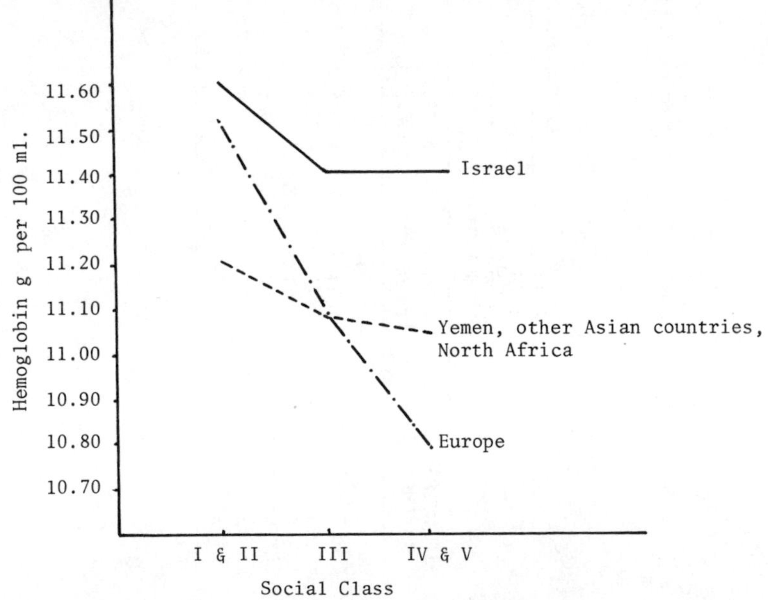

FIG. 29-2. Mean hemoglobin levels of parturient women. Jerusalem 1958–1959. By region of birth according to social class. (Adapted from Kark and associates.[7])

TABLE 29-8. Mean Hemoglobin Level and Anemia Rate by Husband's Occupational Rating and Place of Birth

HUSBAND'S PLACE OF BIRTH	OCCUPATIONAL RATING								
	I and II			III			IV and V		
	No.	Hemoglobin	Anemia (%)	No.	Hemoglobin	Anemia (%)	No.	Hemoglobin	Anemia (%)
Israel	105	11.60	11.4	403	11.41	14.6	85	11.42	9.4
Yemen-Aden	3	(10.83)	(33.3)	25	11.10	20.0	28	10.64	32.1
Other Asian countries	19	11.45	10.5	266	11.08	19.1	537	10 95	24.4
Europe and other countries of European origin	126	11.52	10.3	212	11.10	17.5	31	10.79	29.0
North Africa	13	10.96	7.7	215	11.09	20.0	411	11.22	17.8

(From Kark et al.[7])

TABLE 29-9. Comparison of Social Class and Other Characteristics of Pregnant Women Living in Areas of Jerusalem, 1962

	AREA "B" (THREE NEIGHBORHOODS RATED 1)		AREA "A" (THREE NEIGHBORHOODS RATED 4 AND 5)	
		Percentage		Percentage
Number of women	93		138	
Family income—				
Average per month	381 I.L. (Israeli pounds)		212 I.L. (Israeli pounds)	
Social class				
I and II		51		2
III		47		43
IV and V		2		55
Education				
Never attended school		0		32
Primary school only		20		56
Secondary school or more		80		12
Area of birth				
Israel		54		18
Europe		26		5
North Africa		7		33
Asia (excluding Israel)		12		44

(From Kark et al.[15]*)*

that when social class is held constant the Israeli-born group has a higher mean hemoglobin level and less anemia than other ethnic groups.

Diet in Relation to the Hemoglobin Picture

It has been shown that social class and neighborhood are associated with levels of hemoglobin. The higher the social class and municipal rating, the higher the level of hemoglobin and the lower the rate of anemia. A study was carried out in 1962 by a team that included a nutrition expert in order to elucidate what bearing diet had on these findings. A sample of pregnant women from different areas of Jerusalem was chosen for this investigation. Table 29-9 shows the marked social and economic differences between the women of two groups of neighborhoods, namely area "a," the poorer neighborhood, and area "b," the better-off neighborhood.

A quantitative dietary interview was conducted by a dietician. Each pregnant woman who visited the maternal and child health center was interviewed on three separate days. One interview dealt with her food consumption on the Sabbath and the other two dealt with regular week days. Two of the interviews were carried out at the home of the pregnant women and the other was conducted at the clinic. Hemoglobin tests were also done.

Among those women who had their blood tested for the first time before the third trimester, there were 7 percent in area "a" and none in area "b" with levels of hemoglobin under 10g/100 ml. For those women who had their blood tested for the first time during the third trimester, the rates were 13.5 percent for area "a" and 6.4 percent for area "b."

Table 29-10 shows a comparison of the nutritive value of daily diet

TABLE 29-10. Mean Hemoglobin Levels in Two Areas in Relation to Diet

	BETTER-OFF AREAS "B" (LOW INCIDENCE ANEMIA)	POORER AREAS "A" (HIGH INCIDENCE ANEMIA)
	Mean Hemoglobin g/100 ml	Mean Hemoglobin g/100 ml
First Hb Examination		
Before third trimester	12.12	11.65
Third trimester	11.68	11.09
Nutrients in Daily Diet		
Total protein	72.60 g	69.20 g
Animal protein	43.50 g	31.10 g
Iron	12.40 mg	10.96 mg
Ascorbic acid	106.00 mg	78.00 mg

(From Kark et al.[15]*)*

TABLE 29-11. Differences in Protein, Iron, and Ascorbic Acid in Daily Diet, According to Hemoglobin Level

	NEIGHBORHOODS WITH LOW INCIDENCE OF ANEMIA			NEIGHBORHOODS WITH HIGH INCIDENCE OF ANEMIA		
	Above 12 g/100 ml	Below 12 g/100 ml	*P*	Above 12 g/100 ml	Below 12 g/100 ml	*P*
Total protein (g)	74.20	71.80	—	72.80	63.60	< 0.05
Animal protein (g)	42.10	48.10	—	42.30	29.70	< 0.025
Iron (mg)	12.58	12.40	—	12.84	10.29	< 0.015
Ascorbic acid (mg)	107.00	94.00	—	113.00	77.00	< 0.03

(From Kark et al.[15]*)*

and hemoglobin levels of the pregnant women living in the two groups of neighborhoods.[15]

The findings in Table 29-11 indicate that dietary differences between women living in "poorer" areas are important in determining the differences in Hb levels whereas in "better-off" areas diet in itself is not the differentiating factor. Women with hemoglobin levels of less than 12g/100 ml, living in the poorer neighborhoods, had markedly inferior diets to those of the women living in the same neighborhoods but who had hemoglobin levels above 12g/100 ml. They also had inferior diets compared with those of the women whose hemoglobin levels were also below 12 g/100 ml but who were living in the better-off neighborhoods (area "b").

JERUSALEM PROGRAM

The Jerusalem program was conducted by all the mother and child health centers of the city. It was initiated following a series of preparatory discussions and seminars on the subject of anemia and pregnancy with particular reference to its epidemiology, including the common causes. During these seminars a citywide program was agreed upon. Each pregnant woman attending the center completed a specially prepared questionnaire. Her hemoglobin was measured three times, first at her first attendance, usually

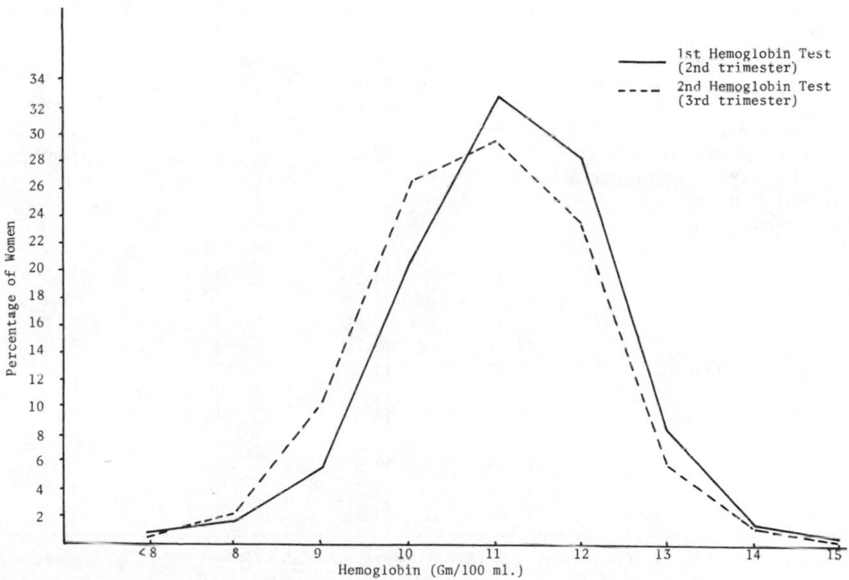

FIG. 29-3. The distribution of prenatal hemoglobin levels of 1,700 parturient women attending Jerusalem maternal and child health centers, 1961–1962.

in the second trimester, the second in the third trimester, and the third immediately after delivery. Those with hemoglobin levels below 10g/100 ml were treated with ferrous sulphate or other suitable iron preparations.

Of the 2,466 women who participated in this program during its first two years, 1961 to 1962, there were 1,700 who had both first and second hemoglobin estimations. The lower distribution of hemoglobin readings in the third trimester is illustrated in Figure 29-3.

Change in the Hemoglobin Picture

The changes were measured by comparing the hemoglobin picture of parturient women delivered in the Hadassah University Teaching Hospital in 1958 to 1959 and 1964 to 1966. Table 29-12 shows the differences between

TABLE 29-12. Mean Hemoglobin Level and Anemia Rate in Normal Deliveries—Comparative Data 1958–1959 and 1964–1966

	MEAN HEMOGLOBIN (g/100 ml)		ANEMIA (PERCENT OF WOMEN WITH ANEMIA)	
	1958–1959	1964–1966	1958–1959	1964–1966
All women	11.19	11.69	20.7	12.8
Normal deliveries	11.18	11.78	18.6	10.8
Husband's occupation				
Grade I and II	11.52	12.08	10.8	7.4
Grade III	11.20	11.76	17.4	11.1
Grade IV and V	11.07	11.56	21.0	14.9
Husband's region of birth				
Europe	11.24	12.05	16.2	5.9
Israel	11.39	11.85	14.1	10.8
North Africa	11.16	11.68	17.5	11.5
Asia (other than Israel)	11.02	11.60	23.1	13.6
Neighborhood of residence in Jerusalem by municipal rating				
1	11.63	12.11	8.6	8.2
2	11.35	11.90	14.8	11.0
3	11.14	11.76	18.4	9.2
4	11.09	11.56	20.2	13.5
5	11.01	11.70	23.2	11.8
5a (Kiryat Harim)	11.60	11.95	12.0	8.8
6	10.94	11.46	20.1	24.0
Outside Jerusalem	11.17	11.53	19.5	13.3
Parity				
1	11.39	11.91	13.4	11.1
2–5	11.18	11.78	18.5	11.3
6 +	11.01	11.56	22.7	13.1

These are hemoglobin levels in parturient women delivered in the Hadassah University Teaching Hospital.
(From Epstein et al.[16])

these two periods using the same variables, namely social class, ethnic group, neighborhood of residence, and parity.[16] These findings indicate a considerable improvement in the hemoglobin picture of the women delivered in Hadassah Hospital. The question arises as to whether this change is due to the treatment administered to this population or whether there were other concomittant changes, such as a rise in standard of living with improvement in diet or changes in the demographic structure.

Social Mobility and Demographic Changes. The improvement was general, affecting women of various neighborhoods in the city as well as in each class. The social class differences in the hemoglobin picture which were present in cases delivered in the Hadassah Hospital in Jerusalem in 1958 to 1959 were still present in those delivered there in 1964 to 1966. The difference between the mean levels of hemoglobin of the upper and lower social groups has remained similar: 0.45 g per 100 ml in 1958 to 1959, and 0.52 g per 100 ml in 1964 to 1966.

In the light of the earlier findings it could be expected that an increase in the proportion of Israeli-born women would have a favorable effect on the hemoglobin picture. In the period under review there has been a change in this respect—almost 40 percent of the more recent group were married to men born in Israel, compared with 20 percent in the earlier group. There was a corresponding decrease in the proportion of Asian and North African women. A second demographic factor of importance is the change in the social class distribution in the two periods, as shown in Table 29-13. This indicates a very clear change in the social

TABLE 29-13. Change in Social Class Distribution

SOCIAL CLASS	1958–1959	1964–1966
I and II	10 %	22 %
III	46 %	60 %
IV and V	44 %	18 %

class ratings of the women delivered in the Teaching Hospital but may not represent a general trend in upward social mobility in the Jerusalem Jewish population as a whole.

Diet Changes. No direct information is available concerning changes in the food intake of pregnant women in Jerusalem. The national food balance sheets published annually by the Israel Central Bureau of Statistics indicate little change in iron consumption. The mean amount per capita per day was 15.5 mg in 1957 to 1958 and 15.9 mg in 1966 to 1967.[17] Other trends however indicate a general improvement in food consumption which may be of relevance to hemoglobin levels. The mean daily consumption of meat protein shows a steady rise from 9.4 g in 1957 to 1958 to 18.8 g in 1966 to 1967 and that of total animal protein from 33.6 to 41.3 g. These figures, being overall averages, have limited relevance to the actual intake of nutrients by specific population groups, such as pregnant women in Jerusalem.

The general national improvement in food consumption may be an important element in the change which was observed in the hemoglobin levels of parturient women in Jerusalem. This is not the only factor involved as is shown by the reports from other parts of the country which indicated continuing high rates of anemia in pregnant women and parturient mothers. There was no change in the proportion of women with hemoglobin levels below 10g/100 ml immediately before birth or in the first stage of labor at the Sharon Hospital between 1955 and 1965 (17.6 and 16.8 percent respectively). Reports from Kiryat Shemona[13] have also shown much anemia, the rate in pregnancy being 22 percent in 1963 to 1965 with similar rates in 1966 to 1967. This was so before a special program of treatment was introduced.[14]

While demographic trends and general nutritional changes may have had an influence on the overall improvement, it is probable that continuing surveillance during pregnancy and the introduction of defined prophylactic and treatment programs have played an important part in changing the hemoglobin picture among parturient women in Jerusalem.

THE NEIGHBORHOOD PROGRAM OF THE HEALTH CENTER IN KIRYAT HARIM

This program for the control of anemia has been developed as an integral part of the service of three maternal and child health clinics of the Department of Social Medicine and is in reality an intensification of what had been initiated in the Jerusalem area as a whole. This more intensive program began in 1963 and continues at present. It has two objectives: (1) to have a continuing epidemiologic surveillance of the hemoglobin level in pregnant women; and (2) to institute a program to reduce the incidence of anemia in pregnant women.

Methods

Hemoglobin investigations are performed as far as possible in the first, second, and third trimesters, the first postnatal day, and at 6 weeks after delivery.

The investigations are made on venous blood including hemoglobin (Klett hemoglobinometer standardized every two months), hematocrit

(Wintrobe Tubes), red cell count (Thomas), and blood smears (Giemsa). These methods were standardized according to those used in the Teaching Hospital laboratory. Apart from the postnatal day hemoglobin estimations carried out in the hospital in which the women delivered, all other bloods are examined by the laboratory at the Community Health Center.

Treatment Program

During Pregnancy. Cases with hemoglobin values of over 12g/100 ml are not treated.

Cases with hemoglobin values of 11 to 12g/100 ml receive one tablet of ferrous gluconate (0.3 g), ferrous sulphate (0.2 g), or ferrocal (0.5 g) daily.

Cases with hemoglobin values of 10 to 11g/100 ml receive three tablets of iron daily.

Cases with hemoglobin levels of less than 10g/100 ml have a hematocrit and full blood count and receive treatment according to the nature of the anemia.

One Day Postnatal. If postnatal hemoglobin is less than 12g/100 ml, treatment is given for anemia. In cases who had anemia during pregnancy, treatment is continued if the level of hemoglobin is less than 13g/100 ml after delivery.

Six Weeks After Delivery. If the hemoglobin level is less than 13g/100 ml, treatment is given.

Review of Program

Review of the program includes (1) the extent to which the blood examinations were carried out at the prescribed times; and (2) changing trends of hemoglobin values and of the incidence of anemia.

The team responsible for the program consisted of an epidemiologist, two physicians, and the coordinating nurse of the health center's maternal and child health service. This team met weekly during the early years of the program in order to review each aspect of progress. The program is now well established, functions smoothly as an integral part of the overall service, and the rate of anemia is very low. For these reasons it is now reviewed once a year in the Epidemiology-in-practice sessions in order to ensure that it is continuing satisfactorily.

In the review of 1970 the extent to which the hemoglobin examinations were carried out was discussed and is shown in Table 29-14. Further examination of these findings showed that women living in the poorer neighborhoods had a higher rate of performance of blood examinations than did those who were better-off or more educated. This was especially

TABLE 29-14. The Extent to Which Hemoglobin Examinations Were Performed

	NO. OF PREGNANT WOMEN IN CARE	PERCENT OF TOTAL
Total of pregnant women	343	
Performance of blood examination		
Second trimester	324	94.5%
Third trimester	301	87.8%
First day after delivery	302	88.0%
Six weeks after delivery	235	68.5%

so in the third trimester hemoglobin (93 percent as compared with 85 percent) and in the blood examinations 6 weeks after delivery (83 percent and 60 percent respectively). The hemoglobin levels were as shown in Table 29-15.

TABLE 29-15. Hemoglobin Levels During and After Pregnancy

TIME OF EXAMINATION	MEAN	SD	PERCENT BELOW 10 g/100 ml
Second trimester	12.67	1.40	1.9
Third trimester	12.30	1.34	2.6
One day after delivery	11.78	1.37	9.6
Six weeks after delivery	13.72	1.21	0.4 (5.1% under 12 g)

Of the 343 women examined during pregnancy there were 11 (3.2 percent) who had a hemoglobin level of less than 10g/100 ml at any stage of pregnancy, and of these there were three cases of thalassemia minor. Of these 11 women, six had anemia in the second trimester and three of these were the cases of thalassemia minor. Excluding these three cases, less than 1.0 percent of women in the second trimester had hemoglobin levels of less than 10g/100 ml.

Evaluation. The same questions asked in relation to the improvement of the hemoglobin picture seen in Jerusalem as a whole may be asked about the very low rate of anemia in the community of Kiryat Harim. Are these changes due to a change in demographic variables such as social class distribution, ethnic origin, or change in diet with improvement in nutrition?

There has been a change in the demography of the area. A higher proportion, especially of the young mothers, are Israeli-born or have had schooling in Israel. The people of this neighborhood have also shared in the improved standard of living of the country.

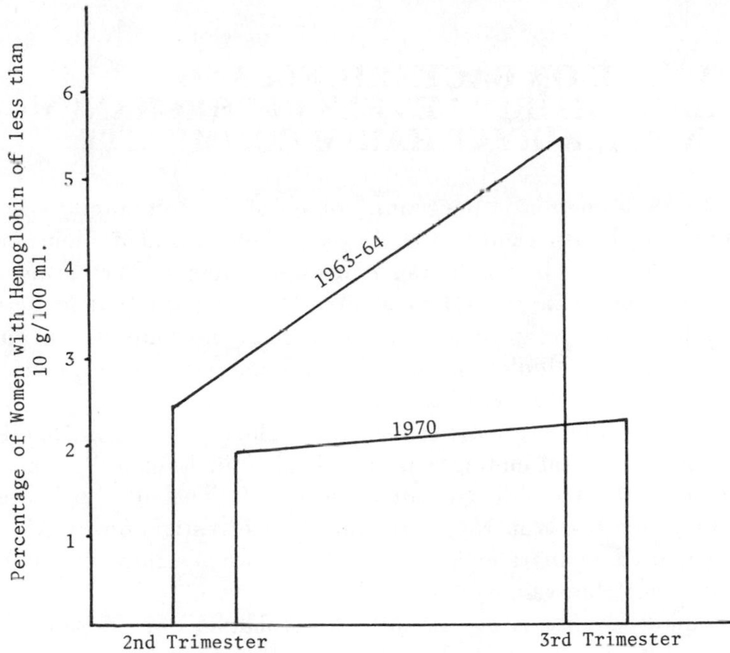

FIG. 29-4. Indicating the difference in percentage of women with anemia in the second and third trimesters of pregnancy—comparing 1963–1964 with 1970.

It is of interest to compare the differences in anemia rates for the second and third trimesters. Whereas in 1963 to 1964 there was a difference of 3 percent between the rates of women with anemia in these trimesters, in 1970 this difference was reduced to 0.4 percent (Fig. 29-4). Social class differences were also very low as indicated by the following figures in Table 29-16. The essential similarity between the better-off and poorer

TABLE 29-16. Hemoglobin Levels in Women of Different Areas of Kiryat Harim

	BETTER-OFF AREA		POORER AREA	
	Mean Hemoglobin	SD	Mean Hemoglobin	SD
Second trimester	12.64	1.16	12.53	1.88
Third trimester	12.32	1.35	12.34	1.28

neighborhoods where this service operates is indicative of the contribution which a program of this kind can make in diminishing the health implications of social class differences.

A NOTE ON BACTERIURIA AND HEMOGLOBIN LEVELS IN PREGNANCY IN THE KIRYAT HARIM COMMUNITY

The low rate of anemia in pregnant women of the community served by the Community Health Center of the Department of Social Medicine encouraged us to look for less common causes of anemia. Furthermore, our own earlier studies in Jerusalem women[15] had shown that in better-off neighborhoods no relation was found between anemia and diet, in contrast to the association with diet that was found in poorer neighborhoods where the incidence of anemia was higher.

A study of the relation between hemoglobin levels and bacteriuria in pregnant women attending a prenatal clinic in England[18] encouraged us to explore the possibility of such an association between bacteriuria and hemoglobin levels in Kiryat Harim. This investigation by Abramson and associates demonstrated an association between significant bacteriuria and low hemoglobin values.[19]

Defining bacteriuria as "definite," "probable," or "possible," they found positive results in 2, 2.8, and 3.1 percent, respectively, of 652 women who had special urine examinations. The definitions used were the following.

Definite bacteriuria: Women with 10^5 or more pathogenic bacteria per ml in *two* urine specimens
Probable bacteriuria: Women who had a single count of 10^5 or more and had then been treated for urinary infection
Possible bacteriuria: Women with a single count of 10^5 or more pathogens per ml who were not treated for urinary tract infection
No bacteriuria: All other women examined

Nonbacteriuric women had a higher mean value hemoglobin than did the women with definite or probable bacteriuria, as shown in Table 29-17.

These differences were not found to be associated with social class, age, parity, or diet. While the results of this study do indicate a significant association between bacteriuria and hemoglobin levels in the pregnant women, the low rate of bacteriuria and the actual difference in hemoglobin levels suggests that bacteriuria is not an important cause of anemia in pregnancy in this community.

TABLE 29-17. Hemoglobin Values in Relation to Presence of Bacteriuria

TIME OF MEASUREMENT OF HEMOGLOBIN		BACTERIURIA		
		Definite and Probable	Definite, Probable, and Possible	No Bacteriuria
Early Pregnancy	Number	27	47	526
	Mean ± SD	12.10 ± 1.22	12.20 ± 1.08	12.48 ± 1.03
	Under 12 gm %	48*	43	28
	Under 11 gm %	22*	15	10
	Under 10 gm %	0	0	2
Late Pregnancy	Number	23	41	531
	Mean ± SD	11.70* ± 1.19	11.84† ± 1.15	12.22 ± 1.11
	Under 12 gm %	57	54	38
	Under 11 gm %	26†	24*	11
	Under 10 gm %	9	7	3
Postnatal	Number	20	35	500
	Mean ± SD	13.67 ± 1.06	13.72 ± 1.10	13.60 ± 1.05
	Under 12 gm %	10	6	5
	Under 11 gm %	0	0	1

*†*Values which differ significantly from those for nonbacteriuric women:* * $P<0.05$; † $P<0.02$.
(From Abramson et al.[19])

REFERENCES

1. Izak G, Rachmilewitz M, Stein Y, et al.: Vitamin B_{12} and iron deficiencies in anemia of pregnancy and puerperium. Arch Intern Med 99:346, 1957.
2. Rachmilewitz M, Izak G, Grossowicz N, et al.: Anemia in pregnancy. (In Hebrew.) Harefuah, 57:81, 1959.
3. Izak G, Rachmilewitz M, Sadowski A, et al.: Folic acid metabolites in whole blood and serum in anemia of pregnancy. Am J Clin Nutr 9:473, 1961.
4. Kark SL: Change and variation in the incidence of anemia in pregnancy in Jerusalem. Isr J Med Sci 2:480, 1966.
5. Sadowski A, Koch W, Toaff R, et al.: Haemoglobin values in pregnant women. J Obstet Gynaec Brit Emp 55:152, 1948.
6. Sadowski A, De Vries A, Bercovici B: Anemia in pregnancy. Acta Med Orient (Tel Aviv) 14:67, 1955.
7. Kark SL, Peritz E, Shiloh A, et al.: Epidemiological analysis of the hemoglobin picture in parturient women of Jerusalem. Am J Public Health 54: 947, 1964.
8. Strauss W, Fattal B, Weiskopf P: Haemoglobin and other blood values in pregnant women. Isr Med J 20:183, 1961.
9. Gitlin M, Bialik O, Flug D, et al.: A community program for the prevention, treatment, and evaluation of anemia in pregnancy. (In Hebrew). Harefuah 75:360, 1968.
10. Halbrecht I, Rubinstein J, Menache R, et al.: Studies on the different aspects of anemia in pregnancy with special reference to the physiological anemia of pregnancy: A survey of 3,896 cases. (In Hebrew). Dapim Refuiim 25:25, 1966.
11. Avivi L, Ilan J, Guggenheim K: Haemoglobin levels in the Jewish rural population of Israel. (In Hebrew.) Briut Hatsibur 5:5, 1962.
12. Bloch A: Routine haemoglobin estimations in mother and child welfare clinics in moshavim and development towns. (In Hebrew). Harefuah 69:75, 1965.
13. Rachmilewitz M, Nitzkin J, Levy S, et al.: Anemia of pregnancy in a rural community of Upper Galilee. Isr J Med Sci 2:472, 1966.
14. Levy S, Rachmilewitz EA, Izak G, et al.: A therapeutic trial in anemia of pregnancy. Isr J Med Sci 4:218, 1968.
15. Kark SL, Abramson JH, Guggenheim K: Diet and haemoglobin levels among pregnant women in Jerusalem. (In Hebrew.) Harefuah 67:247, 1964.
16. Epstein LM, Bialik O, Abramson JH, et al.: Changing haemoglobin picture among parturients in Jerusalem. Isr J Med Sci 6:267, 1970.
17. Central Bureau of Statistics: Statistical Abstract of Israel 1968. No. 19. Jerusalem, Government Press.
18. Giles C, Brown JAH: Urinary infection and anaemia in pregnancy. Brit Med J 2:10, 1962.
19. Abramson JH, Sacks TC, Flug D, et al.: Bacteriuria and hemoglobin levels in pregnancy. JAMA 215:1631, 1971.

30

A Community Program for Promotion of Growth and Development (PROD)

The history of organized maternal and child health work in Israel goes back to 1921 when the first Maternal and Child Health Center was established in the Old City of Jerusalem. By 1971 there was a network of 729 centers throughout the country.[1]

The aims of this service have been stated as follows.

(a) Provision of prenatal, natal, and postnatal care for every mother and full preparation for the birth of every child.
(b) Health protection, health promotion, and health instruction for every child from birth through adolescence.
(c) Prevention, detection, and rehabilitation of handicapped children.[2]

Three of the maternal and child health centers of Kiryat Harim are run by the Department of Social Medicine through its health center in the area. One of these is an integral part of the family practice, with its combined preventive and curative services; the other two do not include comprehensive family care. These latter two are more in line with the traditional maternal and child health centers of the country. The centers are open to all members of the community and were established shortly after settlement began in the Kiryat Harim area.

THE CASE FOR ACTION

Retardation in Physical Growth

The initiation of the project is the result of findings indicating growth retardation among infants and children of poorer neighborhood communities.

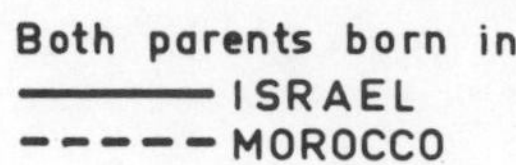

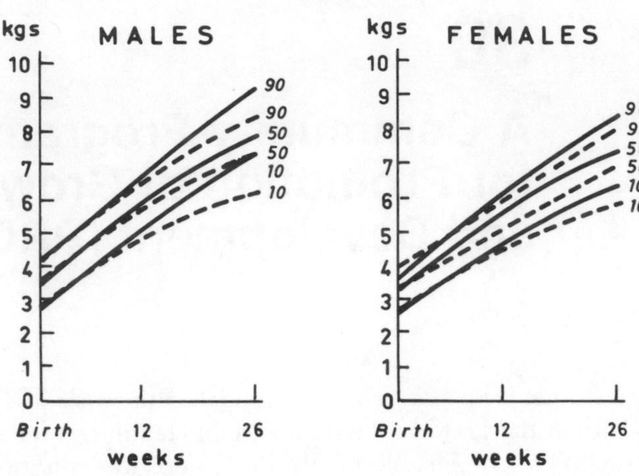

FIG. 30-1. Differences in weight in two groups of Jerusalem infants, 1957 to 1961. (Adapted from Epstein.[3])

The weight growth of two groups of babies born in West Jerusalem during the period 1957 to 1961 was compared. The babies of Israeli-born parents were heavier than those of Moroccan-born parents from the age of 8 weeks to 6 months, despite the fact that the latter were heavier at birth (Fig. 30-1).[3]

At a Community Medicine Conference (CMC) of the Department of Social Medicine, the height and weight growth of the children of two adjacent neighborhoods in West Jerusalem was contrasted. At the age of 3 years a considerable proportion of children in the poorer neighborhoods were below Stuart's Boston third percentile, in contrast to those of the better-off neighborhood. The difference was especially marked in boys, among whom 42 percent of those in the poorer neighborhood were below the third percentile in height (Fig. 30-2). The social class distribution in the two areas differed markedly, the percentages being as shown in Table 30-1.

TABLE 30-1

	SOCIAL CLASS		
	I and II	III	IV and V
Better-off neighborhood (a)	36	57	7
Poorer neighborhood (b)	0	61	39

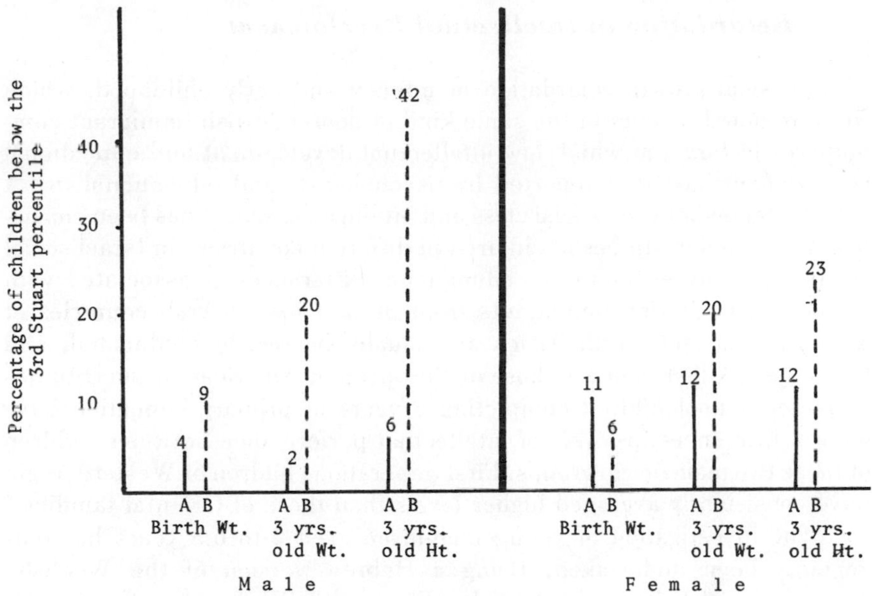

FIG. 30-2. A comparison in weight and height of 170 children born in two adjacent neighborhoods of Kiryat Harim. The percentage of children below the third percentile is shown for children of both neighborhoods for weight at birth and for weight and height of 3- to 4-year olds. A: Predominantly middle-class neighborhood, with 73 percent of parents born in Israel or of European origin. B: Poorer neighborhood, with 97 percent of parents born in North Africa and Asian countries other than Israel. (Adapted from D. Flug. Personal Communication 1970.)

The growth retardation occurs in children of the same neighborhoods in which anemia in pregnancy was common. Anemia in infancy is also a common condition, especially in the poorer neighborhood of this area. Although this low hemoglobin level is readily corrected, it is probably a reflection of more fundamental processes determining growth retardation, namely inadequate nutrition and a higher rate of infection, especially gastroenteritis, in infancy.

In another investigation conducted in Tel Aviv a comparison was made of the height and weight of three groups of children: Moroccan children who had recently immigrated, Israeli-born children of Moroccan-born parents, and children living in a better-off neighborhood of Tel Aviv.[4] The height of recently immigrated Moroccan boys was found to be less than that of Israeli-born boys of Moroccan parents. Both groups of children were living in a poor neighborhood of Tel Aviv. The difference was even more marked when the recently-immigrated Moroccan children were compared with children living in the better-off neighborhood.

Retardation in Intellectual Development

The physical growth retardation in infancy and early childhood, which we have noted, occurs in the same kind of poorer Jewish immigrant communities in Israel in which low intellectual development and educational achievement has been reported by psychologists and educationalists. A direct relation between social class and intelligence scores has been consistently reported in studies of children in different countries. In Israel social stratification by economic or educational differences is associated with ethnic origin. Jewish immigrants from predominantly Arab countries of western Asia and North Africa are usually poorer, less educated, and hence less skilled than are those of European or American origin. Studies of Israeli schoolchildren completing 8 years of primary education have shown differences in levels of intellectual performance between children of these two main origin groups. First-generation children of Western origin have consistently averaged higher levels than those of Oriental families.[5]

The investigation of younger children aged 4 to 6.5 years has only recently been undertaken. Using a Hebrew version of the Wechsler Preschool and Primary Scale of Intelligence (WPPSI), a random sample of children attending preschool, kindergarten, and first-grade classes in Jerusalem, Tel Aviv, and Haifa has been investigated.[6] The sample of 1,072 children was equally distributed between the sexes and between the age groups of 4, 4.5, 5, 5.5, 6, and 6.5 years. Figure 30-3 shows the average IQ scores of children of different ethnic origin and social class (socioeconomic status—SES). The effects of ethnic group and social class are independent of one another. The researchers found encouragement in the fact that children of Israeli-born fathers, of whom at least one-third were of Oriental origin, had IQ scores similar to those of Eastern European origin. Testing this further they found that second-generation Oriental children had an average IQ score of 101.3 compared with an IQ of about 92 for the first-generation children of similar origin. The same comparison for Israeli children of Western origin showed only 4 IQ points increase in the second-generation group.

In the early years after the establishment of the State of Israel there was a mass immigration of Jewish communities from Oriental countries, involving close to 700,000 people between 1948 and 1965. Immediately following this mass immigration one of the central problems that confronted teachers in schools was the scholastic performance of the children of these immigrants. Writing of this phenomenon in 1953, Gina Ortar stated " . . . the proportion of scholastic failure is high and a large percentage of children experience great difficulties in learning to read and write in

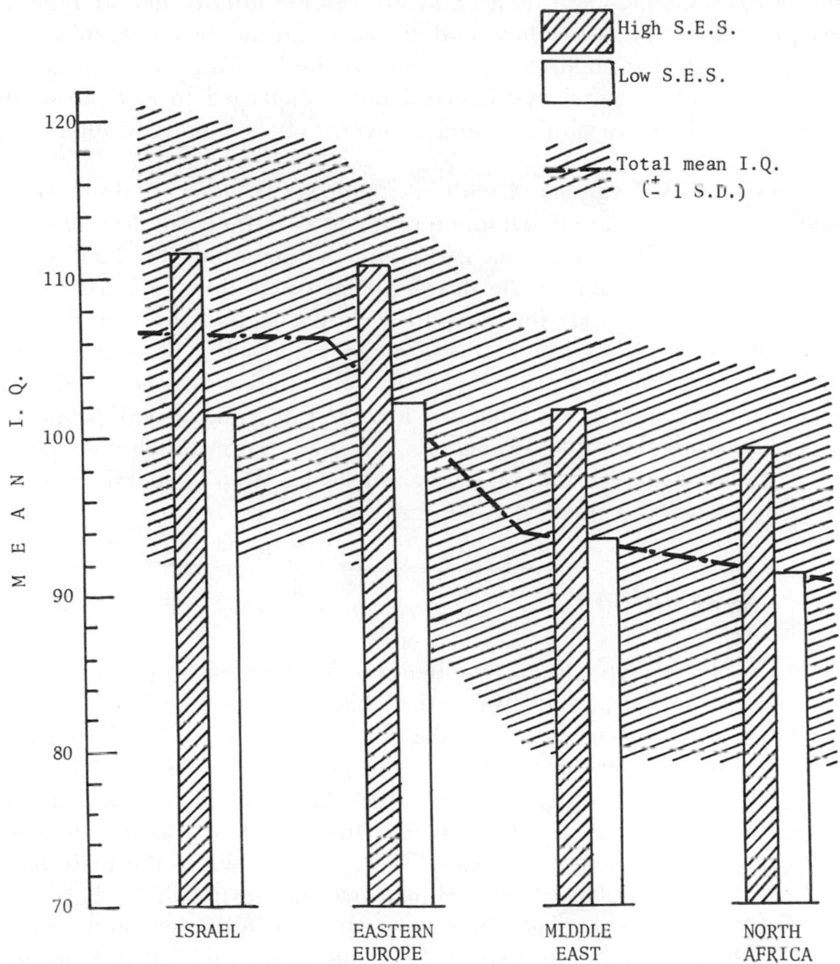

FIG. 30-3. Ethnic and social class differences in intellectual performance in Jewish children aged 4 to 6½ years in Israel. (Adapted from Lieblich and associates.[6])

the first three grades and fail to achieve good overall progress in other study subjects in the higher grades."[7]

She and other workers raised the question as to the reason for this conspicuous failure.[8,9] The problem of mental development has been linked to the need for "social stimulation" of these children in infancy and early childhood. The lack of verbal interaction between mothers and their babies has been commented on. In their discussion of the Kurdish family, Weintraub and Shapira contrast the social and emotional relationship between mothers and their children with the intellectual stimulation they give them. Thus the love and devotion given are contrasted with the observation that children " . . . were seldom spoken to except about elementary and essential matters and not encouraged to ask questions or develop their vocabulary and powers of conceptualization and abstraction."[10]

Following observations of mothers talking with their children, Ortar established a program to teach mothers to speak to their children in order to promote the child's verbal development. A program of this kind would have special importance in the development of children of lower social classes whose mothers are uneducated. Relative backwardness in the verbal development of children of these social classes has been commonly reported. Ortar's studies point especially to a relation between enriching speech and the children's intellectual level.[11] Enriching speech is speech in which not only the actual situation is reflected, but in which it is "made richer" by adding to the content. Instead of saying "Don't touch the stove," say "Don't touch the stove, it is hot and you may get burnt."

Infant Mortality

The lag in physical growth and intellectual development in poorer people must be seen in the perspective of the changing infant and child health picture since the establishment of the State of Israel in 1948. There has been a decline in infant mortality over the period from 1948 to 1970. The decline has varied at different ages in the first year of life, and this is related to different causes of death and the extent to which they have been prevented or treated successfully (Fig. 30-4). While the main ages in which death rates have been reduced are the postneonatal, it will be seen that there have also been important changes in the neonatal period.

The main reduction in death rate is due to a rapid fall in mortality from gastroenteritis, pneumonia, and acute bronchitis. Sex differences in mortality from various causes have usually shown the expected higher male rates. An exception to this was the infant mortality rate from gastroenteritis from 1950 to 1957, the period when there was a mass immigration to Israel of Jews from western Asian and North African countries. During this time the female mortality rates were consistently higher than those of the males and this might reflect a nonconscious sex preference in care (Fig. 30-5).

With this favorable trend in infant mortality rate, public health activity can focus more closely on other aspects of child health, such as further reducing morbidity and preventing retardation in growth and development. It must not be assumed that a declining infant mortality rate in itself indicates favorable growth and development in all segments of the community.

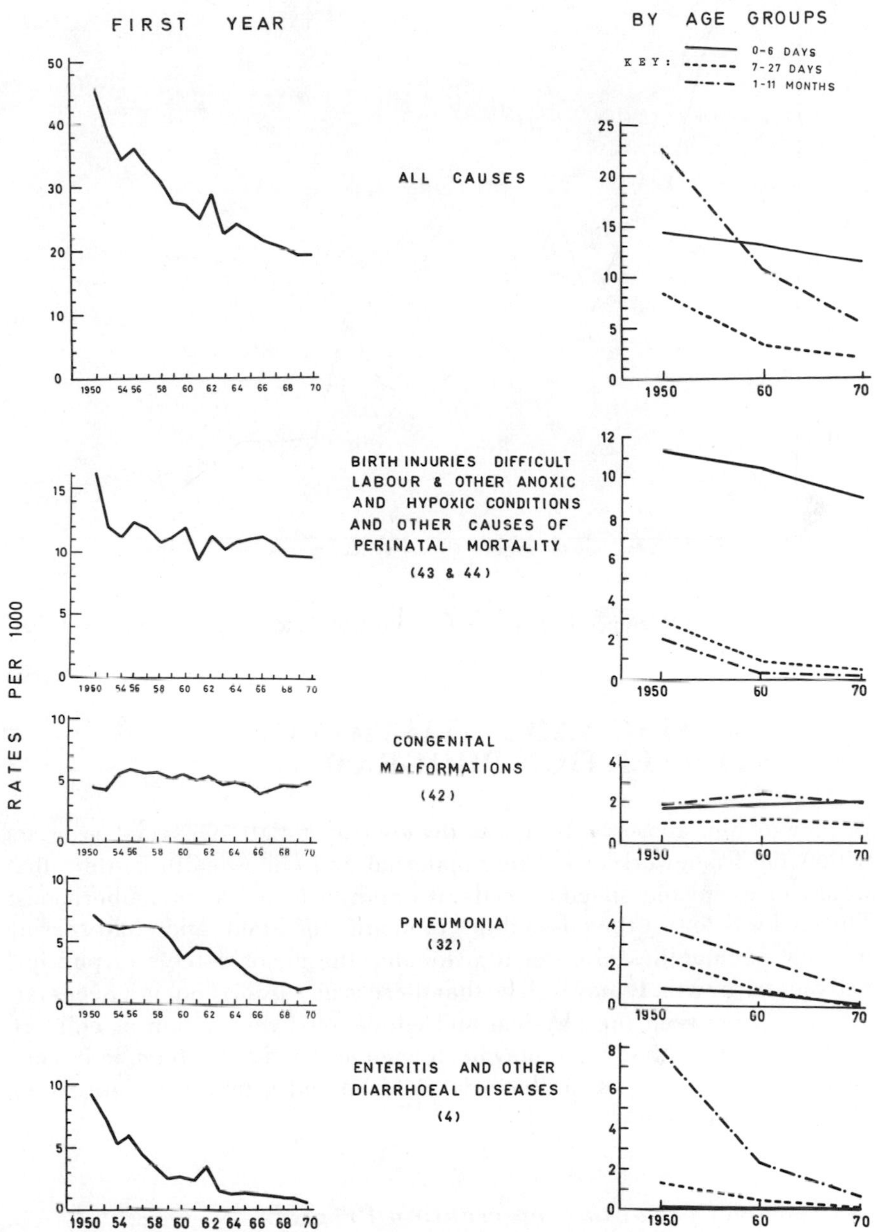

FIG. 30-4. Israel infant mortality rates. Jewish infants, 1950 to 1970.

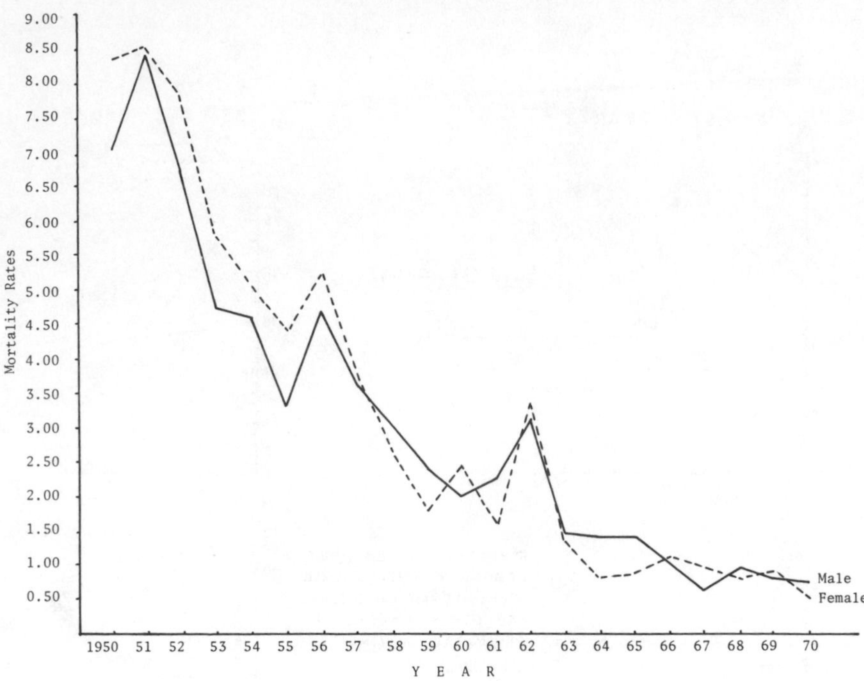

FIG. 30-5. The sex difference in Jewish infant mortality rates of gastroenteritis, Israel, 1950 to 1970.

PLANNING AND INITIATION OF INTERVENTION PROGRAM

In view of the above facts it was decided to initiate a special program within the framework of existing maternal and child health centers that would focus on the specific needs of children in poorer neighborhoods. The goal was to test the possibilities of modifying infant- and child-rearing in such communities in order to overcome the major defects of physical and mental growth. It may well be that there is an association, not necessarily causal, between the physical and educational retardation of children in these communities. What may be defined as a health problem in infancy becomes an educational problem in children and a failure in integration of the adult in society.

Objectives of the Intervention Program

Objectives of the intervention program included the following. (1) Promotion of health through improved nutrition, protection against infection, and social stimulation with emphasis on verbal stimulation in the first instance. (2) Prevention of retardation in physical growth and in behavioral and intellectual development, especially in infants and children of poor and uneducated families.

The overall program is summarized in Figure 30-6.

Methods

Project and Control Communities. The project has been initiated in several neighborhoods in Kiryat Harim. These neighborhoods include families of different social classes—poor, lower middle class, and middle-class professional. There is a clustering of families of similar social class in neighborhoods of the area. These neighboring communities are served by the three departmental maternal and child health centers mentioned earlier. These centers together serve an area in which approximately 400

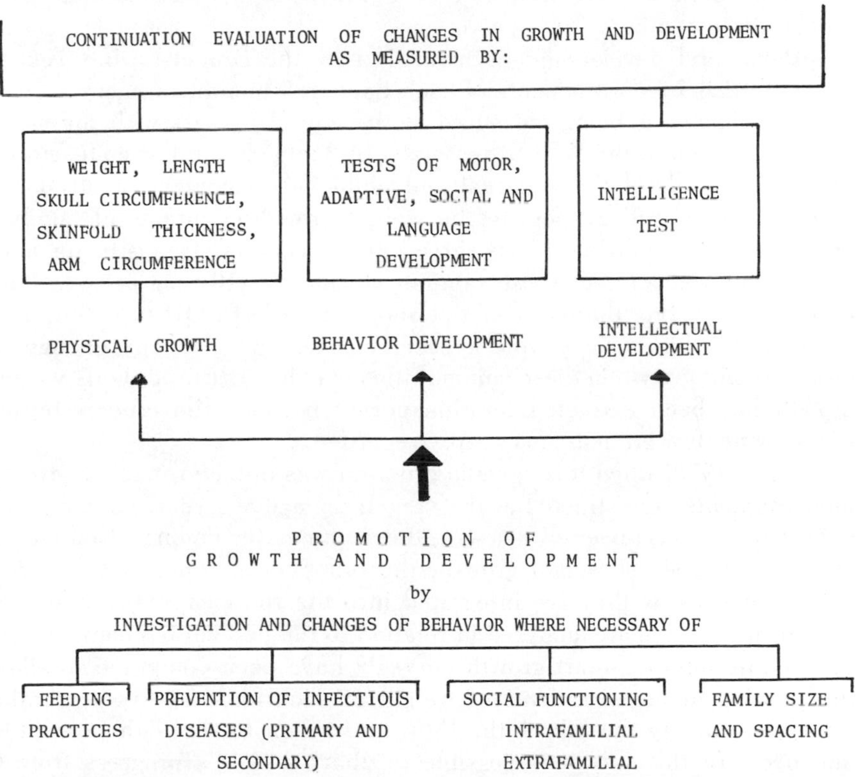

FIG. 30-6. Diagrammatic representation of program for promotion of growth and development (PROD).

births are registered annually; between 95 to 100 percent of mothers use these facilities for their babies. We thus have the opportunity to establish this project on the basis of existing contact with the vast majority of families concerned.

Where necessary the service in these clinics is being modified with respect to methods of interview of mothers and examination of infants and children, as well as with respect to methods of preventive treatment and education.

It is proposed to use comparable communities as control groups in the evaluation of change that may be effected by the intervention program.

Assessment of Growth and Development. The critical variables which we aim to change, and which will therefore be the final decisive points of evaluation of the program, involve physical growth and behavioral and intellectual development.

Physical growth is measured by weight, length, head circumference, triceps skinfold thickness, and arm circumference. The birth weight is obtained from the hospital in which the baby is born. All other measurements are done at 1, 3, 6, 9, and 12 months. Methods are standardized for the three centers.

Behavioral development is measured by the Brunet-Lezine Test.[12] A standardized record is made of each baby at 9 months of age.

Intelligence is being measured at the age of 5 years with the same Hebrew version of the WPPSI test used by Lieblich and her colleagues.[6]

The records of the maternal and child health centers involved are being analyzed with respect to the weight growth of infants of families now living in the neighborhoods served by the centers. This is being done for all children born to these families during the 10-year period, 1960 to 1969, preceding the onset of this more specific PROD program. The objective of this is to provide a baseline against which any change in infant weight growth in these communities may be measured. Only weight growth has been extracted for this period because the other relevant measurements were not consistently recorded.

Since 1970, when this specific program was initiated, babies' growth measurements are extracted as they reach the age of 1 year. Each month-cohort of babies is reviewed as well as the accumulated findings. Commencing with analysis of weight growth, the other measurements are added to the analysis as they are integrated into the routines of the practice. The growth trends are analyzed in relation to the percentile channels that the infants follow. Stuart growth curves[13] have been computed to allow the plotting of measurements of weight of each child in five-percentile intervals, namely the 5th, 10th, 15th, and so on to the 95th percentile and over. In this way it is possible to chart a child's progress from 0 to 3, 3 to 6, 6 to 9, and 9 to 12 months, recording movements as follows.

(1) Any change less than a 10th percentile is scored as no change (0). (2) Any movement more than a 10th percentile is scored plus (+) if upward and minus (−) if downward.

A problem in the use of this method in an on-going practice is the attendance of mothers with their babies, which influences the number of times babies are measured at various ages. At least two measurements are needed to assess the trend of growth in each period. We set a minimum of 8 weeks between any two such measurements within the 3-month periods before their inclusion in the analysis. Of the initial 332 babies reviewed at an Epidemiology-in-practice session of the department, the number of babies with weight measurements at the different periods during the first year as the following:

At birth to 3 months —326 babies
At 3 to 6 months —322 babies
At 6 to 9 months —289 babies
At 9 to 12 months —109 babies

The reviews of such findings are meant to relate growth to independent variables such as social class and education of mother, as well as to the percentile level of the infant at first measurement. Changes seen in preliminary analysis of these 332 infants are shown in Table 30-2. The high percentage of infants increasing their weight channel by more than a 10th percentile in the first 3 months is notable and has led to more intensive investigation of feeding practices during this period. One hypothesis is that decline in breast-feeding is associated with sugar-milk mixtures, which may cause the rapid increase in weight. These preliminary findings showed no consistent sex differences, nor differences by social class and mother's education.

Assessment of behavior development is a routine procedure in the maternal and child health centers. For the purposes of this program, standardization of methods of examination is important and a full record of findings, not only the abnormalities noted, is essential for analysis. In the first instance it was decided to perform this assessment at the age of 9 months, since at this age a high proportion of infants are brought

TABLE 30-2

	AGE PERIOD		
	Between 0 and 3 Months	Between 3 and 6 Months	Between 6 and 9 Months
No. of babies	326	322	289
Change			
Upward (+)	64%	25%	8%
No change (0)	25%	43%	44%
Downward (−)	11%	32%	48%

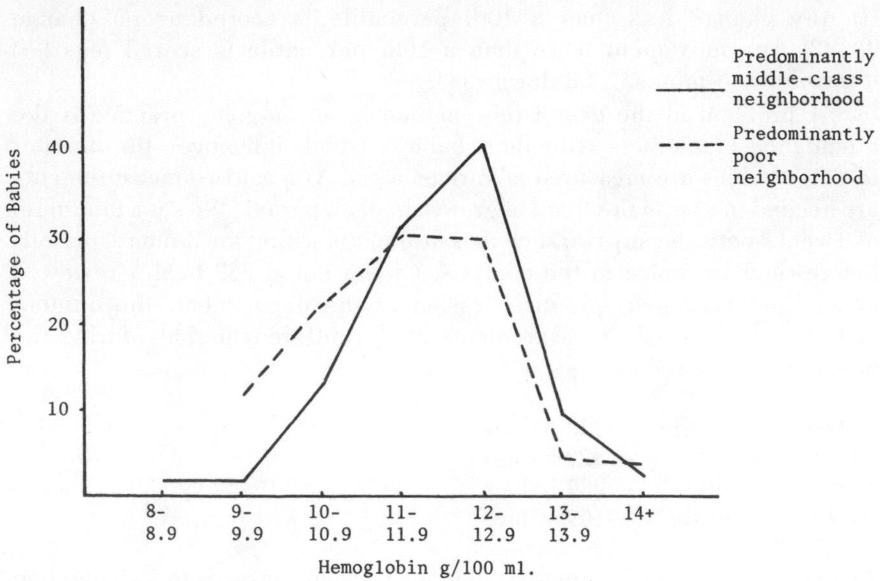

FIG. 30-7. Distribution of hemoglobin levels in 9-month-old babies. A comparison of two neighborhoods, 1968 to 1970.

to the centers for other purposes, such as immunization and hemoglobin evaluation. Furthermore, it is an age at which there is a relatively wide range of behavior, especially adaptive and personal-social behavior.

Study of Relevant Practices.

FEEDING PRACTICES. Severe malnutrition is not seen in infants and children of these communities. Nevertheless, the facts about growth outlined above suggest the need for more careful study of feeding practices. With this object in view a special community study of feeding is under way. The practices of the different communities will thus be compared with one another and related to recommended schedules for infant feeding.

The differences in hemoglobin levels of infants in better-off and poorer families are shown in Figure 30-7. As expected, this difference manifests itself in the anemia rates of these different groups of infants. Comparing a predominantly middle-class neighborhood of our maternal and child health practice with a poorer neighborhood, the percentage of babies with hemoglobin levels below 11g/100 ml at 9 months is shown in Table 30-3.

TABLE 30-3

NEIGHBORHOOD	1968–1969	1969–1970
Middle class	19.7%	16.9%
Poorer	38.3%	33.3%

A program has been developed to treat all children found with anemia at 9 months of age. Details of the program are available to the doctors and nurses of the practice. The program includes blood examinations required and their frequency, indications for treatment, and the preferred medication. A special record of all babies is maintained which includes information on illnesses, specific aspects of the diet, the mother's pregnancy, and demographic data about the family. The program is reviewed once a year at the Epidemiology-in-practice sessions of the department.

INFECTIONS. As shown earlier, gastroenteritis and respiratory illness had been important causes of postneonatal death. This is no longer the situation (Fig. 30-4). In the case of gastroenteritis, the decline in mortality is probably due to a lower incidence of the disease, possibly related to increase in use of refrigerators, as well as earlier and more effective treatment. Nevertheless, frequent mild attacks of gastroenteritis are common, and the frequency and nature of the attacks are being studied together with studies of knowledge and practices in preventing the condition.

SOCIAL INTERACTION. In the first instance particular attention is being given to verbal stimulation.

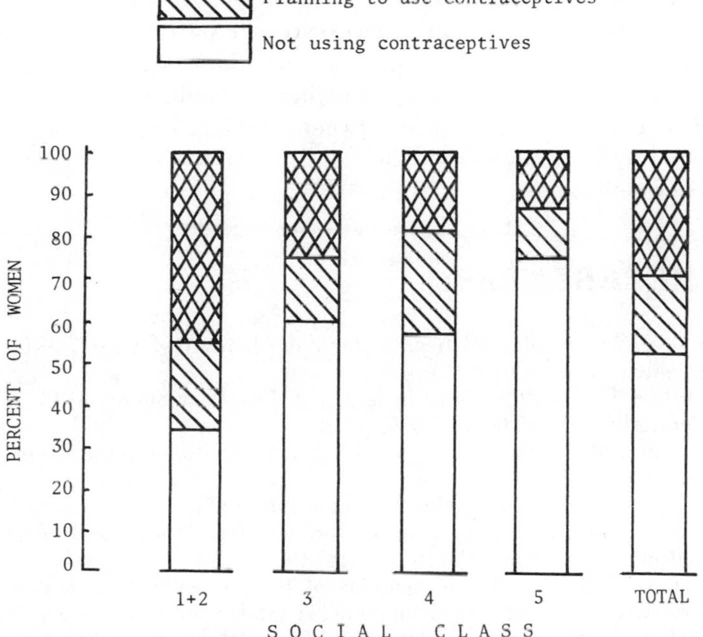

FIG. 30-8. Use of contraceptives by social class in 200 postpartum women. (From H. Kartzman, personal communiction.)

FAMILY PLANNING. Both size of family and spacing between children may be of relevance to the program. With this object in view, the data obtained from 200 postpartum women of this area has been analyzed. The contraceptive practices in this community are illustrated in Figure 30-8. In the majority of cases coitus interruptus had been the contraceptive practice (59.9 percent). There was a small minority of women who used the pill (11.5 percent) or were fitted with an intrauterine device (IUD) (7.5 percent). In one of the communities there was a higher-than-expected use of these contraceptives (46 percent of the women), with 24 percent using the pill and 22 percent the IUD. This was apparently due to the interest of a family physician in this aspect of his practice.

COMPREHENSIVE QUESTIONNAIRE. Further investigations are being conducted regarding knowledge, attitudes, and practices in the different communities. A questionnaire has been designed for self-completion by women attending the mother and child centers. It includes questions about feeding, infections, family planning, and social interaction between mothers and babies. It is mainly a KAP (knowledge, attitudes, and practices) questionnaire which is to be completed by mothers when babies are at various ages.

It is our objective to ensure that the population knows about modern contraceptive facilities and to make these facilities available. At the same time we are hoping to develop an educated opinion on family planning and population control as a whole.

INDICATORS OF SOCIAL FUNCTIONING OF FAMILIES. In planning this PROD program a major deficiency in our knowledge emerged. We do not have a measure of social functioning of families. Such an index is needed to explore associations between child growth and development and the overall functioning of the family. A study to meet this need is now being undertaken.

REFERENCES

1. Central Bureau of Statistics: Statistical Abstract of Israel, 1971. No. 22. Jerusalem, Government Press.
2. Grushka T: Health Services in Israel: A Ten-Year Survey 1948–1958. Jerusalem, Ministry of Health, 1959, p 92.
3. Epstein LM: Standards for weight growth of Israel-born babies. J Trop Pediatr 15:4, 1969.
4. Leiba S, Lunefeld B, Sheba C: Comparative study of growth and development of immigrant children from Morocco, Iran, India, and of Israeli-born children. (In Hebrew.) Harefuah 70:3, 1966.
5. Ortar G: Educational achievements of primary school graduates in Israel as related to their socioeconomic background. Comp Educ 4:23, 1967.
6. Lieblich A, Kugelmass S, Ninio A: Effects of Ethnic Origin and Parental SES on WPPSI Performance of Pre-school Children in Israel. Mimeo report. Israel, Human Development Center, Hebrew Univ of Jerusalem, 1972.

7. Ortar G: A comparative analysis of the structure of intelligence in various ethnic groups. In Frankenstein C (ed.): Between Past and Future—Essays and Studies on Aspects of Immigrant Absorption in Israel. Jerusalem, Henrietta Szold Foundation for Child and Youth Welfare, 1953, p 267.
8. Ortar G, Frankenstein C: How to develop abstract thinking in immigrant children from oriental countries. In Frankenstein C (ed.): Between Past and Future—Essays and Studies on Aspects of Immigrant Absorption in Israel. Jerusalem, Henrietta Szold Foundation for Child and Youth Welfare, 1953.
9. Feitelson D: The socialization of the young in the Kurdish community. (In Hebrew.) Megamot 6:4, 1955.
10. Weintraub D, Shapira M: The family in the process of change. Crisis and Continuity. In Weintraub D (ed.): Immigration and Social Change. Isreal Univ Press, Jerusalem, and Manchester Univ Press, Manchester, 1971, p 166.
11. Ortar G, Carmon H: An Analysis of Mother's Speech as a Factor in the Development of Children's Intelligence. Mimeographed report. Jerusalem, Hebrew Univ School of Education, 1969.
12. Brunet O, Lezine I: Le développement psychologique de la première enfance. Paris, Presses Univ de France, 1951.
13. Stuart HC, Stevenson SS: Physical growth and development. In Nelson WE (ed.): Textbook of Pediatrics, 7th ed. Philadelphia, Saunders, 1959.

31

CHAD Program (Community Syndrome of Hypertension Artherosclerosis, and Diabetes)

THE CASE FOR ACTION

In 1953 attention was drawn to a striking difference in the incidence of acute myocardial infarction between Israelis of different ethnic origin.[1] This observation was made shortly after the mass immigration of Jews to Israel following the establishment of Israel as an independent state. Among hospital patients the diagnoses of myocardial infarction or coronary occlusion was much more common in Ashkenazi patients than in those of Oriental origin. This initial observation was soon followed-up and substantiated in a number of subsequent reports by different investigators. The studies continue, with the primary objective of shedding more light on the causes of these differences.[2–24] The low rate of myocardial infarction was not only reported for Oriental Jewish communities, but is equally striking among the Bedouin of the Negev.[8,18]

From the evidence of several studies it could be expected that the ethnic group differences would narrow in the course of time, i.e., with increasing length of residence of immigrant communities and greater assimilation to the Israeli way of life. Comparing more recent and earlier Yemenite immigrants, Toor and his associates[5] found that the former had consistently lower total serum cholesterol levels in men and women of different ages. Certified death rates from "atherosclerosis" were four times higher in those who had been in the country for a longer time. They felt that the differences between the two immigrant groups of Yemenites were mainly a result of differences in total food intake, particularly fats, which was shown in their comparison of the diets of these groups.

Cohen, in his studies of diabetes and atherosclerosis, had a different view about dietary changes and their health implications. Comparing early and more recent Yemenite immigrants, he reported finding only three cases of diabetes in the recent immigrants from a total of about 5,000 examinations.[15] In contrast to this, in his examination of Yemenites who had lived in Jerusalem for more than 25 years, he found the prevalence rising steeply with age, resembling the findings in Jews of European origin. He reported similar contrasting findings between new Kurdish Jewish immigrants and earlier settlers. With his associates[14] he also investigated and reported on differences between early and more recent Yemenite immigrants, concerning the much higher prevalence of signs of involutional retinal sclerosis and high diastolic blood pressure among the former.

In his considerations of the reasons for these differences, Cohen contrasted the dietary practices in the Yemen, which were reported in interviews by the more recent settlers from the Yemen, with a 1-week dietary study of families who had lived in Israel for over 25 years. While being aware of the questionable data based on recollection, he stresses that there were two outstanding differences between the food consumed in the Yemen and in Israel: (1) Fats: In the Yemen, fats were mainly or solely of animal origin, namely dehydrated butter ("samne"), milk, mutton, beef, and very few eggs. Vegetable oil was rarely used. In Israel the "settled" group consumed animal fats, together with margarine (40 to 50 g daily) and an additional amount of vegetable oil (about 30 g daily—soya, sesame, and olive oil). (2) Carbohydrates: In the Yemen, carbohydrates consisted solely or mainly in starches. *Almost no sugar was used.* In Israel, sugar (sucrose) accounted for 25 to 30 percent of the total carbohydrates.

Cohen concluded that sucrose must be suspected as a cause of the change in occurrence of atherosclerosis and diabetes in these people.[13]

Confirmation of the expected narrowing of differences between various ethnic groups is now available. Coronary heart disease and cerebral vascular disease are important causes of mortality in Israel.

The figures over the period of 1950 to 1970 show a rise in the certification of death from arteriosclerotic heart disease in men and to a lesser extent in women, and a decline in deaths due to vascular lesions of the central nervous system (Fig. 31-1).[26] Since the community of Kiryat Harim consists of people of different origins, especially North Africans and Europeans, it is of interest to follow the trends of these two causes of death in the different ethnic groups of the country (Fig. 31-2). Particularly striking is the steep rise in the death rates from arteriosclerotic heart disease in men of North African origin and the fact that women of North African origin have a higher death rate from this cause than any other women. Both men and women of North African origin also have a much higher death rate from vascular lesions of the central nervous system than do the other ethnic groups. Over the same period of time there has been

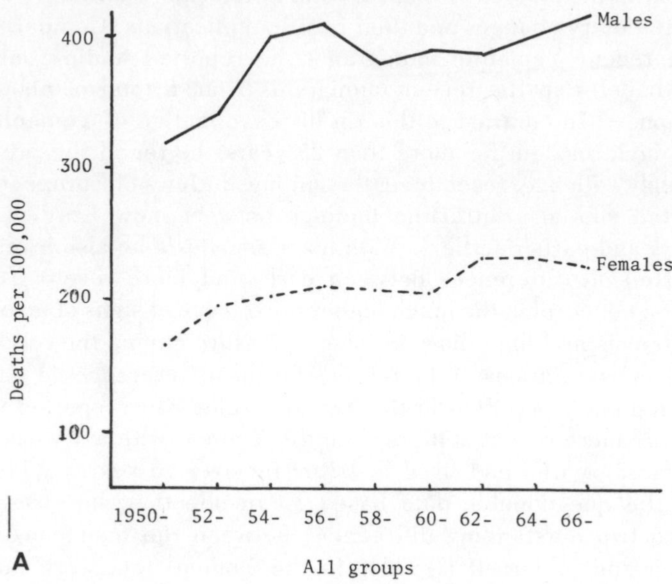

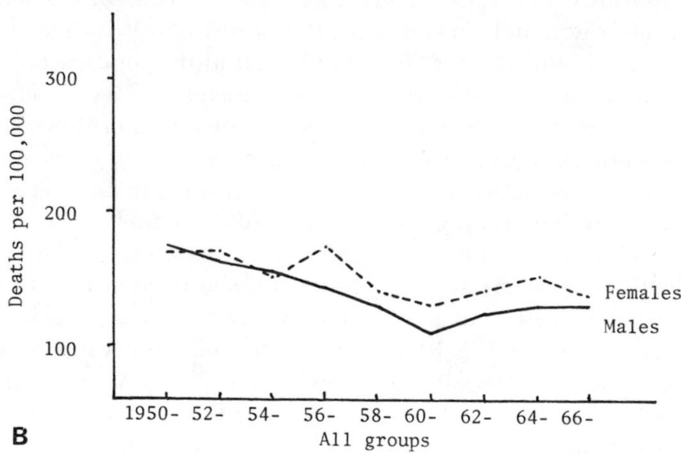

FIG. 31-1.A: Age standardized death rates, ages 25 to 74, from arteriosclerotic heart disease in Israel (Jewish population) by year and sex. B: Age standardized death rates, ages 25 to 74, from vascular lesions of the central nervous system in Israel (Jewish population) by year and sex. (Adapted from Peritz and associates.[26])

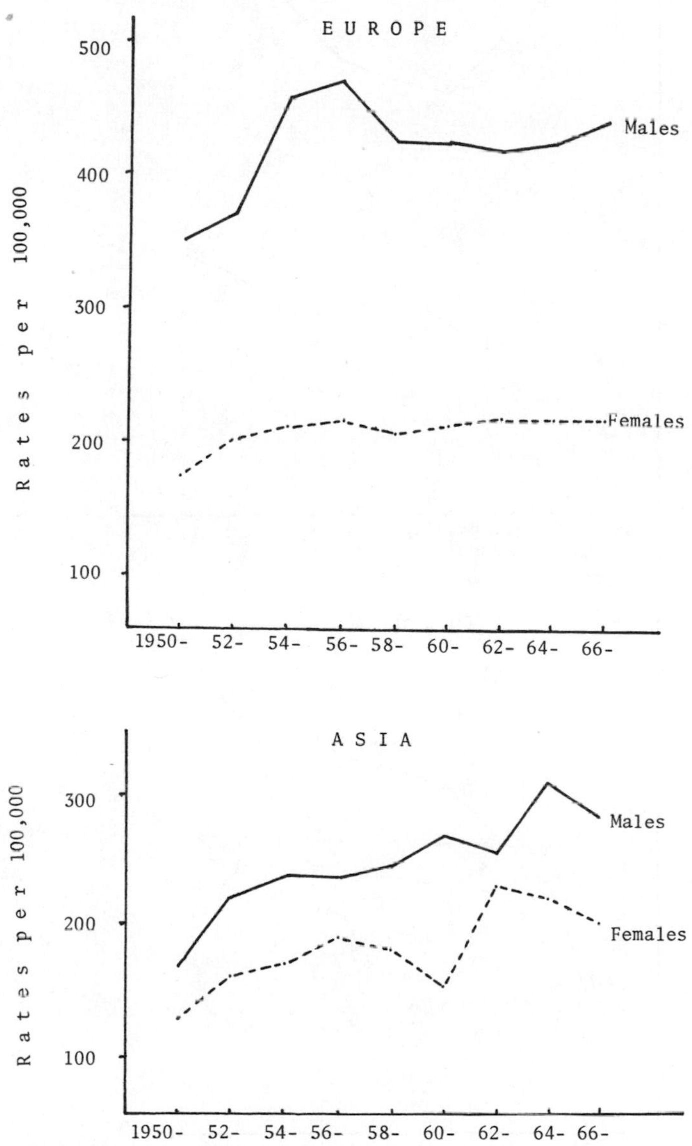

FIG. 31-2. A: Age standardized death rates, ages 25 to 74, from arteriosclerotic heart disease (ICD 7th Revision 420–422) in men and women of different ethnic groups in Israel as shown by place of birth. (Adapted from Peritz and associates.[26])

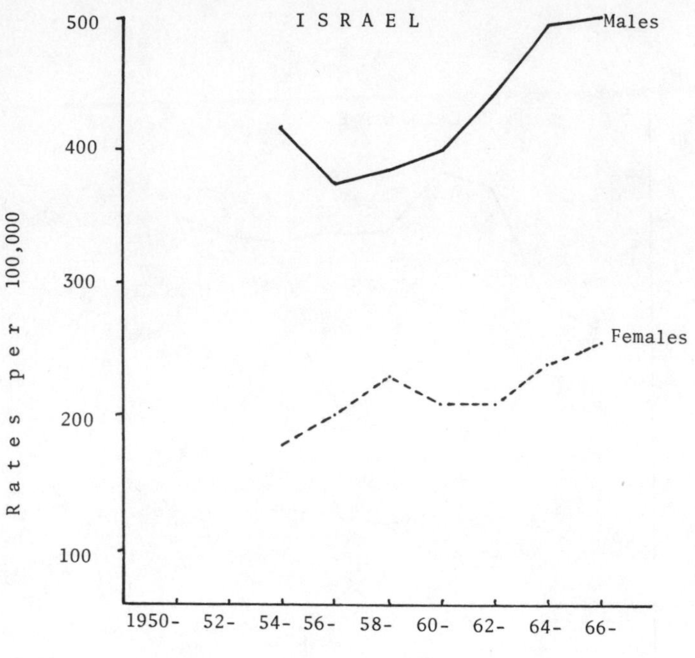

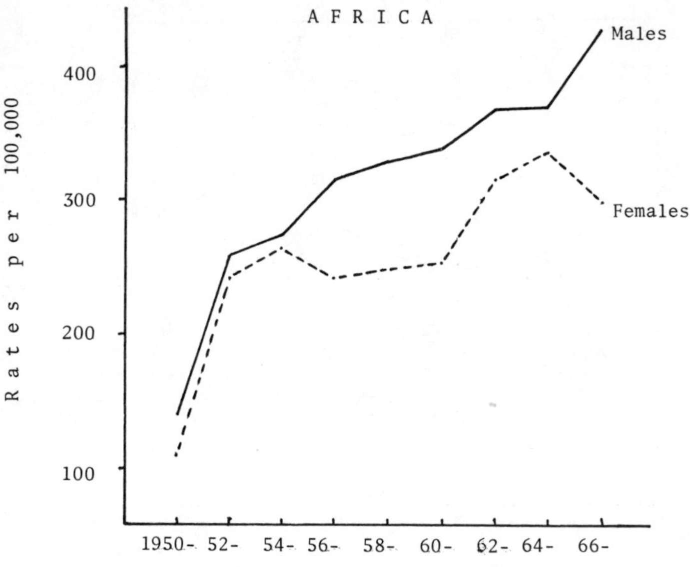

FIG. 31-2. A: (cont.)

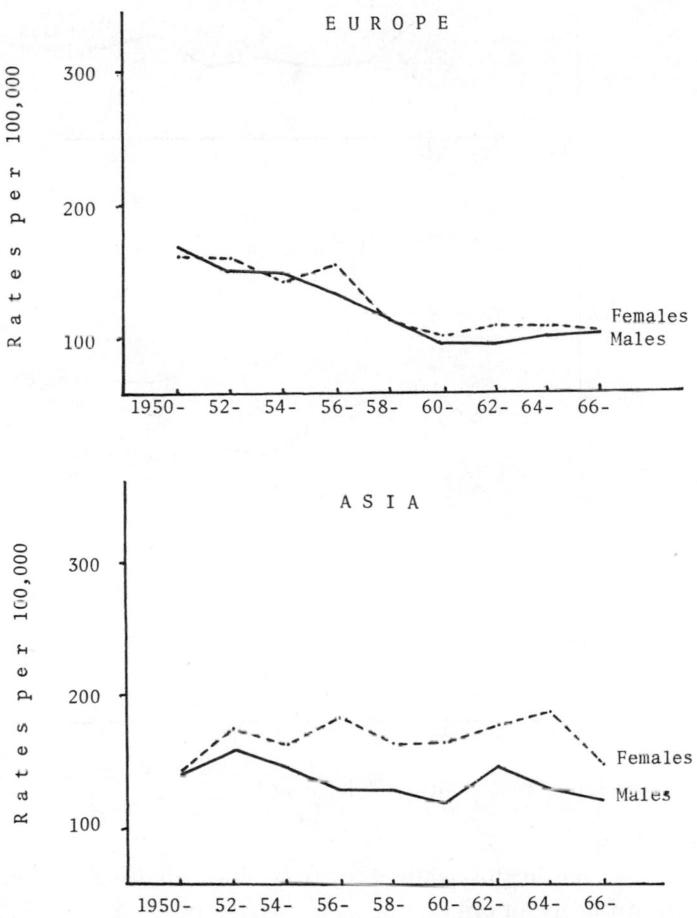

FIG. 31-2. B: Age standardized death rates, ages 25 to 74, from vascular lesions of the central nervous system (ICD 7th Revision 330-334) in men and women of different ethnic groups in Israel as shown by place of birth. (Adapted from Peritz and associates.[26])

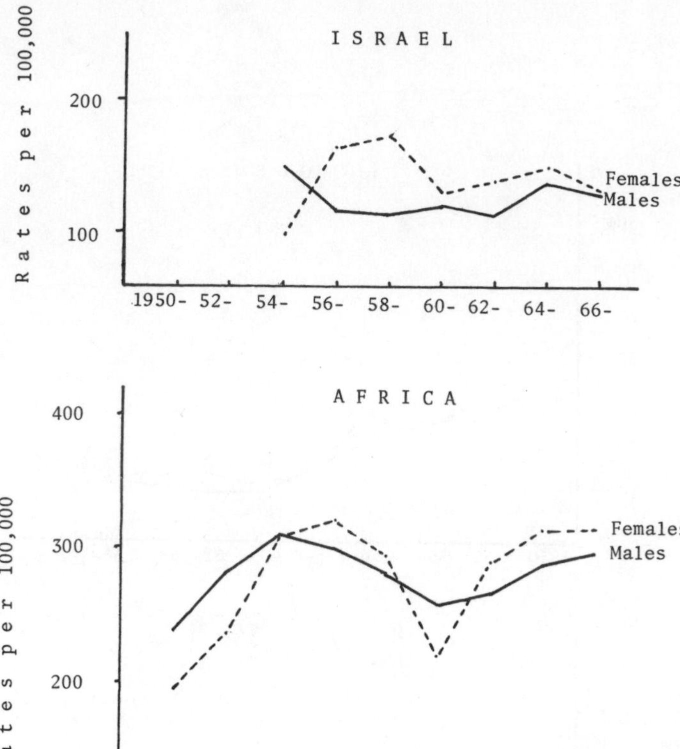

FIG. 31-2. B: (cont.)

a consistent decline in the death rates from this condition for both men and women of European origin.

In addition to these changes in death rates there has been considerable change in dietary habits, as evidenced by the food balance sheet over the years 1950 to 1970 (Fig. 31-3). The changes are in accord with present-day theory on the relation between diet and atherosclerosis.

In the community of Kiryat Harim, death notifications which are maintained by our departmental health center show coronary heart disease and cerebral vascular disease to be among the most important causes of death (Table 31-1). We have therefore introduced a special program designed to reduce the risk for these diseases in that part of the community which is served by the family practice of our health center. To do this it was necessary to conduct a health survey of the whole community. The objectives of community health surveys include screening for cases

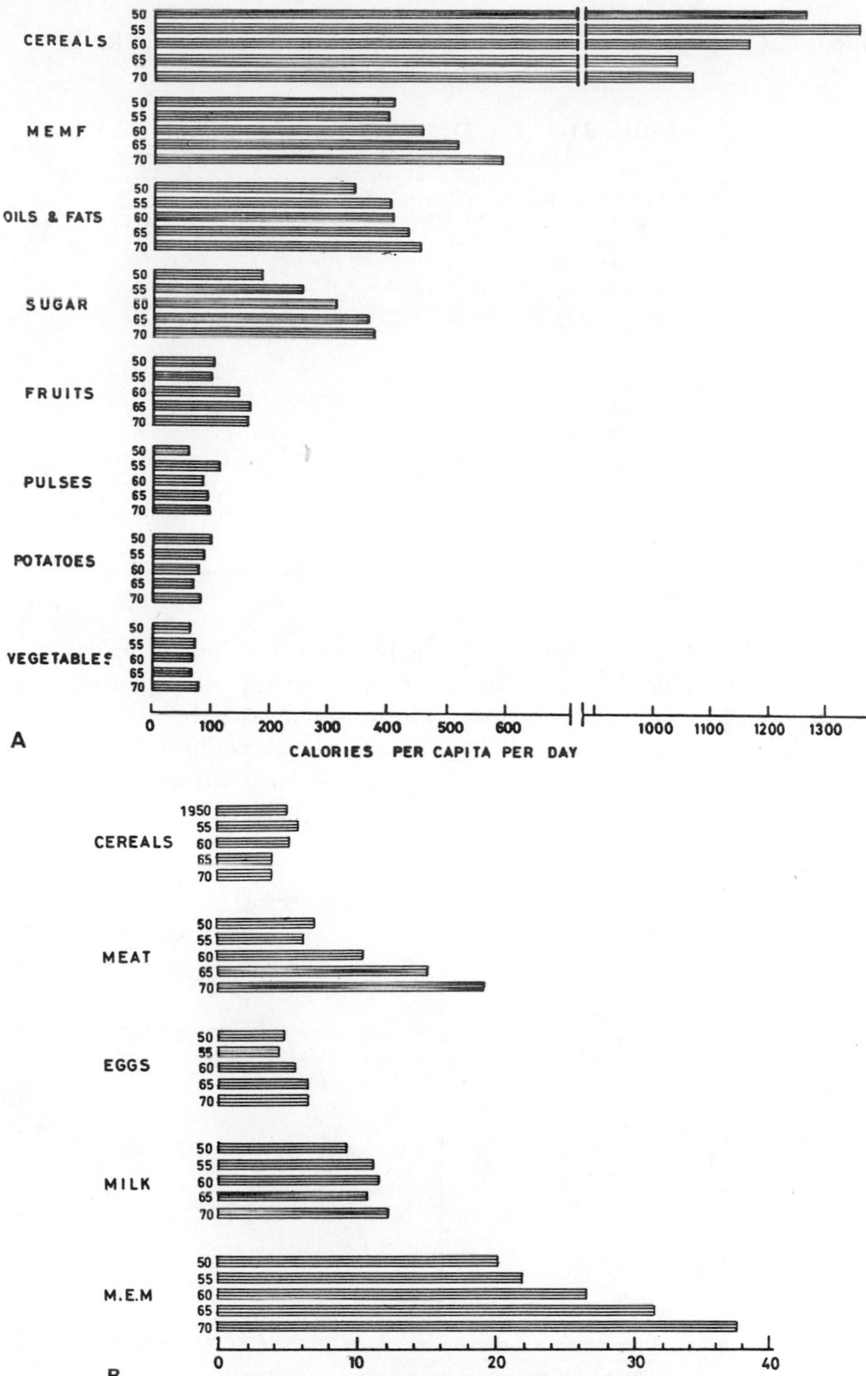

FIG. 31-3. A: The changing food balance sheet of Israel, 1950 to 1970. Calories available per capita per day from different foods. B: The changing food balance sheet of Israel, 1950 to 1970. The contribution of different foods to the fat available per capita per day. MEM: Meat, eggs, and milk. MEMF: Meat, eggs, milk, and fish. (Adapted from Central Bureau of Statistics.[25])

TABLE 31-1. The Deaths Reported in Kiryat Harim for the Year 1971

DISEASE CLASSIFIED ACCORDING TO B-LIST (ICD 8th REVISION)	NO. OF CASES
21 Diabetes	2
28 Ischemic heart disease	18
30 Cerebral vascular disease	7
21, 28	3
21, 30	3
28, 30	6
21, 28, 30	1
27,* 28, 30	1
27,* 28	2
	43
Other causes	43
Total	86

**Hypertensive disease.*

in need of treatment, study of the quantitative continuous distribution of health variables in a community, and testing of hypotheses in epidemiologic research. Screening procedures are used for recognition of treatable conditions for which individuals may not yet have experienced symptoms, or for which they may not yet be under treatment.

In regard to our CHAD program, Figure 31-4 illustrates the difference

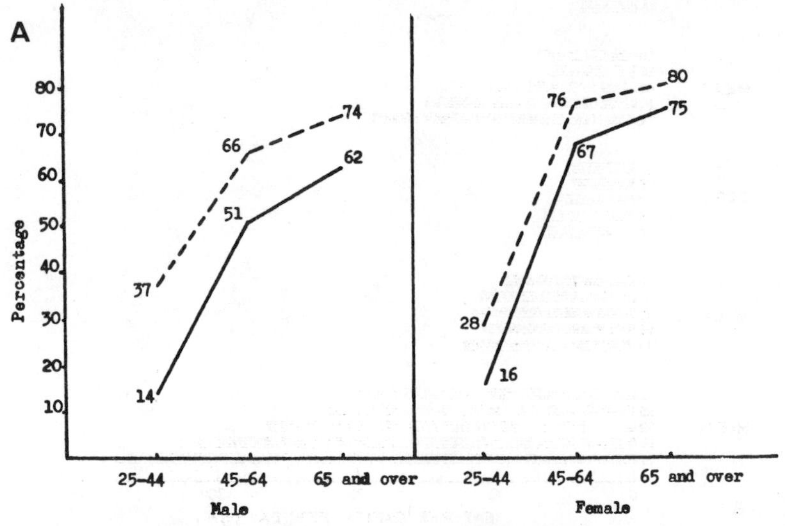

FIG. 31-4. A: A comparison of the known prevalence of diastolic hypertension in a family practice, before and after a community health survey.

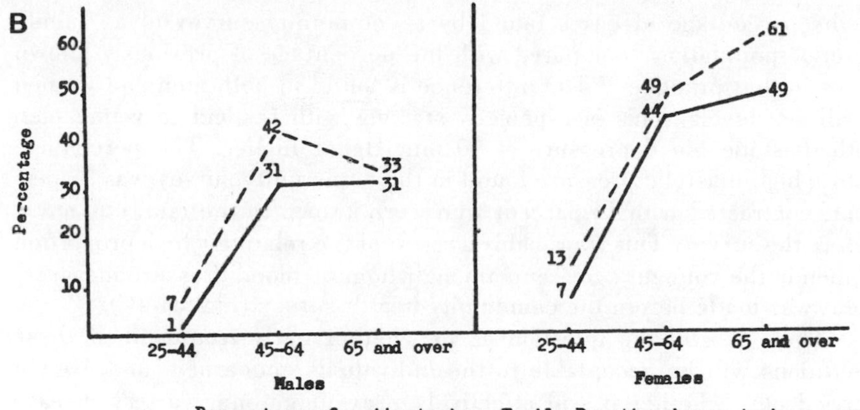

FIG. 31-4 (cont.). B: Comparison of the known prevalence of serum cholesterol level in a family practice, before and after a community health survey. (From Abramson et al.[27])

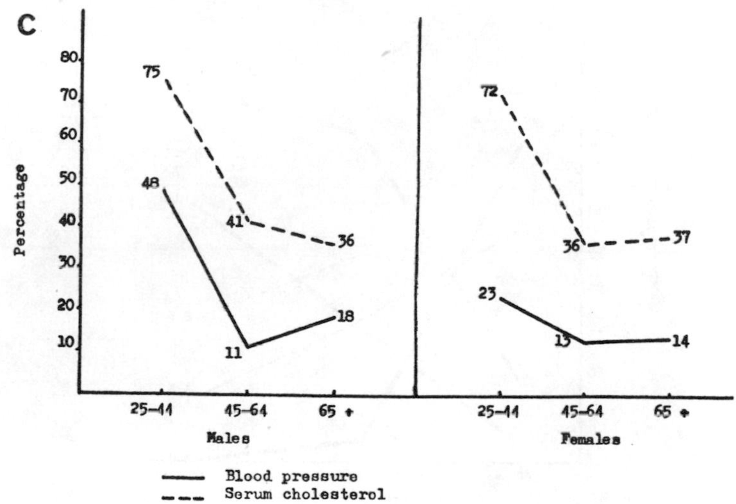

FIG. 31-4 (cont.). C: The percentages of men and women in the family practice who did not have blood pressure or serum cholesterol examinations before the community health survey. (From Abramson et al.[27])

in the percentage of cases found by a community survey of a "family practice population" compared with the percentage of previously known cases in that practice.[27] The difference is found in both men and women at all age levels. This is especially striking with respect to young men with diastolic blood pressure of 90 mm Hg or higher. The percentage with a high diastolic pressure found in the community survey was 37 percent, contrasted with 14 percent who were known to the family practice before the survey. This is probably a result of the relatively high proportion of men in the younger age group among whom no blood pressure measurement was made before the community health survey (Fig. 31-4C).

There is still the question as to whether early treatment of these conditions will be acceptable to the individuals concerned, and even if carried out, whether it will effectively prevent coronary artery disease or cerebral vascular disease.

Present research is providing encouraging results although a great deal remains to be done.

Another important objective not usually stated and seldom used in day-to-day medical practice is that of community diagnosis. In this case the diagnosis is based on the distributions of blood pressure, serum cholesterol, serum glucose, and height-weight curves. This kind of knowledge is illustrated in Figures 31-5–31-8.

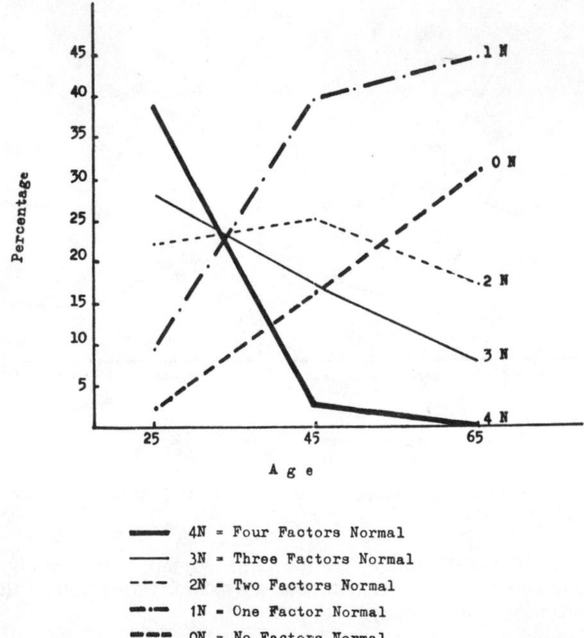

FIG. 31-5. The distribution of findings with respect to four "risk factors" of the CHAD program: systolic blood pressure, diastolic blood pressure, serum cholesterol, and serum glucose levels.

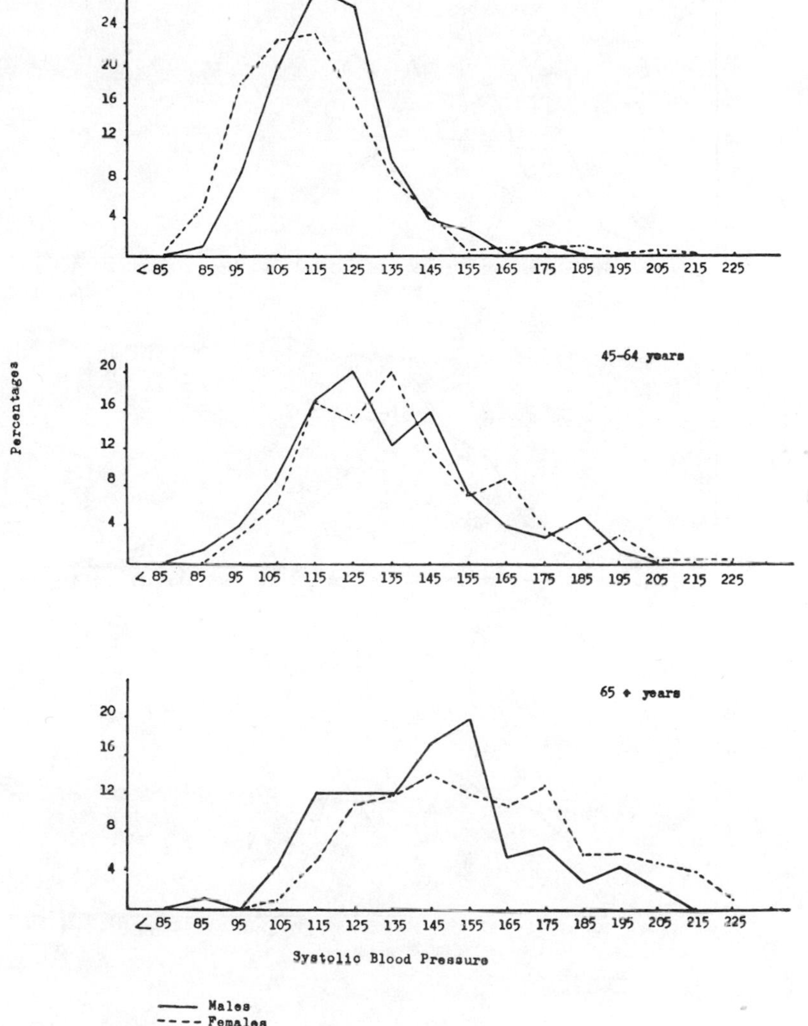

FIG. 31-6. Distribution of systolic blood pressure in a family practice by age and sex. The mean and standard deviation in each age group are as follows.

	25–44	*45–64*	*65 and over*
Male	123.4 (15.1)	138.2 (23.8)	150.2 (24.9)
Female	119.0 (18.9)	142.3 (24.6)	163.9 (28.0)

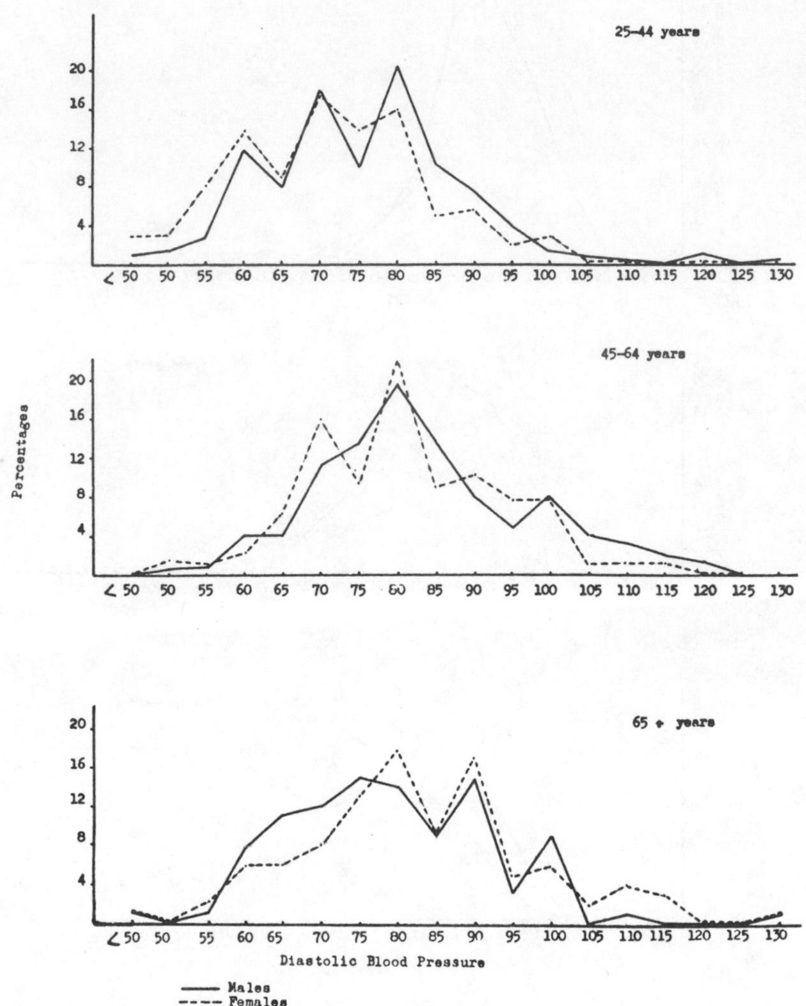

FIG. 31-7. Distribution of diastolic blood pressure in a family practice by age and sex. The mean and standard deviations in each age group are as follows.

	25–44	*45–64*	*65 and over*
Male	73.3 (13.3)	86.0 (14.1)	81.8 (13.7)
Female	74.3 (13.6)	84.2 (13.2)	85.4 (15.2)

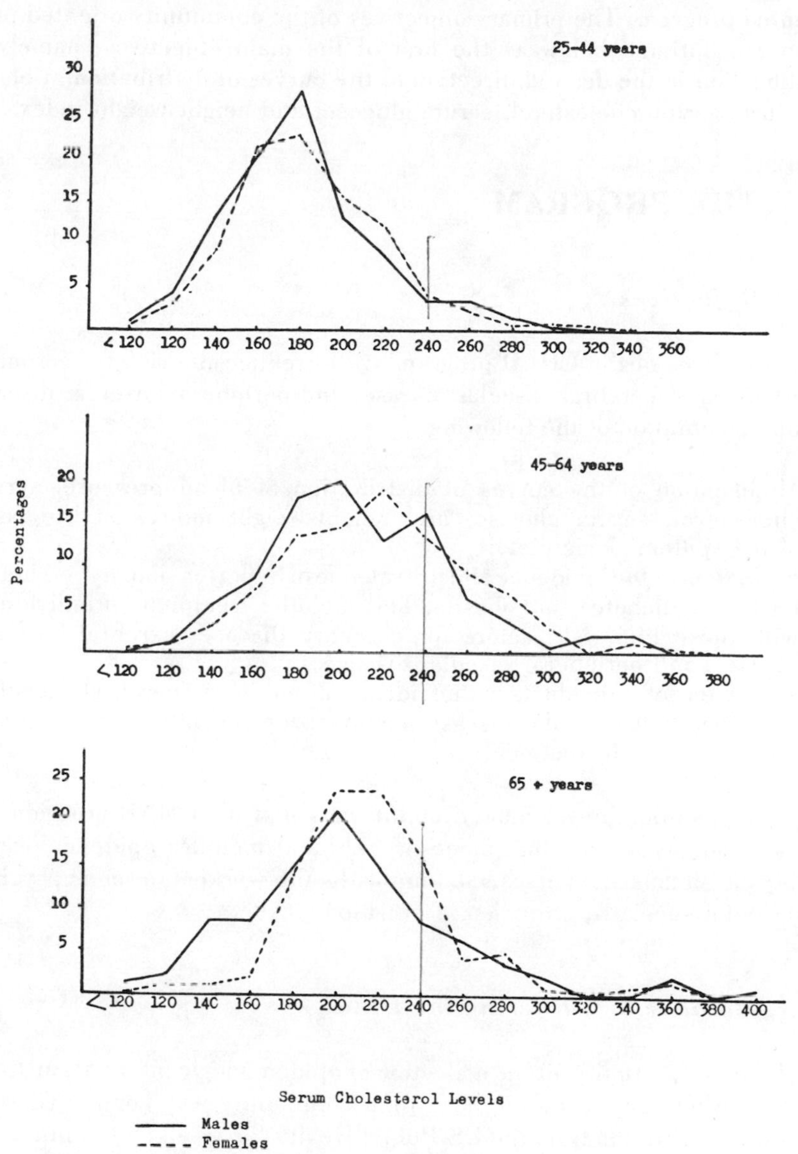

FIG. 31-8. Distribution of serum cholesterol levels in a family practice by age and sex. The mean and standard deviation in each age group are as follows.

	25–44	*45–64*	*65 and over*
Male	190 (36)	221 (45)	217 (52)
Female	195 (36)	229 (45)	229 (39)

The knowledge provided by this analysis is a basis for a community-oriented program. The primary objectives of the community-oriented program are outlined below as the first of the main objectives, namely a modification in the desired direction of the curves of distribution of blood pressure, serum cholesterol, serum glucose, and height-weight index.

THE PROGRAM

Objectives

The objectives of the CHAD program are to reduce the risk for coronary artery disease, cerebral vascular disease, and peripheral vascular disease by implementation of the following.

1. Modification of the curves of distribution of blood pressure, serum cholesterol, serum glucose, and height-weight index, on the basis of the epidemiologic picture.
2. Reduction of the incidence and prevalence of hypertension, hypercholesterolemia, diabetes, and obesity. This includes treatment of individuals with these high-risk factors for coronary disease, cerebral vascular disease, and peripheral vascular disease.
3. Treatment of individuals with evidence of coronary, cerebral vascular, and peripheral vascular disease, emphasizing secondary prevention in the aims of such treatment.

The planning, development, and direction of the CHAD program are carried out by a team that meets weekly and includes epidemiologists, family physicians and nurses, community health workers, a social psychiatrist, and a specialist physician in nutrition.

Methods of Gathering the Data

A valuable opportunity for the collection of epidemiologic information arose in 1968, when a health study of a total community was conducted with the support of funds from the US Public Health Service. This community health study involved interviews with, and examinations of, all the adults and a 50 percent sample of the children in a total population of about 10,000 in a section of Kiryat Harim. The examination included clinical, psychologic, biochemical, electrocardiagraphic, and other investigations. The collection of data began in late 1969, and the first round of examinations

Dwelling unit 120134	Marital status married	Date of examination 29.6.70
Study No. 314047	No. of children 3	Other Significant Findings in C.H.S.
Identity card No. 526318	Living arrangements ?	Personality type ______ Triglycerides 728
Name Hofman, Aron	Social class index 3a	Height 170 Weight 70 Lipoprotein ______
Address Bialik st, 9	Years of schooling 12	Ponderal index 105-109 (11) Insulin 360
Birth date 1897 Sex M	Present occupation clerk (retired)	48.8 Skin-fold thickness 11.2 17.2 20.4 Creatinine 1.6
Country of birth Poland	No. hours work/week 45 hours	Activity index ______ Smoking ______
Year of immigration 1926		

DATE	No. of con-tacts	SELECTION FACTORS				OTHER FACTORS						Hospi-tali-zations (cause)	Past Treatment and Advice											REMARKS
		B.P.	B. Chol.	E. C. G.	Significant findings and diagnoses	BLOOD			Haema-tocrit	Hb.	Weight		DRUGS*										OTHER	
						Sugar	Uric Ac.	Protein					1	2	3	4	5	6	7	8	9	10		
Present		212 106 104	231	1-3-4, 4-1 5-2 2	Diabetes mellitus Peripheral vascular disease M.I. Hypertensive ASCVD	114	6.7	7.0	43	14.5													Fat-free diet	
1955	5	155/90 165/90		✓	Hypertension																			
1956	8	[2] 180/110 180/100																						
1957	1	140/90																						
1958	1	160/95																						
1959	4	[3] 160/90 140/85											2											
1960	7	[4] 190/90 170/110 160/70	238			147																		
1961	24	[16] 190/100 110/60		✓	Coronary insufficiency (anginal signal)	105							1											
1962	14	[19] 170/100 130/70	334- 290	✓		106							1 2					✓						
1963	29	[21] 185/100 130/80	260	✓	Peripheral vascular disease	136-110					71.500		1 2					✓	6	3				
1964	37	[30] 222/120 140/90		✓	Intermittent claudication Hypertensive ASCVD D.M.	106				16.3	71-72.500		1 2					✓	5 6	3				
1965	19	[19] 200/130 140/70	405-350	✓	Post M.I. anginal pain Myocardial syndrome Coronary insufficiency	372-106	5.6	6.5		13.9	70.-		1 2		2		✓	✓	5 6 7	3 1			salt-free diet	
1966	34	[24] 210/110 190/80	455-255			128-110	9.5		44	14.6	72.500		2					✓	7 4	1 3				
1967	37	[13] 200/100 154/78	336-294		Diabetes mellitus, mild Hyp. ASCVD State M.I. - Psychotic episode	133-122	5.8						2		2		✓	✓	7 3 9					
1968	43	[32] 230/110 154/78	350	✓	Onset of left ventricular failure ASCVD	288-127		6.6			70.500		1 2		2		✓	✓	9 6	1				
1969	41	[33] 210/80 165/80			Angina pectoris HASCVD								2						9	2				
1970	33	[2] 210/100 155/70		✓	Angina pectoris	138							2		2			✓	9	2				

* See Appendix to this chapter

FIG. 31-9. CHAD summary of previous record.

was completed in December 1971. In effect, this epidemiologic study involved intensive health examinations of most of the population. Apart from its research objectives, it provided information invaluable to our community-oriented service. The family practice includes a population of some 3,000 of the 10,000 included in the study. It was decided to carry out the CHAD program in four housing projects (shikunim) of the family practice area. The remaining population of some 7,000 would continue with their regular medical care and thus constitute a control group for evaluation of the special CHAD program. A census of each dwelling unit was conducted as part of the community health study, providing similar basic information on the target and control populations. The record of each adult resident (25 years of age or more) in the family practice has been reviewed, including the past and present clinical records of the practice and the findings from the community health study. The data extracted are shown in a sample record of this care program (Fig. 31-9). From this record special individual records for use in the family practice were prepared (Fig. 31-10). This process is summarized below.

CHAD TEAM RECOMMENDATIONS (Summary)

Study No. 314047
Family Name Hofman Personal Name Aron Birthdate 1897
Address Bialik st. 9 Date of Study Examination 29.7.70
Date Entry Program 28.8.71

Diagnoses	Findings	Initial Recommendations	Remarks
Heart, C.V.A. etc.	B.M. P.U.D. M.I.	Treatment for cardiac	
Blood Pressure - S/D	212/104 (7./70) (1961) H/H	condition and B.P. and	
Serum Cholesterol	455 H	diabetes.	
Serum Glucose	231 (6/70)		
- Screening		Treatment for hypertension	
- Diabetes	known diabetes M.	check cholesterol.	
Weight/Ht Index	105 - 109 N		
Uric Acid	6.7 L	Check Uric Acid	
Anxiety			
Personality/Behav.			
Diet			
	ECG 2 (Possible CHD)	Reduce sugars	
Smoking		modify fats.	
Exercise			
Family History			

FIG. 31-10. A: The CHAD team recommendation card.

RECOMMENDATIONS OF C.H.A.D. PROGRAM
FOR THE FAMILY FILE

Surname: Hofman Name: aron Age : 1897 Sex: M

Address: Bialik street, 9

Personal No. in Study: 314047 Date of Examination: 29. 6. 70

Date of delineating his/her program: ____ Date of Interview ____

Diagnoses and other Findings	Recommendations	Remarks (date follow-up)
Heart Disease - A.P. ____		
M.I. ____		
Other ____		
Cerebral Vascular Disease ____		
Peripheral Vascular Disease ____		
Systolic Blood Pressure ____		
Diastolic Blood Pressure ____		
Serum Cholesterol ____		
Glucose Screening ____		
Diabetes ____		
Serum Uric Acid ____		
Height-Weight Index ____		
Anxiety ____		
Behavior Patterns ____		
Diet ____		
Smoking ____		
Physical Activity ____		
Family History ____		
Other ____		

FIG. 31-10 (cont.). B: CHAD record for the family file.

1. Periodic Review
   a. Summary record of relevant findings
      1. Past and present records maintained in file for CHAD Program (Fig. 31-9)
   b. CHAD team review of findings and recommendations passed on to the Family Practice Unit
      1. Recommendations card maintained in file for CHAD program (Fig. 31-10A)
   c. Family physician discussion with family members
      1. Record maintained in family file (Fig. 31-10B)

COMMUNITY HEALTH CENTER
SURVEILLANCE CARD - C.H.A.D. PROGRAM

Name: Hofman Aron Address: Bialik street, 9 Study No. 314047

Examination \ Month	1971 Aug.	Sep.	Oct.	Nov.	Dec.	1972 Jan.	Feb.	Mar.	Apr.	May	June	July
Medical Examination												
Weighing												
Dietetic Interview												
E.C.G.												
Urine text												
Blood:												
Cholesterol	ⓧ			ⓧ			x			x		
Glucose	ⓧ			ⓧ			x			x		
Electrolytes	ⓧ			ⓧ			x			x		
Uric acid	ⓧ			ⓧ			x			x		
Trigliceride												
Other:												
Periodic Evaluation												

x = to be done

ⓧ = done

FIG. 31-10 (cont.). C: CHAD surveillance card.

C.H.A.D. PROGRAM - DRUG TREATMENT

(Record of the Pharmacist)

Serial No. ________ Identification No. ________ Address ________________

Surname ________ Name ________ Sex ________ Birth date ________

DRUGS

DRUG*	1	2	3	4	5	6	7	8**	REMARKS
	Anti-hypertensives	lower choles-terol	Anti-Diabetes	Anti-Arryth-mia	Cardiac Glycosides	Vaso-Dilators	Tranquilizers	Others	
DATE	Thiazides, Rauwolfia, Methyl-Dopa		Orsenon, Diabenese, D.B.I., Insulin	Quinidine	Diaitalis	Nitroglyn			

* Check with X in corresponding square

** This includes vaso-bronchial dilators, anticoagulants, etc.

FIG. 31-10 (cont.). D: CHAD drug card.

d. Decision on treatment and action
e. Follow-up by family physician and nurse, noting adherence to treatment program and progress in individual's health
   1. Surveillance card kept in CHAD clinic card index (Fig. 31-10C)
   2. Drug card maintained in Pharmacy card index. (Fig. 31-10D)

Listings A through D are continuous processes which flow into one another in sequences. In addition, a number of major risk factors have been extracted from the record and shown on a community wall chart.

Preliminary Analysis of the Basic Data

The risk factors to which particular attention is being directed in this preliminary analysis are the systolic and diastolic blood pressures, serum cholesterol, serum glucose levels, and height-weight ratios.

These risk factors are widespread. The distribution of four selected risk factors (systolic blood pressure, diastolic blood pressure, serum cholesterol, and glucose tolerance) is shown in Figure 31-5. These cases comprise the respondents in the community health study, and constitute 85 percent of a 50 percent random sample of all adults in the family practice. The levels regarded as normal or constituting borderline and high risk for coronary disease and cerebral vascular disease are shown in Table 31-2.

Only a minority of persons had all four factors normal (4N), i.e., with no borderline or high-risk factor ever recorded. Even in the age group 25 to 44 years, only 40 percent of the men and 44 percent of the women could be classified as 4N. These percentages dropped markedly in the middle age group, 45 to 64 years, where only 3 percent of men and 9 percent of women were 4N, and no one aged 65 and over could be classified as free of all these risk factors.

Over a half of the total group examined had at least one high-risk factor. In the age group 25 to 44 years, high diastolic blood pressure (95 mm Hg and over) was the commonest high-risk factor, being present in 16 percent of the men and 11 percent of the women. It was also the most common high-risk factor in the middle age group, 45 to 64 years (44 percent of men and 52 percent of women). As expected, the picture changes in older people. In the 65 and over age group, high systolic blood pressure (160 mm Hg and over) was the commonest high-risk factor (70 percent of men and 81 percent of women). The commonest combination of high-risk factors was the systolic and diastolic blood pressure in all age-sex groups. Combinations of three or four high-risk factors were not found in the age group 25 to 44, but were common in the middle age group (25 percent of men and 31 percent of women) as well as in those aged 65 and over (28 percent men and 52 percent women). The high preval-

TABLE 31-2. Levels of Risk for the Four Selected Factors—Systolic Blood Pressure, Diastolic Blood Pressure, Serum Cholesterol, and Glucose Tolerance

FACTOR	NORMAL (N)	BORDERLINE RISK (B)	HIGH RISK (H)
Systolic blood pressure (mm Hg) (highest recorded value)	less than 140	140–159	160 or more
Diastolic blood pressure (mm Hg) (highest recorded value)	less than 90	90–94	95 or more
Serum cholesterol mg percent (highest recorded value)	less than 200	200–239	240 or more
Glucose tolerance— screening, serum glucose mg percent (1 hour after ingestion of 75 g glucose	less than 180	180 or more, or possible diabetes*	Diagnosis of diabetes*

Diabetes is diagnosed as follows: (1) known diabetic under treatment; and (2) following screening test if serum glucose is 180 mg percent or more, a glucose tolerance test (GTT) is done. The GTT is performed as follows: Take fasting serum glucose and then give 1.75 g glucose per kg body weight, to a maximum of 125 g, then measure serum glucose at 60, 120, and 180 minutes after loading. The findings are scored as follows:

	FASTING	*AT 60 MINUTES*	*AT 120 MINUTES*	*AT 180 MINUTES*
Level	*130 mg or above*	*200 mg or above*	*140 mg or above*	*130 mg or above*
Point	*1 point*	*0.5 point*	*0.5 point*	*1 point*

Score: 0.5 point, normal; 1 point, possible diabetes mellitus; 1.5 points, probable diabetes mellitus; and 2 points or more, definite diabetes mellitus.

Criteria based on the Community Health Study of the Department of Social Medicine.

ence of these risk factors in the community and the frequency with which they are found together supports the need for testing a coordinated program to modify the community syndrome.

The distribution curves of the systolic and diastolic blood pressures are shown in Figures 31-6 and 31-7. This distribution is based on data of all adults of the family practice who were examined in the survey. In the younger age group the female distribution is generally lower than that of the male; with increasing age the female distribution is higher than that of the male. There is also a change in the shape of the curves of both male and female. At the younger ages there is a large central tendency with a dome-shaped and relatively steep curve, but with increase in age, the distribution of the blood pressure not only shifts to high levels but the central tendency is smaller with a flatter, more widely dispersed curve.

The change of the curve of distribution of the diastolic blood pressure is similar to that of the curve of systolic blood pressure in that it shows an increase with age. However, there is less change in the shape of the diastolic blood pressure curve.

High blood pressure, systolic and diastolic, is more common in diabetics than in nondiabetics in both sexes. The same is true of obesity and, as expected, arterial vascular diseases are more common among the diabetics. The prevalence of hypercholesterolemia is similar in both diabetic and nondiabetic men, whereas it is more common in diabetic women. The findings for the age group 45 to 64 are illustrative (Table 31-3).

Intervention

This planned intervention program is carried out at two main levels: individual and family on the one hand, and community on the other.

Individual and Family. While each risk factor has been considered separately in some detail, together they constitute a syndrome having certain common features requiring change. Thus dietary change is an important element in almost all cases with a risk factor and the dietary changes required have important common elements.

The programs which have been developed to guide the family physicians therefore include general dietary recommendations and specific programs for hypertension, hyperlipedemia, and diabetes.

DOCTOR AND NURSE CHAD CLINICS. The fact that the risk factors are so often found together led the team to decide that they should be dealt with together rather than in separate specialty clinics. The family physicians, together with the CHAD team, meet weekly to discuss the families who will be invited to the special sessions. A specific family health maintenance plan is prepared for each family to provide a guide for family

TABLE 31-3. Hypertension and Hypercholesterolemia in Diabetics and Nondiabetics Aged 45 to 64 in the CHAD Program

	DIABETICS				NONDIABETICS			
	Male		Female		Male		Female	
	No.	%	No.	%	No.	%	No.	%
Total	28	100	32	100	120	100	166	100
Systolic hypertension	21	75	25	78	32	27	69	41
Diastolic hypertension	20	71	25	78	48	40	68	41
Hypercholesterolemia	11	39	25	78	55	46	80	48
Obesity	11	39	21	66	32	27	76	46
Vascular disease* {CAD, CVD, PVD}	11	39	16	50	18	15	17	10

**CAD, coronary artery disease; CVD, cerebral vascular disease; PVD, peripheral vascular disease.*

or individual action with respect to change in behavior as well as for medication.

The family physicians set a special time for the initiation of patients into this CHAD program. In the first instance, persons with at least one risk factor are invited. Adult members of a family are invited together even if only one of them has a risk factor. Thus, husbands and wives are seen together except in those cases in which the family physician thinks it is better to meet them separately.

At this meeting the relevant clinical, laboratory, and dietary findings are outlined by the family physician and these are then discussed in relation to their cause and possibilities of prevention. Both family physician and nurse participate in these family conferences, discussing and elaborating on the family program needed. Participation of the family in decision making is a major objective at this family conference. The plan usually involves changes in diet, requiring modification of cooking methods as well as eating habits. This follows a dietary study (Burke interview)[28] which is conducted for all persons who are overweight or diabetic, or have raised serum cholesterol levels.

Additional CHAD clinics are conducted by senior family nurses to ensure continuity and compliance in individual and family care.

The Community. While the aims of the community program are similar to those outlined for the individual and family, they are focused on education and changing behavior in the community as a whole in relation to the following four areas.

MODIFICATION OF DIETARY PRACTICES OF THE COMMUNITY. Modification of dietary practices includes reduction of caloric intake, e.g., bread; foods with high saturated fatty acid contents, e.g., butter, sour cream, cream cheese, hard margarine, and meats with high fat content (in this community meat is not consumed in large quantities and therefore does not present a problem); sugar, sweets, cakes, and sweetened soft drinks; and egg consumption. Practices that are encouraged include eating of foods with low saturated fat content, e.g., fish, lean poultry, and low fat milk foods, (instead of high-fat milk foods); and use of unsaturated fatty acid oils.

CHANGE OF SMOKING HABITS IN COMMUNITY. Cigarette smoking should be stopped completely; if this is impossible, switch from cigarettes to a pipe.

INCREASING PHYSICAL ACTIVITY. Encourage the habit of walking as a recreation or walking reasonable distances to work instead of using bus or car.

Without a properly staffed and equipped club for exercises this activity is not undertaken by the health center at present.

ENCOURAGE EFFECTIVE USE OF SERVICES. Ongoing use of doctor and nurse services includes positive response to invitations to the CHAD clinics; participation in the decision making in relation to the care program; compliance with the program; participation in the development of special group activities such as the diabetes club; and discussion groups concerned with changing diet and smoking habits.

In the development of community organization and community health education for these purposes, several investigations were undertaken. The first of these was a basic study of social networks as a foundation for establishing informal discussion groups. In addition, a special questionnaire was designed to determine the knowledge, attitudes, and practices of people regarding the specfic elements of the program that have been outlined above.

The Elements of the CHAD Program

A program such as CHAD has a number of facets, each of which requires specific consideration (Fig. 31-11). At the present time special guides to the following elements of the program have been developed by the CHAD team:

1. Diet and obesity, in their relation to other risk factors
2. Cigarette smoking
3. Blood pressure and hypertension
4. Hyperlipidemia
5. Glucose intolerance and diabetes mellitus
6. The combination of risk factors

Program for the Alteration of Diet. All adults in the community are included in this program and, in particular, any persons found with one of the following conditions: obesity, high cholesterol level, and/or diabetes mellitus.

The fact that so many people need to change their diet has led us to develop a program with a common basis, such as reduction of calories, saturated fats, and sugars. In this framework particular attention can then be focused on the needs of those with particular conditions. The aim has been to make the dietary changes simple, inexpensive, and acceptable to the community.

A food consumption study is conducted at home by a trained nutritionist who interviews the individual concerned. This dietary history includes initial questions about the usual daily pattern of eating. This is followed by more detailed questions about the amounts consumed of the particular food items. Wherever necessary, additional clarifying questions are asked. Household measures and natural-sized colored paintings of foods and food portions are used.

Special attention is paid to the methods of preparing food, in order

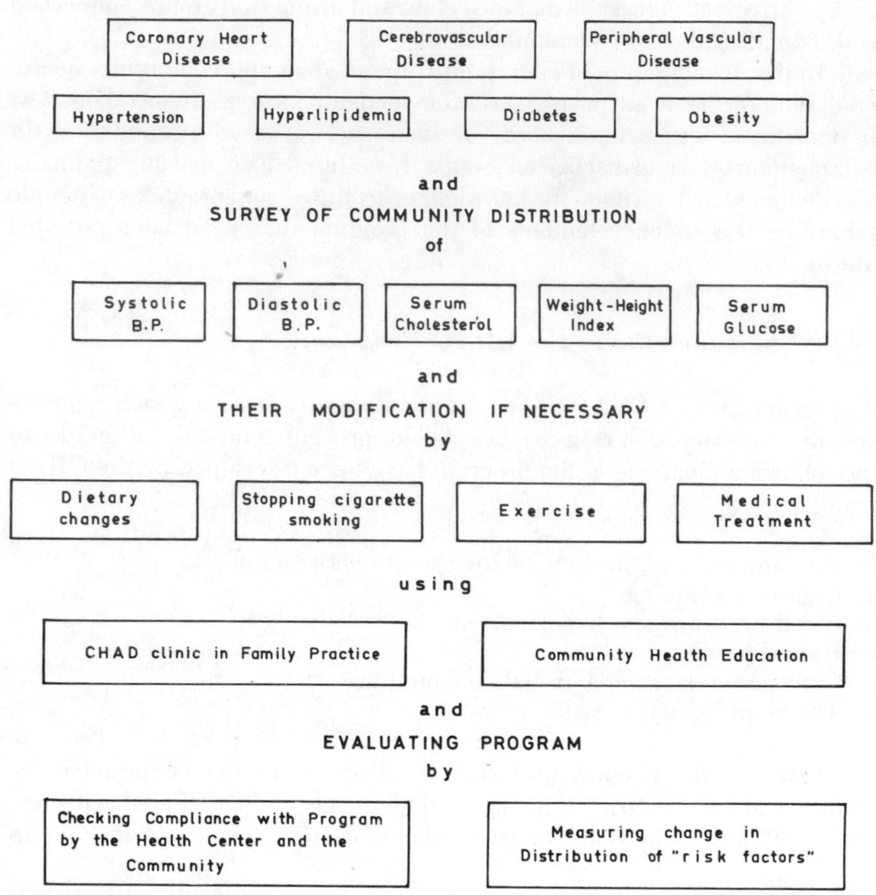

FIG. 31-11. Summary of the elements of the CHAD program.

to obtain the best possible estimates of the components of various dishes as well as the types and amounts of fats and oils consumed. As the study is conducted at a particular time of the year, the subject is also questioned about his usual consumption of the various food items during other seasons. For items where differences are reported, the mean of the two values is used. The nutrient composition of the diet is calculated by computer from the usual weekly consumption of the various individual food components.

Using a computer program, a print-out showing the mean daily intake of nutrients and foodstuffs, the reliability of which has been tested,[29,30] is available to the CHAD team and family physicians a few days after the interview.

The general aim of this program is to encourage preparation of food in a way that reduces the caloric content. Wherever possible, sucrose and foodstuffs rich in saturated fat are considerably reduced or removed from the diet. It is in this way that we aim to replace foods with a high percentage of fat by those with a much lower percentage or total absence of fat.

OBESITY. The percentage of "standard weight" is determined by reference to a table of standards for height and sex. The standards for age 25 have been adopted for all individuals above that age, details of which were published by the US Society of Actuaries.[31]

The classification of persons in CHAD is as follows.

Normal: ±10 percent of the standard weight
Borderline obesity: 10 to 19 percent above standard weight
Obesity: 20 percent or more above standard weight

Weight-for-height tables are available in doctors' and nurses' offices. The aim is to achieve a negative caloric balance by reducing caloric intake and increasing physical activity. The reduction of foodstuffs with a high caloric content is done in relation to the findings of the dietary survey. Thus if the patient's diet lacks variety to the extent that a restriction of a certain food item might cause a deficiency of nutrients, variation of the diet must first be achieved. This can then be followed by the reduction of caloric intake. The addition of various foods to the diet for this purpose should be restricted to those with a low caloric content. Sweetened foods and drinks should be avoided, using noncaloric sweeteners if necessary.

HIGH SERUM CHOLESTEROL LEVEL. If a patient has both obesity and a high serum cholesterol level, the obesity should be dealt with first. In the absence of obesity the total amount of fat in the diet should not exceed 30 percent of the caloric intake. The ratio between saturated and unsaturated fatty acids should be in the range of 1:1.5 or 1:2.

DIABETES MELLITUS. The general guidance for dietary change given above should be observed with particular attention to the avoidance of mono- and di-saccharides.

Program for Stopping Cigarette Smoking. In order to stop cigarette smoking at least two steps are needed. The first is to advise those who already smoke to stop, and the second is to discourage people—especially young people—from acquiring the habit. The extent of cigarette smoking in the community was determined in the community health study, the preliminary findings of which are presented in Table 31-4.

The doctors and nurses in the practice have been discouraged from smoking and there is no smoking in the clinic or offices of the physicians.

TABLE 31-4. Percentage Prevalence of Cigarette Smoking by Age and Sex in a 50 Percent Sample of the "Family Practice" Population

SEX	AGE	NO. OF PERSONS INTERVIEWED	PERCENTAGE SMOKING ANY NUMBER OF CIGARETTES PER DAY	PERCENTAGE SMOKING 20 CIGARETTES PER DAY OR MORE
Male	25–44	102	57	30
	45–64	74	46	16
	65+	39	28	0
Female	25–44	116	34	10
	45–64	97	22	6
	65+	51	12	2

Patients are advised by their physicians to stop smoking. Those who are unable to do so are advised to replace cigarettes by a pipe. It is proposed to establish a community-wide program involving special discussion groups of smokers who wish to stop smoking.

Program for Blood Pressure and Hypertension.

ASSESSMENT OF RISK STATUS. As indicated earlier, the highest blood pressure readings ever recorded by the health center were used for initial assessment of the risk status of an individual using the criteria shown in Table 31-2. In cases where a high- or borderline-risk blood pressure is found on one occasion only, or the patient's blood pressure status is doubtful, repeated measurements of casual blood pressure are done on 10 successive occasions. Wherever possible this is done daily. Following this, the criteria used for assessment of blood pressure as a risk factor are as follows.

1. High (H). Patients are considered high risk if
   a. Either the systolic or diastolic, or both together, are in the category of high risk (systolic 160 or over; diastolic 95 and over) in eight or more of the 10 readings
   b. Six of the 10 readings are high with the remaining four having at least a borderline risk level of systolic (140 to 159) or diastolic (90 to 94) blood pressure
2. Borderline (B). Patients are considered borderline, requiring a further evaluation after a period of 3 months, if
   a. Two or less of the readings were high and the remainder borderline or normal (systolic below 140 and diastolic below 90)
   b. Any combination of borderline and normal readings are taken with no high readings
3. Normal (N). Patients are considered to have a normal blood pressure if

a. The ten consecutive readings are normal for both systolic and diastolic pressures

Table 31-5 adapted from a personal communication of Professor B.

TABLE 31-5

DIASTOLIC BLOOD PRESSURE	SYSTOLIC BLOOD PRESSURE Below 140	140–159	≥160
Below 90	N	B	H
90–94	B	B	H
≥95	H	H	H

Modan of the Chaim Sheba Hospital, Tel Hashomer, summarizes the various possibilities.

GUIDELINES FOR INVESTIGATION OF CAUSE AND EFFECTS OF HYPERTENSION. Guidelines for investigation of the cause of hypertension and of complications have been prepared. They include the following.

1. Investigation of cause of hypertension. Special attention is given to these investigations in younger age groups. They are aimed to exclude secondary hypertension, resulting from renal disease, pheochromocytoma, and so on.
2. Investigation of cases of hypertension to establish the extent of organ damage. In addition to a full history and general examination, this includes ECG, urinalysis, serum urea, electrolytes, serum creatinine and clearance, fundal examination, and chest x-ray.

TREATMENT. Treatment of high blood pressure as a risk factor in persons who have not been diagnosed as having had cerebrovascular disease, coronary artery disease, or other heart disease is as follows.

1. Diet and exercise in persons who are overweight, as outlined in the program for alteration of diet. Where weight reduction or modified diet does not reduce the blood pressure, or when the patient does not adhere to a diet, consideration is given to need for antihypertensive drug treatment.
2. Antihypertensive drug treatment. Consideration is given to the use of antihypertensive drugs in all cases of hypertension, i.e., persons with a high diastolic or a high systolic blood pressure; and persons with a borderline diastolic or systolic blood pressure who may also be candidates for treatment, especially younger persons.

Where the family physician does not give drug treatment he states his reasons. Cases who are not under drug treatment have the same degree of surveillance as those under drug treatment.

A guidesheet has been prepared which includes details of a preferential treatment schedule listing the drugs, their dosage, and functions. This schedule is modified from time to time.

Hyperlipidemia Program. For purposes of this program the serum cholesterol level is estimated and classified as high risk (240 mg percent or more), borderline risk (200 to 239), and normal (less than 200), as shown in Table 31-2.

It has been recommended that clinical management should be directed toward the type of hyperlipoproteinemia rather than just to the measurements relating to hyperlipidemia.[32,33] However, serum triglyceride levels have not yet been used as a routine measure in determining hyperlipidemia in this program. We are at present testing the validity of nonfasting triglyceride levels. If the results of these tests are satisfactory the data gathered on nonfasting subjects will be used.

Dietary management is the first step in treatment and only when diet is not successful and cholesterol levels very high are pharmacologic agents utilized. The program of care of all persons having hyperlipidemia includes the following stages.

FURTHER EXAMINATIONS BEFORE TREATMENT. Further examinations before treatment include dietary interview; assessment of relative body weight in relation to the standard used in the program; and reexamination of cholesterol level (two further investigations are carried out). These are aimed to include determination of the type of lipidemia.

DIETARY ADVICE. If the person is more than 10 percent above his ideal body weight, dietary advice is directed toward reduction in caloric intake.[34] When weight is reduced, the caloric intake should be stabilized at a level that would prevent recurrence of obesity.

Whether the person is obese or not, the advice aims to reduce the saturated fat content of the diet. When necessary, dietary advice should aim at reduction of cholesterol-rich foods.

ROUTINE PROGRESS EXAMINATIONS. Routine progress examinations include the following.

Weighing: Monthly until desired decrease is obtained and then every 3 to 6 months.
Serum cholesterol determination: Every 3 months.
Dietary interview: Six months after the start of the program or earlier if the patient shows no response.

ADDITIONAL PROCEDURES. In cases who do not respond to dietary management, the following additional tests should be carried out.

Fasting triglyceride estimation
Lipoprotein electrophoresis

If the serum cholesterol level has dropped moderately but remains at high-risk levels, further modifications of diet should be made; in addition, drug therapy should be used, e.g., clofibrate (Atromid-S).

Referral for special consultation—cases in whom the serum cholesterol remains above 300 mg percent and those who do not respond satisfactorily to combined dietary and drug treatment, i.e., those who do not change their status at least from high to moderate risk levels.

Program for the Control of Glucose Intolerance and Diabetes Mellitus. The program outlined here is not directed toward cases of juvenile diabetics. For purposes of this program persons are classified as normal, borderline risk, and high risk as shown in Table 31-2. As indicated in the table, patients are classified as "possible," "probable," or "definite" diabetics according to the findings of the glucose tolerance test (GTT).

ROUTINE PROGRESS EXAMINATIONS. In cases of "possible" diabetes the GTT should be repeated in 6 months. If the result is still "possible" it should be repeated annually.

In "probable" and "definite" diabetes a detailed schedule is used for frequency of quantitative estimates of sugar in urine and of weighings, with guidelines to interpretation of findings of treatment.

DIETARY ADVICE. Dietary advice, for persons with maturity-onset diabetes, is considered in the context of the overall need of such patients for alteration of their diet. As previously shown (Table 31-3) a large proportion of these diabetics have one or more of the following: high blood pressure, obesity, or hypercholesterolemia. The dietary advice must take these factors into account and is therefore preceded by a dietary survey. Following this the diet advice is aimed to reduce the level of any of the risk factors.

ORAL HYPOGLYCEMICS. Reports by the University Group Diabetes Program on the effects of hypoglycemic agents on vascular complications in patients with adult-onset diabetes[35,36] has led to our changing the program which was being used. Our decision was to desist from use of these drugs until evidence was forthcoming that the drugs were not harmful.

INSULIN THERAPY. Indications for insulin therapy include the following: when diet fails; if the patient has ketosis; in cases of juvenile diabetes mellitus; and when infections cause poor control of the diabetes. For cases of severe and brittle diabetes, control is initiated in hospital.

Combination of Risk Factors. We have referred to the information that risk factors for coronary artery disease and other atherosclerotic diseases are commonly found together in the same person. With advancing age this becomes more evident (Fig. 31-5). This fact involves careful consideration of treatment in such cases and, as indicated before, it is this that led to the decision to incorporate within the family practice of this community health center a regular combined CHAD session. In this way the family practice focuses on the combination of risk factors in its patients rather than having separate clinics for patients with diabetes, hypertension, hyperlipidemia, and obesity.

REFERENCES

1. Dreyfuss F: Incidence of myocardial infarctions in various communities in Israel. Am Heart J 45:749, 1954.
2. Dreyfuss F, Toor M, Agmon J, et al.: Observations on myocardial infarction in Israel. Cardiologia 30:387, 1957.
3. Dreyfuss F, Hamosh P, Adam YG, et al.: Coronary heart disease and hypertension among Jews immigrated to Israel from the Atlas Mountain region of North Africa. Am Heart J 62:470, 1961.
4. Kallner G: Epidemiology of arteriosclerosis in Israel. Lancet 1:1155, 1958.
5. Toor M, Katchalsky A, Agmon J, et al.: Serum lipids and artherosclerosis among Yemenite immigrants in Israel. Lancet 1:1270, 1957.
6. Toor M, Katchalsky A, Agmon J, et al.: Atherosclerosis and related factors in immigrants to Israel. Circulation 22:265, 1960.
7. Toor M, Born-Bornstein R, Schadel M, et al.: Atherosclerosis in aged Yemenite and European immigrants to Israel. Geriatrics 17:126, 1962.
8. Schwartz MJ, Rosenzweig B, Toor M, et al.: Lipid metabolism and arteriosclerotic heart disease in Israelis of Bedouin, Yemenite, and European origin. Am J Cardiol 12:157, 1963.
9. Agmon J, Schadel M, Toor M, et al.: Diet, fatty acids, and atherosclerosis. Geriatrics 21:159, 1966.
10. Brunner D, Loebl K: Serum lipids in Israel communities. Lancet 1:1300, 1957.
11. Brunner D, Manelis G, Loebl K: Influence of age and race on lipid levels in Israel. Lancet 1:1071, 1959.
12. Cohen AM, Bavly S, Poznanski R: Change of diet of Yemenite Jews in relation to diabetes and ischemic heart disease. Lancet 2:1399, 1961.
13. Cohen AM: Fats and carbohydrates as factors in atherosclerosis and diabetes inYemenite Jews. Am Heart J 65:291, 1963.
14. Cohen AM, Neumann E, Michaelson IC: Involutionary sclerosis and diastolic hypertension. Effect of environmental change. Lancet 2:1050, 1960.
15. Cohen AM: Effect of environmental changes on prevalence of diabetes and of atherosclerosis in various ethnic groups in Israel. In Goldschmidt E (ed.): The Genetics of Migrant and Isolate Populations. New York, Williams and Wilkins, 1963.
16. Ungar H, Laufer A: Necropsy survey of atherosclerosis in the Jewish population of Israel. Pathol Microbiol 24:711, 1961.
17. Librach G: Prevalence of ischemic heart disease among elderly Yemenites and Europeans, residents of homes for the aged in Israel. J Am Geriatr Soc 15:1125, 1967.
18. Groen JJ, Balogh M, Levy M, et al.: Nutrition of the Bedouins in the Negev desert. Am J Clin Nutr 14:37, 1964.
19. Levij IS, Ungar H: Severity of atherosclerosis in Yemenite Jews in relation to their length of residence in Israel. Isr J Med Sci 3:453, 1967.
20. Sacks MI, Vlodaver Z: An autopsy study of myocardial infarction in Israel. Pathol Microbiol 30:570, 1967.
21. Ungar H, Laufer A, Ben-Ishay Z: Atherosclerosis and myocardial infarction in various Jewish groups in Israel. In Goldschmidt E (ed.): The Genetics of Migrant and Isolate Populations. New York, Williams and Wilkins, 1963.
22. Groen JJ, Medalie JH, Neufeld HN, et al.: An epidemiologic investigation

of hypertension and ischemic heart disease within a defined segment of the adult male population of Israel. Isr J Med Sci 4:177, 1968.
23. Medalie JH, Nuefeld HN, Riss E, et al.: Variations in prevalence of ischemic heart disease in defined segments of the male population of Israel. Isr J Med Sci 4:775, 1968.
24. Medalie JH, Kahn HA, Groen JJ, et al: The prevalence of ischemic heart disease in relation to selected variables. Isr J Med Sci 4:789, 1968.
25. Central Bureau of Statistics. Statistical Abstract of Israel 1971. No. 22. Jerusalem, Government Press.
26. Peritz E, Dreyfuss F, Halevi HS, et al.: Mortality of Adult Jews in Israel 1950-1967. Central Bureau of Statistics. Special series No. 409. Jerusalem, 1973.
27. Abramson JH, Epstein LM, Kark SL, et al.: The contribution of a health survey to a family practice. Scan J Soc Med 1:33, 1973.
28. Burke BS: The dietary history as a tool in research. J Am Diet Assoc 23: 1041, 1947.
29. Reshef A, Epstein LM: Reliability of a dietary questionnaire. Am J Clin Nutr 25:91, 1972.
30. Epstein LM, Reshef A, Abramson JH, et al.: Validity of a short dietary questionnaire. Isr J Med Sci 6:589, 1970.
31. Interdepartmental Committee on Nutrition for National Defense: Manual for Nutrition Surveys, 2nd ed. Bethesda, Md, US National Institutes of Health, 1963, Chap. 9.
32. Lees RS, Wilson DE: The treatment of hyperlipedemia. New Engl J Med 284:186, 1971.
33. Fredrickson DS, Levy RI, Lees RS: Fat transport in lipoproteins—An integrated approach to mechanisms and disorders. New Engl J Med 276:34, 94, 148, 215, 273, 1967.
34. National Heart and Lung Institute: The Dietary Management of Hyperlipoproteinemia—A Handbook for Physicians, rev ed. Bethesda, Md, 1970.
35. The University Group Diabetes Program: A study on the effects of hypoglycemic agents on vascular complications in patients with adult-onset diabetes. Diabetes 19 (Suppl 2):747, 1970.
36. Cornfield J: The University Group Diabetes Program. A further statistical analysis of the mortality findings. JAMA 217:1676, 1971.

APPENDIX A

CHAD Program
Coding for Drugs (as of January 1972)

I.* Antihypertensives
II. Cholesterol-lowering drugs
III. Antidiabetics
IV. Antiarrhythmia
V. Cardiac glycosides
VI. Coronary vasodilators
VII. Tranquilizers, sedatives, and hypnotics
VIII. Others
  A. Anticoagulants
  B. Diuretics (other than for antihypertensive therapy)
  C. Vasobronchial dilators and vasodilators (general)

**Within each category a specific list of drugs used is coded.*

Index

Page numbers in **bold**face refer to figures or tables.